THE
INTERVENTIONAL
CARDIAC
CATHETERIZATION
HANDBOOK

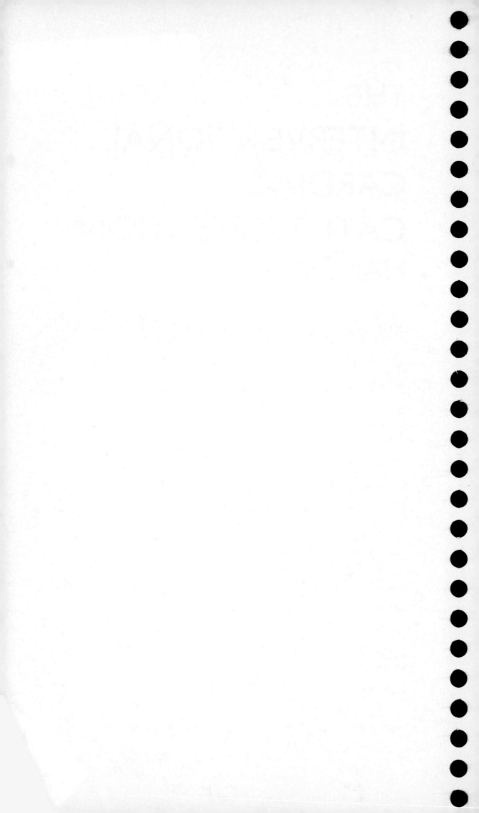

THE INTERVENTIONAL CARDIAC CATHETERIZATION HANDBOOK

First Edition

EDITED BY

Morton J. Kern, MD, FACC

Professor of Medicine
Director, The J. Gerard Mudd Cardiac
 Catheterization Laboratory
St. Louis University Health Sciences Center
St. Louis, Missouri

Ubeydullah Deligonul, MD, FESC

Associate Professor of Medicine
Director, Cardiac Catheterization, Angioplasty,
 and Atherectomy
University of Nebraska Medical Center
Omaha, Nebraska

with 211 illustrations

Special section on stents by
Antonio Colombo, MD

M Mosby

St. Louis   Baltimore   Boston
Carlsbad   Chicago   Naples   New York   Philadelphia   Portland
London   Madrid   Mexico City   Singapore   Sydney   Tokyo   Toronto   Wiesbaden

Vice President and Publisher, Medicine: Anne S. Patterson
Editor: Laura DeYoung
Associate Developmental Editor: Jennifer Byington Geistler
Project Manager: Dana Peick
Production Editors: Stavra Demetrulias, Cindy Deichmann
Designer: Amy Buxton
Manufacturing Supervisors: Betty Richmond, David Graybill

Printed in the United States of America
Composition by TCSystems, Inc.
Project Management by Spectrum Publisher Services, Inc.
Printing/binding by R.R. Donnelley and Sons

Mosby-Year Book, Inc.
11830 Westline Industrial Drive
St. Louis, Missouri 63146

Library of Congress Cataloging-in-Publication Data

The interventional cardiac catheterization handbook / edited by
　　Morton J. Kern, Ubeydullah Deligonul; special section on stents
　　by Antonio Colombo.—1st ed.
　　　　p.　　cm.
　　Companion v. to: The cardiac catheterization handbook /
　　edited by Morton J. Kern. 2nd ed. © 1995.
　　Includes bibliographical references and index.
　　ISBN 0-8151-5032-6 (alk. paper)
　　1. Cardiac catheterization.　　I. Kern, Morton J.　　II.
Deligonul, Ubeydullah.　　III. Cardiac catheterization handbook.
　　[DNLM: 1. Heart Catheterization—methods—handbooks.
WG 39 I61　1996]
RD598.35.C35I58　　1996
617.4'12—dc20
DNLM/DLC
for Library of Congress　　　　　　　　　　　　　　　96-16045
　　　　　　　　　　　　　　　　　　　　　　　　　　　　　　CIP

96　97　98　99　00　9　8　7　6　5　4　3　2　1

CONTRIBUTORS

FRANK V. AGUIRRE, MD

Associate Professor of Medicine
The J. Gerard Mudd Cardiac Catheterization Laboratory
St. Louis University Health Sciences Center
St. Louis, Missouri

RICHARD G. BACH, MD

Associate Professor of Medicine
The J. Gerard Mudd Cardiac Catheterization Laboratory
St. Louis University Health Sciences Center
St. Louis, Missouri

BRUCE A. BERGELSON, MD

Assistant Professor of Medicine
Northwestern University
Northwestern Veterans Administration
Lakeside Medical Center
Chicago, Illinois

EUGENE A. CARACCIOLO, MD

Assistant Professor of Medicine
The J. Gerard Mudd Cardiac Catheterization Laboratory
St. Louis University Health Sciences Center
St. Louis, Missouri

SCOTT CAROLLO, MD

Cardiology Fellow
The J. Gerard Mudd Cardiac Catheterization Laboratory
St. Louis University Health Sciences Center
St. Louis, Missouri

JOHN D. CARROLL, MD

Associate Professor of Medicine
Director, Hans Hecht Cardiac Catheterization Laboratory
University of Chicago Medical Center
Chicago, Illinois

ANTONIO COLOMBO, MD

Interventional Cardiologist
Centro Cuore Columbus
Milan, Italy

THOMAS J. DONOHUE, MD

Associate Professor of Medicine
The J. Gerard Mudd Cardiac Catheterization Laboratory
St. Louis University Health Sciences Center
St. Louis, Missouri

TED FELDMAN, MD

Associate Professor of Medicine
Hans Hecht Hemodynamic Laboratory
University of Chicago Medical Center
Chicago, Illinois

ANTONIO GAGLIONE, MD

Interventional Cardiologist
Centro Cuore Columbus
Milan, Italy

HERBERT J. GESCHWIND, MD

Director
Unite D'Hemodynamique et de Cardiologie
    Interventionnelle
Hospital Henri Mondor
Creteil, France

CAMILLO R. GOMEZ, MD

Interventional Neurology
University of Alabama
Birmingham, Alabama

PATRICK HALL, MD

Interventional Cardiologist
Centro Cuore Columbus
Milan, Italy

JOHN McB. HODGSON, MD

Associate Professor of Medicine
Case Western Reserve School of Medicine
Cleveland, Ohio

THOMAS M. HYERS, MD

Chief, Pulmonary Diseases
St. Louis University Health Sciences Center
St. Louis, Missouri

ALEXANDER KHOURY, MD

Interventional Cardiology Fellow
The J. Gerard Mudd Cardiac Catheterization Laboratory
St. Louis University Health Sciences Center
St. Louis, Missouri

SPENCER KING III, MD

Professor of Medicine (Cardiology)
Director, Interventional Cardiology
Emory University
Atlanta, Georgia

LUIGI MAIELLO, MD

Interventional Cardiologist
Centro Cuore Columbus
Milan, Italy

SHIGERU NAKAMURA, MD

Interventional Cardiologist
Centro Cuore Columbus
Milan, Italy

STEVEN E. NISSEN, MD

Professor of Medicine
Direction, Section of Clinical Cardiology
Vice Chairman, Department of Cardiology
The Cleveland Clinic Foundation
Cleveland, Ohio

STANLEY G. ROCKSON, MD

Assistant Professor of Medicine
Cardiology Division
Stanford University
Palo Alto, California

CARL TOMMASO, MD

Associate Professor of Medicine
Chief, Cardiology
Northwestern Veterans Administration
Lakeside Medical Center
Chicago, Illinois

THOMAS L. WOLFORD, MD

Assistant Professor of Medicine
The J. Gerard Mudd Cardiac Catheterization Laboratory
St. Louis University Health Sciences Center
St. Louis, Missouri

ANDREW ZISKIND, MD

Assistant Professor of Medicine
Director, Maryland Heart Center
Director, Clinical Managed Care
University of Maryland Hospital
Baltimore, Maryland

To Margaret and Anna Rose

M.J. Kern

To the memory of my father

U. Deligonul

FOREWORD

As a companion to *The Cardiac Catheterization Handbook*, we have attempted to provide an introduction to the complex techniques of coronary and peripheral arterial intervention. We have directed the materials toward trainees in interventional cardiology who have completed their basic diagnostic catheterization training and who likely have seen or have been superficially exposed to angioplasty. As in *The Cardiac Catheterization Handbook,* we have also included illustrations and explanations for the more junior cardiologists, nurses, technicians, and associated industry personnel unfamiliar with these techniques who require a background and reference in interventional cardiology.

Several basic aspects of cardiac intervention, such as arterial access and arteriography, are reviewed with the understanding that the detailed descriptions have been provided in *The Cardiac Catheterization Handbook* or other more complete catheterization reference texts. This work emphasizes the approach, indications, contraindications, and methods for performing most of the standard interventional techniques available at the time of publication. This work is not intended to be a comprehensive presentation of all aspects of interventional cardiac catheterization wherein the reader is referred to more definitive works. Likewise, the author's bias is presented with anticipation that most coronary angioplasty methods have stood the test of time and that the approach for stent placement has gained wide acceptance. The brief discussion of laser angioplasty represents the limited experience of most interventionalists with an expensive and evolving technique that has not settled into the daily repertoire of our laboratory.

This work could not have been produced without the steadfast and excellent help of Donna Sander and the inspiration and motivation from the fellows-in-training who continue to make the catheterization laboratory a valuable service for patients and stimulating for both attending and fellowship physicians alike. I would like to acknowledge the contributions of my coworkers in the J. Gerard Mudd Cardiac Catheterization Laboratory, with a special thank you to Margaret and Anna Rose for patience and forbearance in both St. Louis and Paris.

Morton J. Kern

CONTENTS

**4 CORONARY ANGIOPLASTY COMPLICATIONS AND
ANTITHROMBOTIC THERAPY   115**

Richard G. Bach, Ubeydullah Deligonul, Thomas M. Hyers,
and Morton J. Kern

5 STENTS   161

Antonio Colombo, Patrick Hall, Luigi Maiello, Shigeru Nakamura,
Antonio Gaglione, Frank Aguirre, and Morton J. Kern

14 LASER CORONARY ANGIOPLASTY 495

Herbert J. Geschwind

APPENDICES

THE INTERVENTIONAL CARDIAC CATHETERIZATION

HANDBOOK

INTRODUCTION TO INTERVENTIONAL CARDIOLOGY

Spencer B. King, III and Morton J. Kern

The discipline of interventional cardiology is now 17 years old. An extensive database has been developed to be applied by practitioners in the field. Interventional cardiology is a combination of technically mastered skills and extensive knowledge of cognitive information. Several aspects of the cognitive knowledge base are listed below.

Selection of patients for interventional procedures. The physician must have a complete understanding of practice guidelines for angioplasty and related catheter-based interventions, coronary bypass surgery, and medical therapy for coronary artery disease. Practitioners must also have extensive knowledge of the natural history of patients treated for ischemic heart disease by each of these modalities in various subsets. The physician must be well versed on any survival benefit as well as the evidence for symptomatic improvement in various subsets. An understanding of coronary pathoanatomy and pathophysiology is mandatory for selection of the most appropriate treatment option. Specifically, the physician must know:

1. The chance of successful angioplasty or other interventions being performed

2. The chance for benefit to the patient if the procedure is successful
3. The chance of complications
4. The chance of the various types of complications that should be anticipated
5. The methods for addressing complications should they arise
6. The overall risk to the patient

The physician must be able to integrate these facts into judgments that are specific for a given patient. In addition, the interventional cardiologist should understand the indications for balloon valvuloplasty and other evolving interventional techniques.

Performance of interventional cardiology procedures. In no area of cardiology is there a greater need for on-line decision making while performing a procedure. Interventional cardiology procedures are very similar to surgical techniques, and therefore the planning and execution of the procedures require extensive understanding of options and limitations of the technique as well as alternative methods of proceeding if the initial approach fails. In addition, one must be prepared to take measures to avoid complications and to cope with those complications effectively should they arise. Extensive experience with the choice and selection of different types of guiding catheters, guidewires, balloon catheters, and the host of FDA-approved new interventional devices is required. The knowledge base required to perform procedures effectively must not only include many of the items listed below, but, in addition, knowledge of the physical and material properties, the handling characteristics of guiding catheters, their ability to be positioned within aortic structures in order to provide platforms of adequate support to perform interventional procedures, and the special handling characteristics of a multitude of guidewires are essential. Techniques for bending and shaping guidewires and torquing them throughout the three-dimensional coronary circulation are necessary. A complete understanding of the characteristics of balloon catheters, including their profile, trackability, pushability, and the compliance characteristics of the balloon material, is essential for performing successful procedures without complications. Understanding plaque composition and its response to directional and extraction atherectomy cutting, the proper techniques for enabling cutting into plaque while avoiding resecting deep tissue components in the unaffected portion of the coronary artery, and the ability to size rotational atherectomy devices so as to abrade and ablate tissue while avoiding circumferential torsion or the release of excessive particulate matter are crucial. Techniques of administering laser energy and understanding the effect of that energy on tissue removal and the subsequent needed speed for advancement of laser catheters must be understood by interventional cardiologists using laser devices. Success in placing coronary stents requires understanding the relationship of the internal lumina of guiding catheters that will accommodate stents, the proper positioning of catheters, the guidewire support needed to place the stent in the coronary circulation in different locations, the proper sizing of the stent to the recipient artery, and techniques for tailoring the stent into place and assuring proper expansion of the stent, as well as uniform stent wire contact with the arterial wall.

Most complications can be prevented, or at least minimized, with proper planning and selection. When complications arise, prompt recognition and decisions to minimize the consequences and identify the etiology of the complication require knowledge and experience. The appearance of newly forming thrombus, dissection, wall hematoma, and coronary vasospasm all require an understanding and recognition of the processes. Although intravascular imaging may not be routine, it is emerging as a useful technique for detecting intravascular pathology. An understanding of the potential contribution of angioscopy, intravascular ultrasound, and translesional physiology as added tests in selecting cases should be part of the interventional cardiologist's knowledge base.

In addition to the cognitive areas involved in on-line decision making throughout a procedure, clinical decisions will also involve selection of arteries to be treated and special morphologic features that influence the selection of interventional devices. The timing and strategy of applying interventional techniques are critical to assure continued perfusion of viable myocardium during procedures. If obstructive complications should occur, an incorporated cognitive database for on-line decision making during procedures is mandatory for physicians performing procedures on a broad range of patients.

Expanded knowledge of intravascular catheter techniques and their risks. The knowledge required for technical performance of interventional procedures greatly exceeds that required for diagnostic catheterization. The proper selection of guide catheters may be quite large, with potential for vascular trauma. Their correct use must be mastered. Knowledge is acquired only through performance of many procedures under expert supervision through which one can learn the proper use of guidewires, balloons, and all of the new interventional devices that have been developed. The potential complications, including knowledge of how to manage dissections, thrombus formation, severe myocardial ischemia, emboli, and so on, must also be part of the knowledge base of the interventional cardiologist.

Expanded understanding of coronary anatomy and physiology. Although the general coronary anatomy is a component of the three-year cardiology curriculum, a dramatically expanded knowledge base is required to perform interventional procedures optimally. The relationship of the coronary artery ostia within the aortic root and the multiple anatomic variations must be understood. One must also comprehend the coronary anatomy in three dimensions and the physiology of coronary flow in both the normal circulation and diseased states as it is altered by large vessel obstructions and obstruction in the resistance vessels that occur as a result of the intervention.

For example, decision analysis integrating angiographic data often requires supplemental views before deciding on coronary intervention. These radiographic projections are dependent on many details not analyzed during routine diagnostic procedures, including lesion length, eccentricity, filling defects suggesting thrombus, parent vessels' angulation, bifurcation point location, plaque mass position relative to bifurcation points, and many others that influence the six crucial questions listed above. The effect of arterial spasm or microembolization on coronary flow must be well understood. The pharmacology of altering the responsiveness of large epicardial coronary arteries compared to the microcirculation must be understood. Knowledge of coronary anomalies, coronary steal, and the function of collaterals and how these flow dynamics affect myocardial perfusion is important. Physiologic parameters required include pressure gradients across the coronary obstructions and the phasic blood flow velocity alteration as measured with intravascular Doppler techniques. The latter also includes physiologic and pharmacologic techniques to assess maximum coronary flow reserve in a given coronary region.

Expanded understanding of atherosclerosis. The knowledge base must include complete understanding of plaque formation, morphology, and response of arteries and other conduits to various types of injuries. The alteration of the plaque with various interventional technologies and the different types of injuries produced by FDA-approved devices such as balloons, directional and extraction coronary atherectomy, laser, rotablator, transluminal extraction catheter, and stents must be understood.

Expanded understanding of imaging modalities. There should be extensive understanding of different imaging modalities, especially related to quantitative coronary arteriography and its pitfalls and endovascular methods of imaging such as angioscopic examination and intravascular ultrasound studies.

Expanded understanding of the vascular healing response. The understanding of the biologic process of vascular healing and restenosis must be expanded. The interventional trainee should appreciate the impact of the mechanical stretch on the arterial system, the effect of the depth of vascular injury, the occurrence of elastic recoil, the process by which fibrointimal proliferation, migration of cells, and matrix formation, as well as chronic vascular constriction, produce the restenotic lesion. The influence of growth factors, vasoactive substances, oxidative stress, and genetic signals in this healing process must be understood.

An expanded understanding of the dynamics of the quantitative arteriography posttreatment is crucial. The physician must understand the concepts of coronary lumen change due to acute gain, late loss, and net gain, as well as minimal lumen diameter measurements and the relation of posttreatment minimal lumen diameter to late minimal lumen diameter. Decisions that permit the physician to achieve maximum minimal lumen diameter without producing complications must be understood. Clinical factors and lesion-related factors associated with biologic processes in the plaque itself must be understood in order to be able to discriminate those lesions that have increased risk of acute closure or restenosis from those with reduced risk. For example, lesion location such as the proximal anterior descending, the aorto-ostial location, and the mid-graft lesion have very different biologic substrates, which influence the long-term outcome of interventions.

Expanded knowledge of management of acute myocardial infarction. There should be an understanding of the selection for thrombolysis versus acute catheterization leading to either primary angioplasty, angioplasty combined with intracoronary thrombolysis, or urgent bypass surgery. One should understand data supporting decisions in the high-risk subgroups (e.g., cardiogenic shock) that might benefit from urgent catheterization as opposed to intravenous thrombolysis alone. Clinical judgment based on the knowledge of when to intervene by understanding myocardial viability, stunning, hibernation, and the mass of myocardium affected is critical to integrating these factors.

Expanded knowledge of the management of acute hemodynamic alterations. Knowledge of management of patients with acute instability, especially the use of drugs, devices, balloon pumps, cardiopulmonary support, selection for emergency surgery, and emergency pacing, must be well understood.

Expanded knowledge of the hemostatic system. There must be complete understanding of the clotting cascade, the platelet function, thrombolysis, and the function of antithrombins and antiplatelet agents. Knowledge of the methods of intravascular thrombolysis and methods of mechanical thrombus alteration or removal must be understood. New methods of altering clot formation, such as antiplatelet antibodies, specific antithrombins, and peptides, must be mastered. There must be understanding of the biomaterials implanted in coronary arteries and heart chambers and unique methods to control thrombosis on implanted metal stents and other devices. Also, one should be familiar with the new field of site-specific drug delivery using porous balloons, hydrogel-coated balloons, and polymeric coatings on stents.

Expanded knowledge of the management of hemorrhagic complications. Management of hemorrhagic complications, including techniques for femoral artery compression, knowledge of percutaneous techniques for recognizing and closing pseudoaneurysms, understanding of puncture site closure devices, and potential complications of these devices must be understood. The physician must also have a heightened recognition of bleeding complications from various sites, including retroperitoneal, gastrointestinal, pulmonary, and cerebral, a thorough understanding of the tests to measure hemostatic state, and the weaknesses of these various tests. Decisions about the proper use and selection of patients for urgent vascular surgery consultation are essential in the practice of interventional cardiology.

Expanded knowledge of radiation safety. Understanding of radiation physics and measures to assure optimal radiation safety are necessary, given the dramatically increased exposure time that occurs during interventional cardiology procedures and the serious radiation-related complications. Methods of reducing radiation exposure to the patient, the technical staff, and the physician must be understood at a high level.

Expanded understanding of valve disease. Understanding of the anatomy and physiology of valve disease should be expanded. There must be an appreciation of the short- and long-term responsiveness of valvular tissue to balloon valvuloplasty. There should be an in-depth knowledge of the literature concerning long-term results from mitral valvuloplasty, aortic valvuloplasty, and pulmonary valvuloplasty. The physician should comprehend and be able to integrate the factors that predict success or failure of these techniques, including semiquantitative scoring systems for prognostic classification. Also, the relative merits of balloon valvuloplasty versus surgical commissurotomy or valve replacement must be understood.

Although every interventional cardiologist will not be performing every interventional procedure, these physicians should have a broad understanding of the field so as to be effective consultants to other cardiologists.

The rapid expansion of the fund of knowledge that undergirds interventional cardiology has been recognized by the American College of Cardiology,* which has issued guidelines requiring at least one extra year of training. The American Board of Internal Medicine is considering a certificate of added qualification in this field.

---

* Pepine CJ, Babb JD, Brinker JA, et al.: Task Force 3: training in cardiac catheterization and interventional cardiology. In: Guidelines for training in adult cardiovascular medicine: core cardiology training symposium (COCATS), *J Am Coll Cardiol* 25:1-34, 1995.

I

CORONARY ANGIOPLASTY

Morton J. Kern, Ubeydullah Deligonul, and Scott Carollo

INTRODUCTION

On September 16, 1977, Andreas Gruentzig performed the first percutaneous transluminal coronary angioplasty (PTCA). Until then, coronary artery bypass surgery was the only alternative to medicine for the treatment of coronary artery disease.

Over the last 15 years, improvements in equipment and technique have resulted in a dramatic growth of PTCA as a successful method of coronary revascularization. In 1992, approximately 400,000 patients underwent PTCA in the United States alone. Coronary angioplasty is the treatment of choice for discrete single-vessel coronary lesions in patients with good left ventricular function and plays a role in complex revascularization in patients with multivessel coronary artery disease and depressed left ventricular function. Despite widespread clinical application of PTCA, objective investigations comparing revascularization by PTCA or coronary artery bypass graft (CABG) surgery to medical therapy have been limited. In a Veterans' Administration study, PTCA was shown to be more effective than medical therapy in relief of angina in single-vessel coronary disease, but incurred a higher initial cost and a higher frequency of complications. Randomized comparisons of multivessel PTCA versus CABG outcomes are currently being conducted. Beyond patient selection issues, appropriate techniques for percutaneous coronary revascularization remain a case-by-case challenge for the cardiologist.

It is estimated that over 1 million cardiac catheterizations were performed in the United States in 1996. As cardiac catheterization is increasingly performed, patients known to be at an increased risk for complications (elderly, New York Heart Association Functional Class IV, left main coronary artery disease, valvular heart disease, ejection fraction <30%, severe coexisting medical diseases) will require evaluation for coronary angioplasty and associated nonsurgical revascularization techniques. Experience with newer interventional revascularization techniques has identified niche applications for specific devices (Fig. 1-1).

Overview of Method

PTCA was derived from techniques and procedures similar to those used for diagnostic cardiac catheterization. Local anesthesia is used for the insertion of arterial sheaths through which specialized guiding catheters engage coronary artery ostia in the same manner as those used for diagnostic coronary angiography. Under fluoroscopy, a guiding catheter is inserted into the femoral or brachial artery and is advanced to the ostium of the narrowed artery of the heart.

For the most common method (Fig. 1-2), a balloon catheter is loaded with a thin, steerable guidewire (0.014-0.018 in. diameter). The balloon is loaded into the guiding catheter. The guidewire is advanced into the coronary artery and positioned across the stenosis well into the distal part of the artery. The balloon catheter is then advanced over the guidewire and positioned across the stenotic area. Tracking the balloon over the guidewire into correct position within the stenosis requires experience in manipulating and controlling the three movable component parts (guide catheter, balloon catheter, and guidewire) in harmony.

After the balloon catheter is positioned correctly, the balloon is inflated to 4-10 atm several times for periods from 45 sec to several minutes. The inflation and deflation of the balloon in the blocked artery compresses the arterial stenosis and restores blood flow to the area of the heart previously deprived by the stenosed artery. If no complications occur, a

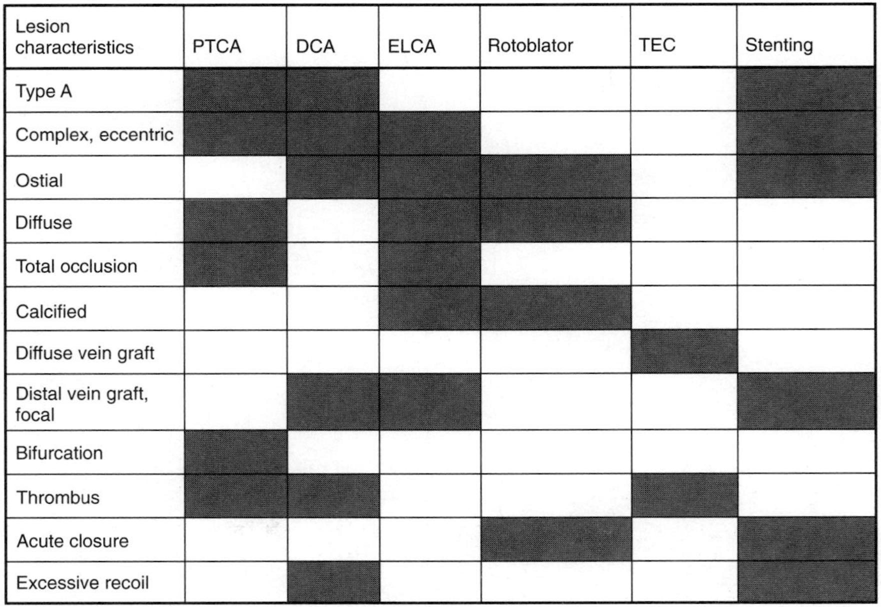

Lesion characteristics	PTCA	DCA	ELCA	Rotoblator	TEC	Stenting
Type A	■	■				■
Complex, eccentric	■	■	■			■
Ostial			■	■		■
Diffuse	■		■	■		
Total occlusion		■	■			
Calcified			■	■		
Diffuse vein graft			■		■	
Distal vein graft, focal	■	■		■		■
Bifurcation						
Thrombus	■				■	
Acute closure						■
Excessive recoil		■				■

Fig. 1-1. Niche applications of interventional techniques. *DCA,* Directional coronary atherectomy; *ECLA,* excimer coronary laser angioplasty; *TEC,* transluminal extraction catheter. Dark boxes indicate most appropriate applications. (From Deligonul U et al.: Interventional techniques. In: Kern MJ, editor: *Cardiac catheterization handbook,* St. Louis, 1995, Mosby, p 531.)

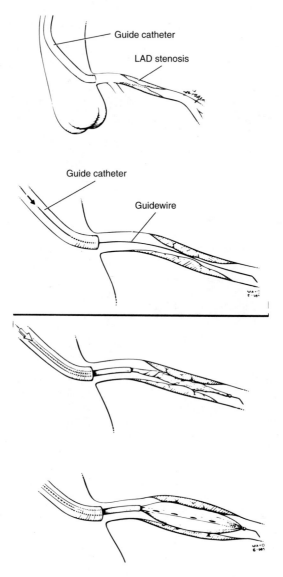

Fig. 1-2. Technique of positioning angioplasty balloon catheter across a coronary stenosis. LAD, Left anterior descending coronary artery. (From Vlietstra RE, Holmes DR Jr.: *PTCA: percutaneous transluminal coronary angioplasty*, Philadelphia, 1987, F. A. Davis, p 13.)

limited hospital stay (1-2 days) can be anticipated. The patient commonly returns to work shortly (<7 days) thereafter.

Mechanisms of Angioplasty

Several mechanisms of angioplasty have been proposed.

Disruption of plaque and the arterial wall.   The inflated balloon exerts pressure against the plaque and the arterial wall, causing fracturing and splitting. Concentric lesions fracture and split at its thinnest and weakest points. Eccentric lesions split at the junction of the plaque and the arterial wall. Dissection or separation of the plaque from the medial wall releases the splinting effect that is caused by the lesion and results in a larger lumen. This is the major effective mechanism of balloon angioplasty.

Loss of elastic recoil.   Balloon dilatation causes stretching and thinning of the medial wall. Stretching causes the medial wall to lose its elastic properties. The degree of elastic recoil loss is affected by the balloon size/artery size ratio. Almost all vessels that have undergone PTCA have a reduction of vessel lumen due to elastic recoil.

Redistribution and compression of plaque components.   During angioplasty, balloon pressure causes denudation or stripping of vascular wall (endothelial) cells, and the extrusion or pushing out of plaque components. There may be some molding of the softer lipid material, but this effect accounts for a very small part of the overall effect of angioplasty.

INDICATIONS FOR PTCA (see Guidelines AHA/ACC Task Force Report, *Circulation*; 88:2987-3007, 1993)

Specific anatomical and clinical features for each patient should be considered in applying angioplasty. The likelihood of failure and risk of complications with abrupt vessel closure, vascular morbidity, mortality, and restenosis should be weighed against specific factors favoring a successful dilatation. Restenosis and incomplete revascularization must also be weighed against the consequences of angioplasty failure.

PTCA Indications

1. Angina pectoris causing sufficient disability to warrant coronary artery bypass graft surgery in spite of optimal medical therapy

2. Mild angina pectoris with objective evidence of ischemia (abnormal stress test or abnormal stress thallium) and coronary lesion in a vessel supplying a large area of myocardium
3. Unstable angina
4. Acute myocardial infarction in patients who have contraindications to thrombolytic therapy or who have evidence of persistent or recurrent ischemia despite thrombolytic therapy (in some institutions, direct PTCA without thrombolytic therapy is used as the primary therapy)
5. Angina pectoris after coronary artery bypass graft surgery
6. Symptomatic restenosis after successful PTCA

Three clinical classifications of indications have been established by the AHA/ACC Task Force:

- *Class 1:* Conditions generally agreed upon in which coronary angioplasty is justified. A class 1 indication does not mean that angioplasty is the only acceptable therapy.
- *Class 2:* Conditions in which there is divergence of opinion with respect to the justification, value, and appropriateness of angioplasty.
- *Class 3:* Conditions for which there is agreement that coronary angioplasty is not ordinarily indicated.

The indications are summarized as follows:

I. Single-vessel coronary artery disease
   A. Class 1
      1. Significant stenosis in a major epicardial artery subtending a large area of viable myocardium with evidence of severe myocardial ischemia during exercise testing
      2. Resuscitation from cardiac arrest after sustained ventricular tachycardia in the absence of myocardial infarction
      3. Patients who must undergo high-risk noncardiac surgery (e.g., aortic aneurysm, peripheral vascular bypass, carotid artery surgery), if symptoms or objective evidence of ischemia are present. These patients should have lesion or lesions associated with a high likelihood of successful dilatation and be at low risk for morbidity and mortality.

B. Class 2

Single-vessel significant stenosis subtending moderate sized area of myocardium with:

1. Objective evidence of myocardial ischemia
2. Low risk of abrupt closure
3. Low risk for morbidity and mortality

C. Class 3

1. Mild or no symptoms, not medically treated
2. Small myocardial area at risk (very distal lesions)
3. No objective evidence of myocardial ischemia
4. Borderline lesions (40%-60% diameter reduction)
5. Moderate or high risk for procedurally induced morbidity and mortality

II. Multivessel coronary disease

A. Class 1

1. One significant lesion in a major epicardial artery that will result in nearly complete revascularization because additional lesion(s) subtend small or nonviable myocardium
2. Patients with a large area of viable myocardium at risk
3. Objective evidence of severe myocardial ischemia
4. Survival after resuscitation from cardiac arrest or ventricular tachycardia in the absence of myocardial infarction
5. High-risk noncardiac surgery candidate with objective evidence of ischemia

B. Class 2

1. Similar to class 1, but patients have only a moderate-size area of viable myocardium
2. Objective evidence of myocardial ischemia
3. Two or more major epicardial arteries, each of which subtends at least a moderate-sized area
4. Subtotally occluded vessel requiring angioplasty wherein the development of total occlusion might result in severe hemodynamic collapse due to left ventricular dysfunction

C. Class 3

1. Multivessel disease with only a small area of viable myocardium
2. Chronic total occlusions in epicardial vessel subtending large areas of myocardium
3. High risk for procedural morbidity and mortality

Other conditions involving direct coronary angioplasty for evolving myocardial infarction or unstable angina are addressed in Chapter 8.

Contraindications to PTCA

1. Unsuitable coronary anatomy (e.g., left main, severe diffuse distal disease)
2. High-risk coronary anatomy in which closure of vessel would result in patient death
3. Contraindications to coronary bypass graft surgery (some patients have PTCA as their only alternative to revascularization)
4. Bleeding diathesis (low platelet count, peptic ulcer disease, coagulopathy, and so on)
5. Patient noncompliance with procedure and post-PTCA instructions
6. Multiple PTCA restenoses

Complications of PTCA (see Chapter 4)

1. Death (<1%)
2. Myocardial infarction (<3% to 5%)
3. Emergency coronary artery bypass grafting (<5%)
4. All complications that can occur during diagnostic cardiac catheterizations can also occur during PTCA:
   a. Access-site bleeding, especially with larger sheaths and prolonged anticoagulation
   b. Contrast-media reactions
   c. Cerebral vascular accident, myocardial infarction, and so on
5. Vascular injury (e.g., pseudoaneurysm of femoral artery)
6. Restenosis (see Chapter 7)
   Note: Restenosis at the site of PTCA occurs in approximately 30% of patients after successful PTCA and may lead to recurrence of anginal symptoms. Typically, restenosis occurs most frequently within the initial 6 months after PTCA. This biologic effect is *not* considered a complication but rather a clinical part of angioplasty.

PTCA EQUIPMENT

Percutaneous transluminal coronary angioplasty equipment consists of three basic elements: the guiding catheter, the balloon catheter, and the coronary guidewire (Fig. 1-3, Table 1-1). The cost of PTCA equipment is shown in Table 1-2.

The Guiding Catheter

A special large lumen catheter is used to guide the coronary balloon system or interventional device to the vessel of the lesion to be dilated.

Functions of the Guiding Catheter (Fig. 1-4)

A guiding catheter serves three major functions during angioplasty: balloon catheter delivery and guidance; backup support for balloon advancement; and pressure monitoring.

Balloon catheter delivery and guidance. The guiding catheter provides a method for delivery of the balloon catheter to the coronary ostium. If the guiding catheter is not seated properly in a coaxial manner, it may not be possible to transmit the force needed to advance the balloon across the stenotic area.

Artery visualization with adequate contrast injection through the guide catheter is critical to position the balloon and depends on the residual catheter lumen with the associated angioplasty device in place. A guiding catheter must be large enough to permit adequate contrast administration with the balloon catheter in place to opacify the target vessel. Large, nonballoon angioplasty devices in some guide catheters (directional coronary atherectomy [DCA], transluminal extraction catheter [TEC], stents) may not allow adequate vessel opacification during procedural angiography.

Operators should select an internal guide catheter lumen diameter large enough to allow adequate contrast flow around the balloon catheter to obtain a clear angiographic image of the lesion being dilated during the angioplasty. As balloon catheters have become smaller, the size of internal diameter of the guiding catheter has become less important for achieving adequate visualization. A large guide catheter lumen, however, is critical to facilitate easy passage of stents, atherectomy devices, and large reperfusion balloon catheters.

Backup support for balloon advancement. Support or "backup" for balloon catheter advancement is achieved after seating (cannulating) the guide catheter in the coronary ostium. The guiding catheter provides the necessary backup platform to push the balloon catheter over the guidewire through the artery and across the stenosis.

Inadequate backup support will result in failure to cross

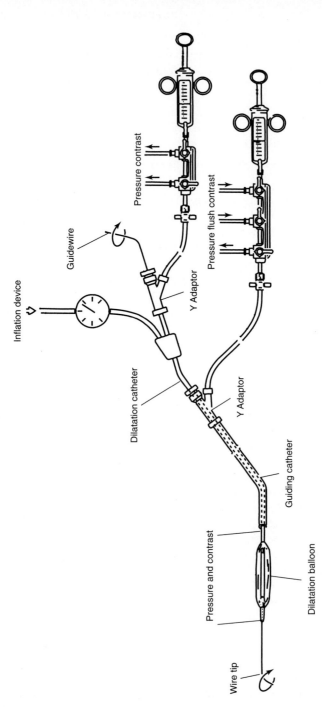

Fig. I-3. Components of PTCA system. (From Tilkian AG, Daily EK: *Cardiovascular procedures: diagnostic techniques and therapeutic procedures*, St. Louis, 1986, Mosby.)

Inflation device

Guidewire

Pressure contrast

Y Adaptor

Pressure flush contrast

Dilatation catheter

Y Adaptor

Guiding catheter

Pressure and contrast

Dilatation balloon

Wire tip

TABLE 1-1.   Advantages and limitations of angioplasty balloon types

Advantages	Limitations
Over-the-wire	
Distal wire position	Two experienced personnel required
Distal port available for pressure measurement or contrast media injection	Larger profile
Accepts multiple guidewires	
Rapid exchange	
Distal wire position	Excellent guiding catheter support
Enhanced visualization	Exchanging balloons at hemostatic valve can be technically demanding
Low-profile balloons	Poor balloon tracking if wire lumen not flushed with heparinized saline
Single-operator system	
Fixed wire	
Enhanced visualization	Lack of full-length guidewire through the catheter lumen
Single-operator system	Inability to recross lesion without removing system
Flexibility	
Access to distal lesions	
Use with small guiding catheters	
Low-profile balloons	

From Kern MJ, editor: *The cardiac catheterization handbook,* ed 2, St. Louis, 1995, Mosby.

a lesion and an unsuccessful procedure. Backup support requires a combination of correct coaxial (in-line with the artery ostium) alignment, as well as the ability to provide carefully controlled advancement of the guiding catheter into the coronary ostium.

The improved quality and size of currently used balloon catheters have reduced the need for robust backup support in many situations. For more complex and technically difficult lesions, the choice of an appropriate guiding catheter for adequate support and lesion visualization remains essential (see Chapter 3). Although commercially formed catheters are generally adequate, occasionally a guiding catheter will need to be reshaped in the catheterization laboratory using a heat gun for successful coronary cannulation and backup support.

TABLE 1-2.   Approximate costs of coronary angioplasty equipment

Equipment	Cost ($)
Balloon dilatation catheter	350–700
Guiding catheter	60–110
Guidewire	85–105
Exchange guidewire (300 cm)	130
Extension for guidewire	105
Indeflator	75
Y connector	20–30
Sheath introducer	20
Torque tool	5
Nonballoon devices	
Stent	1200–1600
Directional atherectomy catheter	1300
Rotablator	1200
Transluminal extraction catheter	1200
Laser catheter	1500

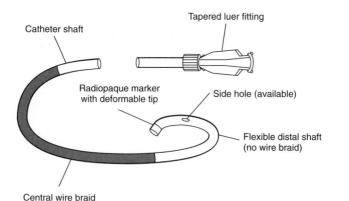

Fig. 1-4.   Construction of a guiding catheter. The features noted differentiate from diagnostic catheters. (From Avedissian MG, et al.: Percutaneous transluminal coronary angioplasty: a review of current balloon dilation systems, *Cathet Cardiovasc Diagn* 18:263, 1989.)

When there is insufficient backup or a very tight stenosis, the guiding catheter may be disengaged from the coronary ostium and backed out into the aortic root. When pressure is applied to the balloon during attempts to cross the lesion, repositioning the guide catheter in a stepwise fashion as the balloon is advanced may overcome this loss of support. Aggressive intubation of the coronary ostium may damage the vessel, stopping the procedure prematurely.

Deep seating of the guide catheter is the result of manipulating the guide catheter over the balloon catheter shaft past the aorto-coronary ostium and farther into the vessel, to obtain increased backup support for crossing difficult lesions. This maneuver typically is used as a *last resort* because of the increased chance of guide catheter-induced dissection of the left main or proximal vessel.

Pressure monitoring.   The guiding catheter measures aortic pressure during the case. Pressure wave damping may occur during coronary artery engagement. Pressure measured proximal to the stenotic area is compared to distal transstenotic pressure for assessment of lesion severity.

Guide Catheter Construction

Catheter shaft.   Compared to the diagnostic catheters, the guiding catheters have thinner walls, larger lumens, and stiffer shafts. A large catheter lumen is achieved at the expense of catheter wall thickness and thus may result in decreased catheter wall strength, less torque control, or catheter kinking. The guiding catheters are stiffer to provide backup support during the balloon catheter advancement into the coronary artery and, therefore, respond differently to manipulation than diagnostic catheters. The guiding catheter tip is not tapered, occasionally causing pressure-wave damping upon engaging the coronary ostium more often than with similar-size diagnostic angiographic catheters. Some guide catheters have relatively shorter and more flexible tips to decrease catheter-induced trauma.

Side holes.   Guiding catheters with small side holes permit blood to enter the coronary artery when the ostium is small. Side holes are used when the guide catheter either partially or totally occludes blood flow into the coronary artery. The guide catheter coronary occlusion is usually noted by arterial pressure waveform "damping." Side holes in the catheter allow for coronary blood to flow into the vessel, eliminating or reducing ischemia when the guiding catheter is seated satisfactorily. However, side holes may lead to inadequate artery visualization from loss of contrast media exiting the catheter before entering the artery. Although side holes may provide reliable aortic pressure, coronary flow and pressure can still be compromised during the angioplasty procedure. The guide catheter and side holes act as a second stenosis at the coronary ostium.

Small-shaft-diameter guide catheters. No. 8 French guiding catheters are currently the most frequently utilized size, although coronary angioplasty has been performed through diagnostic No. 5 and 6 French catheters using fixed-wire balloon systems. Use of smaller-diameter guide catheters, conceptually, will result in fewer vascular complications and allow earlier ambulation of patients. However, this advantage is offset by a compromised quality of coronary angiograms with smaller catheter lumen sizes. Small-size French guide catheters do not allow for the use of perfusion catheters, often required for dissections or acute occlusions. In Europe, stent placement through No. 6 French guide catheters from percutaneous femoral, brachial, and radial arteries is common practice.

Tip configuration. Because a guiding catheter can traumatize the coronary artery being intubated, a softer plastic tip has been advocated to minimize potential trauma during catheter manipulation. Soft tip configurations are available for many guide catheters.

BALLOON DILATATION CATHETER SYSTEMS
Types of Balloon Catheters

There are three types of angioplasty balloon catheters (Fig. 1-5): over-the-wire, monorail, and fixed-wire balloon catheters. The advantages and limitations are summarized in Table 1-1.

Over-the-wire angioplasty balloon catheters. A standard over-the-wire angioplasty balloon catheter (Fig. 1-5) has a central lumen throughout the length of the catheter for the guidewire and another separate lumen for balloon inflation. These balloons are approximately 145-155 cm long and can be used with guidewires of various dimensions

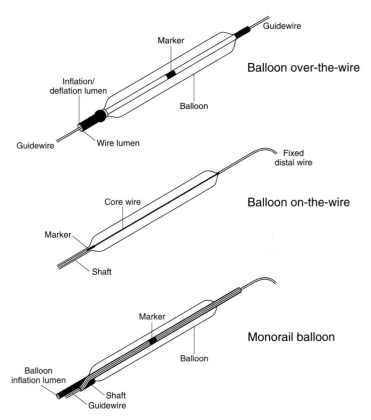

Fig. 1-5.   Three common types of coronary balloon angioplasty catheter designs. (Modified from Freed M, Grines C, editors: *Manual of interventional cardiology,* Birmingham, Mich, 1992, Physician's Press, p 29.)

(0.010-0.018 in.). The balloon catheter may have a guidewire lumen that is large enough for pressure measurement and distal contrast injection with the wire in place.

In these systems, the guidewire and the balloon catheter move independently. The major advantage is the ability to maintain artery access with the guidewire beyond the lesion while exchanging one balloon catheter for another. Using standard technique, after the balloon is tracked over the wire, the wire may be removed from the balloon if distal injections or pressure measurements are needed, or the wire may be removed to be reshaped and reintroduced through the central lumen. A regular guidewire length (145 cm) can be extended (300 cm) to help maintain distal position while the balloon catheter is completely withdrawn over the guidewire and another balloon catheter is exchanged and introduced over the same guidewire for additional dilatations. An alternative method of balloon catheter exchange is to replace the guidewire with a 300-cm exchange-length guidewire.

Over-the-wire catheters can accept multiple guidewires, which allows for exchanging additional devices that may require stronger, stiffer guidewires. Most ultralow-profile angioplasty balloon catheters currently do not permit distal pressure measurement or contrast injection.

Over-the-wire angioplasty balloon catheters have few limitations. These catheters are, in general, slightly larger than the rapid-exchange (monorail) and fixed-wire catheters, and their use with smaller-size (6F) guiding catheters may be more difficult. Despite the very low balloon profile, over-the-wire balloons may also need very good guide catheter backup support. In some laboratories, additional personnel may be required to facilitate long guidewire exchanges.

Rapid-exchange (monorail) angioplasty balloon catheters. "Rapid-exchange" monorail balloon catheters were developed to improve exchanging angioplasty balloon catheters by single operators. Rapid-exchange catheters have only a variable length of the catheter shaft containing two lumens. One lumen runs the entire length of the catheter and is used for balloon inflation. The other lumen, which extends only a portion of the catheter shaft, houses the guidewire. Because only a limited portion of the balloon requires dual lumens, rapid-exchange catheters are smaller, improving contrast visualization of the artery.

Rapid-exchange balloon catheters address certain inherent limitations of over-the-wire catheters. First, over-the-wire balloon exchanges require a long (or extension) guidewire, an unnecessary maneuver for the rapid-exchange type. Second, a single operator can use rapid-exchange balloon catheters without the aid of other assistants to maintain distal guidewire position.

Limitations of monorail catheters include the need for excellent guiding catheter support and difficulty with simultaneous manipulation of the guidewire, balloon catheter, and guiding catheter. There may be excessive blood loss at the rotating hemostatic valve during removal of the balloon catheter or during the balloon removal (back-out) maneuver. Additionally, the balloon may be difficult to track across the guidewire if the distal catheter lumen was not properly flushed with heparinized saline solution. Care must also be exercised when the balloon and guidewire are advanced through the guiding catheter to the coronary ostia. If the monorail balloon is advanced in front of the wire, the wire may come out of its short lumen, necessitating reassembly of the balloon and guidewire. When monorail catheters with relatively short "rails" are used in distal grafts, the free portion of the guidewire in the aorta may loop and kink during balloon catheter pullback, a problem which may be difficult to diagnose when a nonradioopaque wire is used.

Perfusion balloon catheters.   The perfusion catheter is a variant of the conventional monorail balloon catheter system with multiple side holes proximal and distal to the balloon, communicating directly with the central lumen of the catheter, allowing arterial blood to flow through the proximal side holes, down the central lumen, and out of the distal side holes with the balloon inflated in the lesion. This catheter permits perfusion of the myocardium during balloon inflation. Currently, the Advanced Cardiovascular Systems (ACS), Inc. (Mountainview, Calif.) systems are the only balloons available that provide this type of distal perfusion catheter. Two sizes are available, termed 60S and 40S. The 60S is meant to supply approximately 40-50 cc/min of blood during inflations; the 40S has a lower profile and allows less flow (30-40 cc/min). The perfusion catheter is of particular value when the patient is unable to tolerate the ischemia induced with routine balloon inflations. A perfusion catheter is selected to reduce severe angina, hypotension from compromised ventricular function, or when prolonged inflations are required (as with a dissection). Its disadvantages are related to its bulky size, which makes it difficult (if not impossible) to track through the tortuous arterial segment and limited artery opacification.

Fixed-wire angioplasty balloon catheters.   The fixed-wire catheter has the balloon mounted on a central hollow wire with a distal flexible steering tip. The proximal end of the catheter consists of a single nonremovable port connected to a thin metal tube (hypotube). A core wire extends from the hypotube to the end of the distal steerable tip. This assembly is coated with a thin plastic shaft that enhances flexibility. Fixed-wire balloons have only one enclosed lumen for balloon inflation.

The on-the-wire balloon catheter is a fixed system, where the wire cannot be advanced independent of the balloon and the balloon cannot be exchanged without removing the entire system. Since the wire is attached to the distal end of the balloon, there is no central balloon lumen, resulting in a lower total profile than with an over-the-wire system. Its principal advantages relate to its low profile, enabling passage through very tight stenoses, and good contrast visualization of the lesion being dilated around the balloon catheter.

The small shaft size provides excellent coronary visualization. Because the balloon is mounted on the distal guidewire, the device can easily be used by a single operator. Fixed-wire balloon catheters are particularly useful for distal lesions, subtotal stenoses, and lesions located in tortuous vasculature. Additionally, they may be particularly beneficial when small (<6F) guiding catheters are used.

The limitations of fixed-wire catheters include lack of the inherent safety advantage of over-the-wire and rapid-exchange systems because the balloon is mounted on a guide-wire. To exchange this catheter for a different balloon size, the catheter is removed completely and the lesion is recrossed with a new balloon catheter. A narrowed or dissected lesion may not permit recrossing or advancement of another balloon catheter. Further attempts at balloon recrossing may even close the vessel. The lack of a distal lumen prevents measuring of distal pressure or injection of contrast media. An angioplasty guidewire can be introduced alongside the fixed-wire balloon catheter before removing the catheter to assist in placing another balloon, but extra caution to minimize vessel disruption and guidewire displacement is needed.

Balloon Catheter Construction Materials

The plastic material of the balloon determines its compliance and tensile strength. The main differentiation among balloons is related to compliant or noncompliant materials. Inflation of a compliant balloon above nominal pressure (i.e., a set pressure for a known balloon size) will lead to further expansion of the balloon approximately 10%-20% over the rated diameter. Noncompliant balloons, on the other hand, remain very close to their rated diameter, even when inflated several atmospheres above nominal pressure. The advantages and disadvantages of balloon materials remain controversial. A compliant balloon may be more cost effective and result in fewer balloons being used in a given case. However, a compliant balloon may result in oversizing, particularly on second and third inflations, resulting in dissections. The complication rate of such mechanisms has not been tested in randomized clinical trials.

Most balloons are coated with low-friction surface polymers that facilitate lesion crossing. The advantages of the various polymers are related to specific applications for various balloon mechanics.

Balloon Mechanics

The mechanical aspects of balloon angioplasty apply the following fundamental principles.

1. According to Laplace's law, wall stress increases with radius. At a given pressure, a larger balloon undergoes more wall stress than a smaller balloon, promoting balloon rupture. The arterial segment next to the lesion has a larger luminal radius than the lesion. Thus, artery sites adjacent to the lesion may be traumatized.

2. At high pressures, balloons weaken over time. The balloon burst pressure may be decreased during subsequent inflations of the same balloon. When inflating a balloon above the rated burst pressure, consider limiting the number and duration of inflations.

3. Balloon diameters always increase with increasing pressure. Noncompliant balloons will grow in diameter by <10% over nominal pressures. Compliant balloons may increase >20%. The balloon diameter-pressure relation is usually linear, reflecting the compliance characteristics. Figure 1-6A shows the balloon during inflation. Figure 1-6B shows graph for pressure versus diameter.

4. Balloons do not return to the original dimensions when deflated. At any given pressure, the balloon diameter during a subsequent inflation will be larger than during the first inflation. When dilating two lesions with a compliant balloon, consider approaching the smaller lesion first.

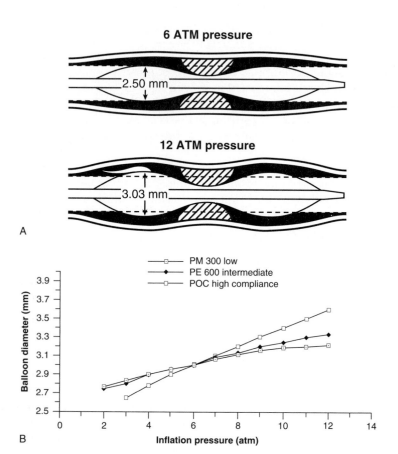

Fig. 1-6. **A,** Balloon size changes proposed to occur during increasing inflation pressure when using compliant balloon material. (With permission from: Clinical issues in angioplasty balloon material: a review of the literature regarding polyethylene terephthalate (PET), USCI Division of C. R. Bard, Inc.) **B,** Diameter–pressure relationships of three balloon materials. All three balloons have nominal size 3.0 mm at 6 atm. (From Raymenants E, et al.: *Cathet Cardiovasc Diagn* 32:303-309, 1994.)

Selection of Balloon Material and Catheter Size

The selection of balloon material is subjective. Conventional wisdom regarding balloon material selection is summarized in Table 1-3. The balloon size is selected to achieve a 1 : 1 size match with the vessel. Balloon-to-artery ratios >1.2 : 1 are associated with increased complications.

The balloon size is determined using the distal arterial reference segment diameter as gauged by the guiding catheter size (e.g., 7F guide = 2.31 mm, 8F = 2.64 mm, 9F = 2.97 mm, 11F = 3.63 mm). Visual estimation of balloon size is less accurate than quantitative angiographic approaches, but it is the method utilized by most interventionalists.

Balloon Length

Longer balloons (30 or 40 mm) are useful for dilating long or diffuse narrowings. Short (10-15 mm) balloons are used for stent reexpansion to avoid stretching the uninvolved vessel wall.

Selection of an appropriate balloon catheter for angioplasty should consider the design characteristics as well as the ana-

TABLE 1-3. Conventional wisdom of balloon material selection

Pick a *noncompliant balloon* if you have . . .	Pick a *compliant balloon* if you have . . .
An *a priori* requirement for exact sizing (not to be exceeded)	An *a priori* expectation of up-sizing balloon
Absolute knowledge of final diameter wanted	Suspicion that absolute dimensions are subject to change
A hard, calcific lesion (need high pressure)	A soft, expansile lesion
No severe bend points	A need for less straightening at bend points
Readiness to use additional balloons	Desire to use fewer balloons
Fear of "dogbones"*	Belief that "dogbones" are not an issue

* The identation in the middle of an inflated balloon that is caused by the unexpected stenotic material. It appears as a dog's bone shape.
From Bach RG, et al.: Dog bones, dumbbells, and dissections: sizing up angioplasty balloons, *Cathet Cardiovasc Diagn* 32:310–311, 1994.

tomic problems to ensure a technically and clinically successful procedure.

Balloon Inflation Strategies

Stenosis resolution occurs when the balloon pressure eliminates the balloon indentation caused by the stenosis. Unstable
or thrombotic lesions are associated with a lower stenosis
resolution pressure than chronic, stable lesions. Most coronary lesions respond to inflation pressures <10 atm. In a large
study of 3398 PTCAs, Kahn and Hartzler found that only
0.6% failed due to undilatable lesions. Morice et al. observed
stenosis resolution pressures of <10 atm in 89% of 4000 patients, and of <13 atm in 99%.

High balloon inflation pressures.   High inflation pressures may be associated with better early angiographic results. Lehmann et al. found that with undersized noncompliant balloons (balloon : artery ratio 0.9), increasing the pressure
from 5 to 10 atm expanded the luminal cross-sectional area
by an additional 25% over that achieved with inflations of
up to 5 atm. However, optimal angiographic results may not
produce the best clinical results. Beatt et al. found that the
greatest improvements in lumen diameter at the time of angioplasty correlated with the highest restenosis rates. High
pressures in compliant balloons may produce an oversized
balloon-to-artery ratio, which has been associated with an
increased incidence of dissection and complications.

Low balloon inflation pressures.   Coronary angioplasty
using low inflation pressures has become a popular approach.
Low-pressure inflations may reduce complications. Most procedures may start with low pressures, but operators often
feel compelled to use higher pressures to achieve satisfactory
angiographic results.

Optimal inflation pressure strategy.   When standard
pressures fail to dilate a lesion, alternative techniques include
switching to a high-pressure balloon, a hugging balloon, a
parallel wire (focused force), or a nonballoon technique such
as rotational or laser atherectomy. Upsizing to a larger balloon
and dilating at low pressures may also be effective. Excessive
inflation pressures should be avoided due to risk of rupturing
or overdilating vessels.

Duration of inflation.   Inflations may be brief (<60 sec),
intermediate (60-180 sec), or long (>180 sec). No consensus

on the optimal duration inflation exists. The length of inflation is usually limited by the patient's tolerance of ischemia. Most physicians use inflation times of between 1 and 3 min. Studies comparing outcomes for 1-min versus 5-min inflations note that there is no difference in acute complication and immediate angiographic results, and 6-month restenosis rates were similar for both techniques.

Issues in Choosing Equipment for Simple Coronary Angioplasty

Simple coronary angioplasty includes the majority of type A and B lesions in the AHA/ACC lesion classification (see Chapter 3). Important technical considerations for selecting appropriate angioplasty systems include balloon catheter profile, trackability, pushability, and ease of exchange.

Balloon profile.   The size of the deflated balloon (profile) has been emphasized in balloon design and selection. The majority of both on-the-wire and over-the-wire systems are currently <1 mm in diameter. Nonetheless, angioplasty balloons are now all small (profile size of 0.035 and 0.033 in.), so there may not be any practical difference among catheters. Manufacturer-reported deflated angioplasty balloon profiles may not always be accurate. The smaller profiles of the new over-the-wire systems have reduced the main advantage (very low profile) of fixed-wire systems. However, in the unusual situation where, in spite of adequate guide catheter support and placement of a wire across the lesion, a balloon cannot be advanced across the lesion, a fixed-wire system often can be successful. Balloon profile alone is not the only factor assisting a balloon to track across a lesion.

Catheter trackability.   Trackability is the ability to advance the balloon catheter through the vessel to reach the lesion. Trackability is a function of both the wire and the balloon. A stiffer guidewire will allow easier trackability. Although balloon catheters are marketed based on their ability to track and conform to the vessel, trackability is difficult to measure in an objective manner.

Catheter pushability.   Pushability is the ability to transfer force through the shaft of the balloon. This feature is also difficult to measure objectively. There may be little difference in the pushability of the majority of the standard systems.

Resistance to balloon catheter forward motion may occur due to guidewire–balloon friction, balloon–guide catheter friction, or balloon–artery friction.

Ease of catheter exchange.   The monorail catheter system is the quickest and easiest to exchange. The standard over-the-wire balloon requires the placement of a long guidewire, the attachment of an exchange system to the end of the guidewire, or a guidewire trapping system (Trapper, SciMed). A rapid-exchange system reduces x-ray exposure time, because fluoroscopy is not required if the wire is fixed during catheter removal.

Balloon compliance.   Compliant balloons increase in size with increased pressure, limiting exchanges and necessity for extra balloons. The theoretical disadvantages include risks that balloon oversizing may lead to dissection.

Guidewire compatibility.   Although the vast majority of lesions can be crossed using a 0.014-in. guidewire, occasionally, a 0.018-in. wire is needed to cross a very severe stenosis or a tight angulation point or for extra support for stent placement. A balloon catheter that is 0.018-in. guidewire compatible has an advantage in these circumstances.

Perfusion balloon catheters.   Perfusion of a distal vessel during balloon inflations may be necessary in certain situations. However, the higher-profile perfusion balloon catheters must be considered and may be difficult to insert the required location. Also, perfusion balloon catheters tend to be stiffer and more difficult to negotiate in tortuous segments.

High-inflation-pressure capability.   The construction material of the balloon determines both its compliance and its tensile strength. The majority of lesions will dilate at balloon pressures of <8 atm. Occasionally, however, high (>20 atm) balloon inflation pressures are required, particularly for calcified lesions. Most balloons are rated to maintain their integrity at <12 atm.

Noncompliant balloons that can exceed 14 atm are especially useful for complete stent deployment and apposition to the vessel wall, a feature associated with improved outcome.

ANGIOPLASTY GUIDEWIRES

Coronary guidewires are very small caliber (0.010-0.018-in.) steerable wires, advanced into the coronary artery or branches beyond the lesion to be dilated. A J tip of varying degree usually is shaped by the operator, allowing steerability in negotiating side branches and tortuous artery curves (Fig. 1-7).

The characteristics of guidewires are determined by the core and tip. The shorter the distance between the central core and the distal wedge tip, the more rigid and torquable the wire will be. Differences in core construction affect guidewire handling. Important considerations when selecting a guidewire include diameter, coating, torque control, steerability, flexibility, malleability, radioopacity, and trackability. Diameters for coronary guidewires usually range from 0.010 to 0.018 in. Larger guidewires have better torquability and steerability and provide more support, while small-diameter wires are more trackable. Certain balloon catheters are not 0.018-in. guidewire compatible and can be used only with a 0.014-in. guidewire. Custom tip shaping will help steer the guidewire. Several helpful shapes are shown in Table 1-4.

Characteristics for Guidewire Selection

The selection and placement of a guidewire distal to the stenosis depend on the clinical situation and the operator's experience and skills. The following terms are applied to angioplasty guidewires.

Stiffness. The overall stiffness of the guidewire contributes to specific performance. Softer wires are safer and easier to advance into the tortuous branches. Stiffer wires give better torque control and are useful for crossing difficult or total occlusions. Extra stiff guidewires provide better support for intracoronary stent placement.

Steerability. The ability to advance the wire successfully through tortuous segments and side branches by steering rotation of the wire from positions proximal to the balloon is the most important feature of the guidewire.

Flexibility. Flexibility relates to the distance from the tip of the central core to the distal tip of the wire. It is important in avoiding vascular trauma when crossing and recrossing lesions.

Malleability. Malleability is the ability to attain and maintain a desired tip shape. Repeated attempts with different wire tip configurations may be required to cross distal

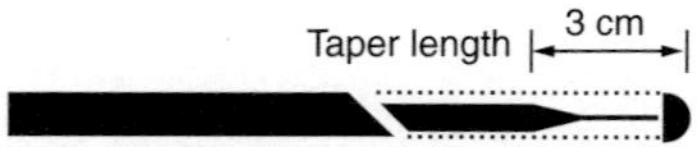

Standard tip flexibility

Catalog number	Diameter, inches	Length, cm	Taper length, cm	Tip shape
502-596	0.014	175	3.0	Straight
502-595	0.014	300	3.0	Straight

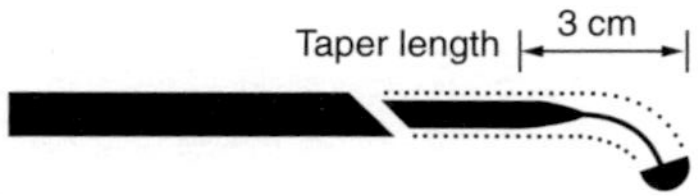

Taper length |— 3 cm —|

Standard tip flexibility

Catalog number	Diameter, inches	Length, cm	Taper length, cm	Tip shape
502-597	0.014	175	3.0	J-Curve

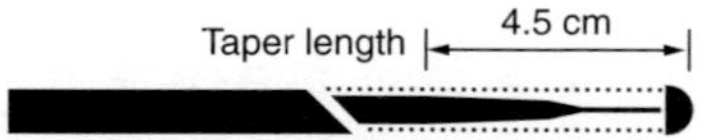

Taper length |— 3 cm —|

High tip flexibility

Catalog number	Diameter, inches	Length, cm	Taper length, cm	Tip shape
502-598	0.014	175	4.5	Straight

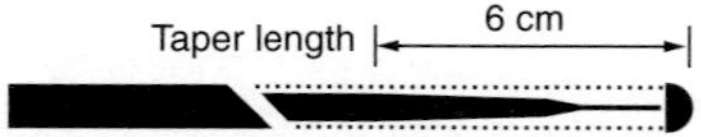

Taper length |——— 4.5 cm ———|

Very high tip flexibility

Catalog number	Diameter, inches	Length, cm	Taper length, cm	Tip shape
502-599	0.014	175	6.0	Straight

Taper length |———— 6 cm ————|

Fig. 1-7. Guidewire construction and flexibility. (Courtesy Cordis Corporation, Miami, Fla.)

segments. Some guidewires are preformed to match specific standard coronary anatomy. Guidewire shaping is accomplished by bending the wire between the thumb and index finger, or by rolling the guidewire tip over a needle. In general, the length of the distal end should approximate half the diameter of the vessel. A large bend may not reach the target takeoff. When steering the wire into an abruptly angled branch, a double bend is helpful (Table 1-4).

Radioopacity. Visualization of the guidewire is provided by the platinum coil wrapped around the distal parts of the wire. The advantages of a radioopaque wire include better ability to see and maneuver the wire. However, a wire that is too highly visible may obscure useful angiographic detail, particularly small coronary dissections. A variety of different coatings are now used on guidewires, leading to increased ease of wire movement within the balloon catheter.

Exchange length and extension guidewires. An exchange guidewire is similar to those mentioned above, except that its length is 280 to 300 cm. This long wire replaces the initial wire when exchange of the balloon catheter is necessary (e.g., upsizing balloon or insertion of perfusion catheter). Alternatively, and more conveniently, a 120-145-cm extension wire can be connected to the initial guidewire to allow balloon catheter exchanges. Some specially designed balloon catheters with only a distal wire lumen (monorail system) allow exchange over a regular-length guidewire. A magnet designed to hold the regular-length guidewire in place while the balloon is advanced or pulled back is available.

Trapper exchange system. Another technique involving a guidewire trapping exchange balloon system (SciMed) has become available, allowing an exchange without the use of a long guidewire. The Trapper guidewire exchange system uses a special short balloon-on-a-wire that is not long enough to leave the end of the guide catheter. When it is inflated, it traps the guidewire against the inside wall of the guide catheter, permitting the balloon catheter to be pulled off without moving the guidewire. A different size balloon catheter can then be advanced over the wire, the trapper deflated, and the balloon catheter readvanced into the artery. Air or thrombus embolization into the coronary artery has been encountered with the Trapper system.

TABLE I-4. Guidewire tip curves which can facilitate difficult anatomic problems during PTCA

No. of angulations	Configuration of the tip	Location of the lesion	Characteristics of the coronary anatomy	Rationale
Single	*Angle is mild or moderate* RD is smaller than the diameter of the LMCA (tip is similar to commercial J curves).	Proximal RCA, Cx or LAD	Vessels are straight, take off of the branches is shallow, difference in diameter of the LMCA and a narrowed branch is not marked	Lesions are easily reached with only minimal manipulations
Double	*Proximal and distal angles are mild or moderate* Total RD approximates the diameter of the LMCA. Distal RD is similar to the diameter of the narrowed branch	Proximal or mid RCA, LAD, and Cx	Vessels are mildly tortuous; branches take off with mild to moderate angles; difference between the diameter of the LMCA and diameter of the narrowed branch is not marked	Proximal angle adds RD to improve entry into the branches of the large proximal vessels; distal angulation allows easier manipulations in the smaller distal branches
	Shallow distal angle Proximal angle is steeper; total RD is unchanged from the above	Proximal, mid, or distal RCA, Cx, and LAD	Tight stenoses; trifurcation or two opposing branches originating from the same segment (e.g., septal and diagonal branches of the LAD)	The shallow distal angle with small RD has tendency to remain centrally located, avoid sidebranches and traverse lesions easier
	Steep distal angle With short arm and small reaching distance. Proximal RD is unchanged	Distally, primarily in the obtuse marginal or diagonal arteries	Vessels have sharp bends and kinks; narrowed branches have sharp angles; the difference in diameter of the LMCA and the narrowed branch is *very marked* (e.g., the diagonal branch taking off sharply and subsequently curving resembling a small letter "h")	Steep distal angle is required to enter the sidebranches at the proper angle and improves advancement of the wire around a steep curve

	Long proximal arm required	If the LMCA has large diameter and the LAD or Cx have a sharper angle of origin (more common with Cx)	Longer proximal arm adds RD, thus improving entry into the large proximal vessels (LAD or Cx)
	Very long proximal arm Distal arm is shallow	Severe stenosis of the proximal Cx (rarely LAD)	The vessel has a take off of 90° or more from the LMCA with subsequent posterior curve; the lesion is severe, located immediately distal to the bend
			The very long proximal arm permits the distal angle to function "independently," facilitating the vertical entry into the lesion
	Both arms are long Total RD is large but usually smaller than the diameter of the large vessels	Large vessels—e.g., severely arteriosclerotic abdominal aorta or iliac arteries	Large RD is required to enter eccentrically located lumen, often from the aneurysmal areas
Triple or multiple 	*Angles are moderate* Distal arm is shorter; total RD is large	Mid or distal in all major vessels	The difference in diameter of the LMCA and a narrowed branch is *very marked*; the LAD or Cx originate *steeply*
			Transition from the long to short arm and advancement of the wire around a sharp angle of the proximal vessel are smoother

From Voda J: Angled tip of the steerable guidewire and its usefulness in percutaneous transluminal coronary angioplasty, *Cathet Cardiovasc Diagn* 13:204-210, 1987.

A magnetized guidewire with a strong magnet can secure the guidewire in place while the balloon catheter is withdrawn and another is inserted over the wire being held by the magnet.

Accessory Equipment for Balloon Catheter Placement

Adjustable hemostasis and rotating Y-connector valve. The Y connector is attached to the guide catheter to permit introduction of the balloon catheter into the guide while allowing injection of contrast agent through the guide catheter. The end of the Y connector has a rotating adapter. The Y connector is an accessory device that minimizes bleeding through the guide catheter while the balloon catheter is inserted. The Y connector permits the injection of contrast and pressure monitoring through the guiding catheter, regardless of balloon catheter position. When attached to a balloon catheter, pressure around a guidewire can be measured.

Balloon inflation device.   A disposable syringe device delivers pressure to inflate the balloon on the angioplasty catheter. A pressure gauge or display indicates the precise inflation pressure in atmospheres or psi. Typically, the balloon is inflated with sufficient pressure (4-12 atm) to fully compress the stenosis indentation ("dumbbell") of the partially inflated balloon. Occasionally, some lesions involved with calcium or highly fibrotic may require very high inflation pressures (>14 atm) to expand the lesion and eliminate the "dumbbell." Overinflation of the balloon increases the risk of dissection and balloon rupture.

Guidewire torque (tool) device.   A small cylindrical pin vise clamp slides over the proximal end of the steerable guidewire, permitting the operator to perform fine manipulations of the guidewire.

Guidewire introducer.   A very thin, needlelike tube with a tapered conical opening helps the guidewire to be inserted into balloon catheters and through Y adapters.

Long arterial sheaths.   Long-length (23-cm) femoral arterial sheaths allow one to repeatedly negotiate a tortuous iliac artery more easily than with the standard 10-cm sheath used for diagnostic catheterization. A long sheath may also improve the torque control for guiding catheter maneuvers.

CORONARY BALLOON ANGIOPLASTY:
THE CLINICAL PROCEDURE

I. Pre-PTCA workup
  A. Noninvasive testing for ischemia
    1. Electrocardiogram
    2. Exercise stress testing with/without thallium as indicated. Alternative means of demonstrating ischemia, such as pharmacologic stress with adenosine or dipyridamole, may suffice.
    3. Two-dimensional echocardiogram (as indicated for left ventricular function or valvular heart disease)
  B. Coronary angiography
  Note: Order of tests depends on clinical presentation. An objective demonstration of ischemia is important. If there is no prior physiologic assessment of intermediately severe lesions (40%-70%), use translesional pressure/flow measurements (see Chapter 10).

II. Pre-PTCA preparation
  A. Patient preparation
    1. Cardiothoracic surgeon consultation, particularly for multivessel disease or patients with decreased left ventricular function
    2. Appropriate laboratory work (type and cross-match, complete blood count [CBC] and platelet, prothrombin time [PT], partial thromboplastin time [PTT], electrolytes, blood urea nitrogen [BUN], creatinine)
    3. Patient and family information
  B. Premedication before coming to the laboratory
    1. Aspirin (325 mg PO)
    Note: Failure to administer aspirin before angioplasty is associated with a two to three times higher acute complication rate.
    2. Persantine (75-100 mg PO, optional)
    3. Calcium antagonist (diltiazem, 30 mg PO, or nifedipine, 10 mg PO, amlodipine, 5 mg PO)
    Note: Avoid doses that produce hypotension.
  C. Patient preparation in catheterization suite
    1. ECG (inferior and anterior wall leads): 12-lead (radiolucent) ECG
    2. Skin preparation; both inguinal areas

3. Venous access for temporary pacing (for large right coronary or dominant circumflex arteries or high-risk cases)
4. Premedications
   a. Diazepam (5 mg IV or PO)
   b. Benadryl (25 mg IV or PO)
   c. Demerol (25-50 mg IV) before balloon inflation
   d. Heparin (10,000 U or 100 U/kg IV bolus; 1000 U IV/hr; activated clotting time [ACT] should be >300 sec)
D. Guiding coronary arteriograms (perform after giving 100-200 μg nitroglycerin intracoronary)
   1. Confirm coronary vessel size and collateral supply (if any)
   2. Guiding shots to use as reference maps for guidewire and balloon positioning.
III. Angioplasty balloon dilation procedure
   A. Seating guiding catheter
      1. Guiding catheter selected for angle of vessel take-off and optimal backup support
      2. Cannulation of target vessel; check for arterial pressure "damping"; if present, consider side holes
   B. Insertion of balloon catheter
      1. Size of angioplasty dilatation catheter to fit vessel (based on normal reference; balloon/artery ratio <1:1.2)
      2. Steerable guidewire with appropriate tip softness (pin vise connected to guidewire)
      3. Balloon catheter loaded with guidewire. Assembly is inserted through hemostasis valve (Y connector) or guide catheter.
      4. Flush catheter systems for pressure monitoring (when applicable)
   C. Crossing the lesion with the wire and balloon
      1. Maintain seating of guiding catheter.
      2. Pass guidewire beyond lesion as far distal as possible.
      3. Advance dilatation balloon into center of lesion.
   D. Dilating the lesion
      1. Maintain centering of the balloon
      2. Using adequate inflation pressure (to remove lesion indentation [dumbbell]) and time (60-120 sec, as tolerated).

  3. Deflate balloon. Withdraw balloon, leaving guide-wire in place.
 E. Assess immediate result with angiography
  1. Enlarged artery lumen ($\leq$40% residual lesion), no thrombus
  2. Good angiographic flow
  3. Observe for lesion stability
   Note: Patient should have no residual ischemia.
 F. Postangioplasty arteriograms
  1. Removal of balloon catheter and wire
  2. Obtain target vessel arteriograms (after additional IC nitroglycerin)
  3. Evaluate contralateral collateral supply arterio-grams (optional)
IV. Discharge from catheterization suite after angioplasty
 A. Secure arterial and venous sheaths in place. Apply sterile bandages.
 B. Instruct patient and family members on postan-gioplasty outcome, expected course, and potential problems (e.g., bleeding).
 C. Notification of departments
  1. Intensive care (or other appropriate patient-care area)
  2. Operating room and surgical team
  3. Lab and ECG
  4. Referring physician
 V. Hospital floor postangioplasty care
 A. Sheath care and removal after angioplasty (see Chapter 2)
 B. Postangioplasty medications
  1. Calcium antagonists (diltiazem, 30 mg PO, tid; nifedipine, 10 mg PO, tid; amlodipine, 5 mg PO, qd)
  2. Aspirin (325 mg PO, qd)
 C. Discharge teaching
  1. Adherence to medications and testing
  2. Early symptoms of restenosis and contributing fac-tors (e.g., smoking, diet)
 D. Discharge activity postangioplasty (home)
  1. Return to activities of daily living
  2. Exercise treadmill test (usually performed 2-6 months after angioplasty)
  3. If symptoms or signs of recurrent ischemia, see physician for repeat coronary angiography

Femoral Sheath Management (see Chapter 2)

Femoral sheaths are often removed 4-6 hours after discontinuation of heparin when the ACT is <140 sec or PTT <50 sec. Uninterrupted anticoagulation may be required in some patients having complicated postangioplasty angiographic results, including extensive coronary dissection, evidence of intraluminal filling defects, or thrombus. In these patients, heparin infusion is decreased by 50% before sheath removal. ACT ranges between 140 and 170 sec are acceptable for sheath removal and assessment of femoral artery hemostasis. A pressure dressing or C clamp can be applied. Patients remain recumbent for 8-24 hours following sheath removal, depending on the level of heparinization and procedure.

Use of Pacemakers During Angioplasty

A temporary transvenous pacemaker insertion was used routinely in the early period of coronary angioplasty, especially for right coronary artery stenoses. Temporary pacing is rarely required for the simple angioplasty in patients without bundle branch block. Temporary pacing is indicated:

1. In patients with high-risk conditions
2. In patients with bundle branch associated with a large dominant right coronary artery occlusion
3. During rotational atherectomy, due to the frequency of transient heart block of the procedure

   Note: Temporary pacemakers should be positioned carefully so that perforation of the right ventricle does not occur in the setting of heparinization. A 5F balloon-tipped flotation pacemaker is satisfactory to accomplish this goal with minimal trauma and confidence in the pacing when required.

CORONARY ANGIOPLASTY FOLLOW-UP
Medical Therapy After Angioplasty

Antivasospastic drugs. Vasoconstriction during or after coronary angioplasty is treated with calcium channel entry blockers, especially when the history suggests potential active vasoconstriction with coronary artery disease or frank variant (vasospastic) angina. Calcium channel entry blockers are given for approximately 2 weeks to 3 months after angioplasty to counter any propensity for spasm after angioplasty and to reduce ischemia due to incompletely revascularized regions.

Calcium channel blockers do not prevent restenosis. Commonly used calcium channel blockers may be of any of the three classes and include Nifedipine, amlodipine, Diltiazem, and Verapamil in standard antianginal doses. Caution must be used to prevent adverse effects known to occur when these drugs are used in combination with beta blockers or in patients with depressed left ventricular function or conduction defects.

Anticoagulant drugs. The angioplasty-damaged arterial wall may cause acute thrombotic coronary occlusion. Thrombus at the angioplasty site may also contribute to restenosis.

1. *Heparin:* Treatment with intravenous heparin (10,000 unit bolus, 1000-1200 U/hr infusion) for 4-48 hours after angioplasty diminishes the likelihood of acute thrombotic occlusion after the procedure. Longer periods (48-72 hours) of intravenous heparin may be needed in patients with preexisting intraluminal thrombus or thrombus formation during angioplasty, angioplasty for acute myocardial infarction, or extensive coronary dissection with or without stent placement.

2. *Dextran:* Dextran does not prevent acute thrombotic occlusion after angioplasty. Some patients may have an allergic reaction to dextran.

3. *Warfarin:* Orally administered anticoagulants (warfarin) after angioplasty are not more effective than aspirin for preventing restenosis or abrupt closure. The restenosis rate was not better for coumadin-treated patients as compared to aspirin-placebo control patients (Emory University).

Antiplatelet agents. Platelets are a major factor in the vascular injury response to balloon angioplasty. Platelet-derived growth factors contribute to the proliferation of smooth muscle cells and fibrocellular response that are found in restenoses. Platelet deposition on balloon-damaged intima is partially inhibited by selected antiplatelet regimens.

Recommended antiplatelet regimens include aspirin (80-365 mg/day) and dipyridamole (75 mg/day), or aspirin alone. Acute reocclusion is more frequent in patients who have not received aspirin before angioplasty.

Ischemia testing after angioplasty. Exercise treadmill testing or radionuclide scintigraphy is performed 2-6 weeks after angioplasty to establish a baseline status. Most ischemic tests are sufficiently specific and selective to screen asymptomatic patients for restenosis. The use of angiography to determine restenosis is mandatory only in investigative studies (for example, assessment of antiplatelet agents) and in subgroups of patients known to have high restenosis rates (those with prior restenosis or saphenous vein grafts, or chronic total occlusions). Angiography, and potentially repeat angioplasty, is reserved for patients with positive results of functional tests or a recurrence of symptoms.

Rarely, a very early (within the first few days) exercise test may precipitate acute coronary occlusion at the dilatation site. False positive results are seen at the early (1-month) tests. Patients with incomplete revascularization will have positive tests more often.

Return to work after angioplasty. Most patients are able to return to work weeks after angioplasty. Factors preventing rapid return to work include prolonged convalescence, job availability after a prolonged absence, socioeconomic factors, and persistent symptoms. In general, however, in the asymptomatic patient after successful single-vessel coronary angioplasty, the patient may return to full activity, including work, within 7-10 days. A functional (ischemic testing) evaluation for patients with multivessel coronary angioplasty or incomplete revascularization after angioplasty will indicate the limi-

TABLE 1-5. Employment rates before and after PTCA in 1150 patients expected to have good results after dilation*

Result of PTCA	No. of patients	Employment rate (%) Before	After	Mean duration to return to work (days)
Successful	775	100	85.8	7
Unsuccessful, followed by bypass grafting	262	100	81.3	73
Unsuccessful, followed by medical therapy	113	100	83.1	13

* These patients were age 60 years or younger and had full-time or part-time employment at baseline.
From Vlietstra RE, Holmes DR Jr: *PTCA: percutaneous transluminal coronary angioplasty,* Philadelphia, 1987, F. A. Davis.

TABLE 1-6. Recommendations for clinical competence in percutaneous transluminal coronary angiography: Minimum recommended number of cases per year

	Bethesda Conference	Society for Cardiac Angiography	ACC/ AHA	ACP/ACC/ AHA	ACC/AHA (1993)
Training					
Total number of cases	125	125	125	125	125
Cases as primary operator	75	75	75	75	75
Practicing					
Number of cases per year to maintain competency	—	50	52	75	75

tations, if any, on work status. Table 1-5 shows typical anticipated employment rates after PTCA.

TRAINING AND GUIDELINES FOR CORONARY ANGIOPLASTY

The demonstrated clinical benefit and continuing technical
advances of interventional procedures have led to higher success rates since the inception of coronary angioplasty. The
need for appropriate training and guidelines for the performance of the procedure is obvious. In assessing the appropriate training requirements and indications for coronary
angioplasty, the task force has established guidelines. Guidelines for the training and practice of coronary angioplasty
have been summarized in a report from the joint task force
from the American Heart Association and American College
of Cardiology on the assessment of diagnostic and therapeutic
cardiovascular procedures (Table 1-6).

In summary, documentation of training in a structured
fellowship program during which a minimum of 125 coronary
angioplasty procedures including 75 performed with the
trainee as primary operator is required to ascertain competence in the procedure according to the Bethesda Conference,
American College of Physicians, American College of Cardiology, and the American Heart Association recommendations
of the joint task force.*

Although the majority of operators fail to meet the requirements for maintenance of competence, which is a minimum
of 75 coronary angioplasty procedures per year as primary
operator, the committee recommendations believe that the
proliferation of small-volume operators should be limited by
appropriate institutional review. Maintenance of competence
for an institution is ≥200 coronary angioplasty procedures
annually as an established minimum performance level for
quality and safe care. Exceptions to minimum requirements
are based on documentation of high-quality performance of
appropriate procedures within each institution.

* *J Am Coll Cardiol* 15:1469-1474, 1990.

SUGGESTED READINGS

AHA Task Force Report: Guidelines for percutaneous transluminal
    coronary angioplasty: a report of the American College of Cardiol-

ogy/American Heart Association Task Force on Assessment of Diagnostic and Therapeutic Cardiovascular Procedures (Subcommittee on Percutaneous Transluminal Coronary Angioplasty), *J Am Coll Cardiol* 12:529-545, 1988.

Avedissian MG, Killeavy ES, Garcia JM, et al.: Percutaneous transluminal coronary angioplasty: a review of current balloon dilatation systems, *Cathet Cardiovasc Diagn* 18:263-275, 1989.

Beatt KJ, Luijten HE, Suryapranata H, et al.: Dilatation parameters: the paradox of optimal improvement in stenosis by PTCA and restenosis (abstr), *Eur Heart J* suppl 10:3, 1989.

Bonzel T, Wollschläger H, Meinertz T, et al.: The steerable monorail catheter system—a new device for PTCA (abstr), *Circulation* 74:II-459, 1986.

Bush CA, Ryan JM, Orzini AR, Hennemann WW: Coronary artery dilatation requiring high inflation pressure, *Cathet Cardiovasc Diagn* 22:112-114, 1991.

Corcos T, Favereau X, Poirot G, et al.: Orion, an improved balloon on a wire system: initial experience, *Cathet Cardiovasc Diagn* 20:103-107, 1990.

Cowley MJ, Dorros G, Kelsey SF, van Raden M, Detre KM: Acute coronary events associated with percutaneous transluminal coronary angioplasty, *Am J Cardiol* 53:56C-64C, 1984.

Detre K, Hulubkov R, Kelsey S, et al.: Percutaneous transluminal coronary angioplasty in 1985-1986 and 1977-1981. The National Heart, Lung, and Blood Institute Registry, *N Engl J Med* 318:265-270, 1988.

Feld H, Valerio L, Shani J: Two hugging balloons at high pressures successfully dilate a lesion refractory to routine coronary angioplasty, *Cathet Cardiovasc Diagn* 24:105-108, 1991.

Ferguson JJ, Parnis SM, Fuqua JM: Equipment technology—inaccuracies in manufacturer-reported deflated PTCA balloon profiles, *Cathet Cardiovasc Diagn* 25:101-106, 1992.

Freed M, Grines C: Saphenous vein graft and internal mammary artery PTCA: saphenous vein graft disease, *Manual of Interventional Cardiology,* Birmingham, Michigan, 1992, Physician's Press, pp 163-170.

Freed M, Grines C: Simple and complex angioplasty—equipment selection, *Manual of Interventional Cardiology,* Birmingham, Michigan, 1992, Physician's Press, pp 15-32.

Gruentzig A: Transluminal dilation of coronary-artery stenosis, *Lancet* 1:263, 1978.

Gruentzig A, Senning A, Siegenthaler WE: Nonoperative dilatation of coronary artery stenosis: percutaneous transluminal coronary angioplasty, *N Engl J Med* 301:61-68, 1979.

Holmes DR Jr, Cohen HA, Vlietstra RE: Optimizing the results of balloon coronary angioplasty of nonideal lesions, *Prog Cardiovasc Dis* 32(2):165-168, 1989.

Holmes DR Jr, Vlietstra RE, Smith HC, et al.: Restenosis after percutaneous transluminal coronary angioplasty: a report from the PTCA registry of the NHLBI, *Am J Cardiol* 53:77C-81C, 1984.

Israel DH, Marmur JD, Sanborn TA: Excimer laser-facilitated balloon angioplasty of a nondilatable lesion, *J Am Coll Cardiol* 18:1118-1119, 1991.

Ivanhoe RJ, Weintraub WS, Douglas JS, et al.: Percutaneous transluminal coronary angioplasty of chronic total occlusions, *Circulation* 85:106-115, 1992.

Johnson LW, Lozner EC, Johnson S, et al.: Coronary arteriography 1984-1987: a report of the registry of the Society for Cardiac Angiography and Interventions. I. Results and complications, *Cathet Cardiovasc Diagn* 17:5-10, 1989.

Kahn JK, Hartzler GO: Frequency and causes of failure with contemporary balloon coronary angioplasty and implications for new technologies, *Am J Cardiol* 66:858-860, 1990.

Kern MJ, Talley JD, Deligonul U, et al.: Preliminary experience with 5 and 6 French diagnostic catheters as guiding catheters for coronary angioplasty, *Cathet Cardiovasc Diagn* 22:60-63, 1991.

Lau KW, Sigwart U: Novel coronary interventional devices: an update, *Am Heart J* 123:497-506, 1992.

Lehmann KG, Le HM, Feuer JM, et al.: Influence of inflation pressure on stenosis reduction during coronary angioplasty (abstr), *Circulation* 80:II-372, 1989.

Martinez A, Pichard A, Little T, et al.: Probe "balloon on a wire" ultra-low profile coronary catheter: results of PTCA in 107 patients, *Cathet Cardiovasc Diagn* 18:222-226, 1989.

Meier B, Gruentzig AR, King SB, et al.: Higher balloon dilation pressure in coronary angioplasty, *Am Heart J* 107:619-622, 1984.

Mooney MR, Mooney JF, Longe TF, et al.: Effect of balloon material on coronary angioplasty, *Am J Cardiol* 69(17):1481-1482, 1992.

Morice MC, Lafont A, Sami Y, et al.: Do high pressure-resisting lesions increase the risk of coronary angioplasty? (abstr), *Circulation* 86:I-786, 1992.

Myler RK, Mooney MR, Stertzer SH, Clark DA, Hidalgo BO, Fishman J. The balloon on a wire device. A new ultra-low-profile coronary angioplasty system/concept, *Cathet Cardiovasc Diagn* 14:135-140, 1988.

Nichols AB, Smith R, Berke AD, et al.: Importance of balloon size in coronary angioplasty, *J Am Coll Cardiol* 13:1094-1100, 1989.

Pande AK, Meier B, Urban P, et al.: Magnum/Magnarail versus conventional systems for recanalization of chronic total occlusions: a randomized comparison, *Am Heart J* 123(5):1182-1186, 1992.

Participants in the National Heart, Lung, and Blood Institute Conference on the Evaluation of Emerging Coronary Revascularization

Technologies: evaluation of emerging technologies for coronary revascularization, *Circulation* 85(1):357-361, 1992.

Results of the first national survey on the practice of coronary angioplasty (monograph), USCI/C. R. Bard, Billerica, Mass, 1992.

Roubin GS, Douglas JS, King SB, et al.: Influence of balloon size on initial success rate, acute complications, and restenosis after PTCA, *Circulation* 78:557-565, 1988.

Ryan TJ, Faxon DP, Gunnar RM, et al.: Guidelines for percutaneous transluminal coronary angioplasty: a report of the American College of Cardiology/American Heart Association Task Force on Assessment of Diagnostic and Therapeutic Cardiovascular Procedures, *Circulation* 78:486-502, 1988.

Ryan TJ, Klocke FJ, Reynolds WA: Clinical competence in percutaneous transluminal coronary angioplasty: a statement of physicians from the ACP/ACC/AHA Task Force on Clinical Privileges in Cardiology, *J Am Coll Cardiol* 15:1469-1474, 1990.

Schmitz HJ, Meyer J, Kiesslich T, Effert S: Greater initial dilatation gives better late angiographic results in percutaneous coronary angioplasty (abstr), *Circulation* 66:II-123, 1982.

17th Bethesda Conference: Adult Cardiology Training, November 1-2, 1985, *J Am Coll Cardiol* 7:1191-1194, 1986.

Simpson JB, Baim DS, Robert EW, Harrison DC: A new catheter system for coronary angioplasty, *Am J Cardiol* 49:1216-1222, 1982.

The Society for Cardiac Angiography: Guidelines for credentialing and facilities for performance of coronary angioplasty, *Cathet Cardiovasc Diagn* 15:136-138, 1988.

Stack RS, Quigley PJ, Collins G, et al.: Perfusion balloon catheter, *Am J Cardiol* 61:77G-80G, 1988.

Talley JD, Joseph A, Killeavy ES, et al.: Multicenter evaluation of a new fixed-wire coronary angioplasty catheter system: clinical and angiographic characteristics and results, *Cathet Cardiovasc Diagn* 22:310-316, 1991.

Talley JD, Joseph A, Kupersmith J: Preliminary results utilizing a new percutaneous transluminal coronary angioplasty balloon catheter, *Cathet Cardiovasc Diagn* 20:108-113, 1990.

Villavicencio R, Urban P, Muller T, et al.: Coronary balloon angioplasty through diagnostic 6 French catheters, *Cathet Cardiovasc Diagn* 22:56-59, 1991.

Willard JE, Sunnergren K, Eichhorn E, Grayburn PA: Coronary angioplasty requiring extraordinarily high balloon inflation pressure, *Cathet Cardiovasc Diagn* 22:115-117, 1991.

Yazdanfar S, Ledley GS, Alfieri A, et al.: Parallel angioplasty dilatation catheter and guide wire, *Cathet Cardiovasc Diagn* 28:72-75, 1993.

2

ARTERIAL AND VENOUS ACCESS AND HEMOSTASIS FOR INTERVENTIONAL PROCEDURES

Ubeydullah Deligonul, Eugene A. Caracciolo, and Morton J. Kern

VASCULAR ACCESS

Vascular access for interventional procedures is the most common cause of patient morbidity that prolongs hospitalizations. Routine vascular access employing standard Seldinger technique for femoral artery and vein entry is similar to that used for diagnostic catheterization. The techniques and methods have been described in detail elsewhere, but will be reviewed in this chapter with specific emphasis on approaches for interventional procedures.

The access site and methodology should follow from the planned intervention, whereby the site and type of access (either percutaneous femoral or cutdown by brachial) are determined in anticipation of the anatomic and pathologic conditions under discussion. Review of the previous difficulties encountered by other operators is helpful so that time can be saved in avoiding these known time-consuming pitfalls.

Assessment of all peripheral arterial pulses before the procedure and at the completion of the procedure is mandatory.

Percutaneous Femoral Artery Approach

Because of the large diameter of interventional equipment, the femoral artery approach is preferred to that of the brachial artery, although brachial artery access is advantageous under certain circumstances.

Conditions. Conditions in which a brachial arterial access should be considered include:

1. Claudication
2. Absent distal pulses
3. Femoral bruits
4. Prior femoral artery graft surgery
5. Extensive inguinal scarring from previous procedures
6. Surgery or radiation treatment
7. Excessively tortuous iliac artery and lower abdominal aorta
8. Abdominal aortic aneurysm
9. Severe back pain or inability to lie flat
10. Patient request

Technique. The technique of cannulation is identical to that described for diagnostic arterial vascular access, in which the operator locates the artery (Fig. 2-1), administers local anesthesia, and creates a skin incision followed by subcutaneous tunneling (see *The Cardiac Catheterization Handbook,* Chapter 2). Single wall puncture is highly desirable (Fig. 2-2). Multiple arterial punctures in a patient taking anticoagulation drugs will be a source of bleeding and potential complications, including femoral pseudoaneurysm or A-V fistula in the postprocedural period. Once the artery has been punctured, standard 0.35- to 0.38-in. guidewires are inserted, and the vessel is cannulated with the sheath and dilator assembly. The sheath dilator is then removed and the sheath flushed. Long sheaths (23 cm) have been commonly used for interventional procedures because of the extra support provided to early guide catheters, reduced arterial trauma in the straight segment of the iliac arteries, and ease of negotiating tortuous segments with guide catheters. For patients with excess girth, a Doppler-tipped needle may be helpful to puncture the artery without multiple attempts.

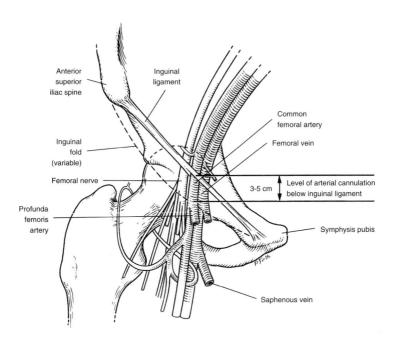

Fig. 2-1. Inguinal anatomy and guidelines for correct vascular access. (From Kulick DL, Rahimtoola SH, editors: *Techniques and applications in interventional cardiology,* St. Louis, 1991, Mosby, p 2.)

When an interventional procedure is performed less than 3 days after the diagnostic study, puncturing the same groin may be associated with a higher incidence of bleeding and infection complications.

Percutaneous Femoral Vein Puncture

In a manner similar to the femoral artery access, the femoral vein is located medial to the femoral artery. The skin is anesthetized; an incision is made; a subcutaneous tunnel is obtained; and vein puncture is performed in a routine fashion with standard guidewire; and sheath-dilator technique used to introduce a femoral venous sheath. Indications for femoral venous sheaths in patients undergoing interventional procedures vary. Routine venous access is indicated for all patients having procedures of the dominant circumflex and right coronary artery for pacemaker access, should one be needed. In

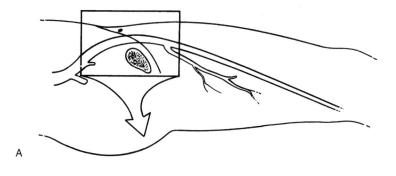

A

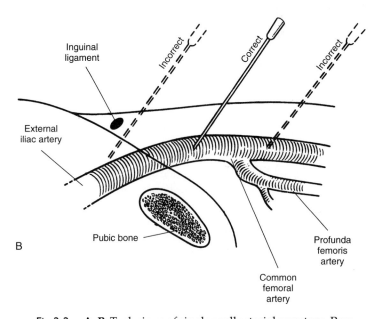

B

Fig. 2-2.   **A, B,** Technique of single-wall arterial puncture. Para-sagittal cross-sectional diagram of inguinal region at level of femoral artery. Correct needle entry position is below inguinal ligament and above femoral artery bifurcation. Correct access is particularly critical for procedures. (From Kulick DL, Rahim-toola SH, editors: *Techniques and applications in interventional cardiology,* St. Louis, 1991, Mosby, p 3.)

patients at high risk, a venous access and pulmonary catheterization may prove very useful.

Brachial and Radial Artery Approach

In general, percutaneous brachial artery puncture for interventional procedures with catheters larger than 8 French is probably undesirable, since control of bleeding in the postprocedure period in patients who are continued on anticoagulation may be difficult. The size of the brachial artery determines the size of the sheath and guide catheter that can be inserted safely. Brachial artery cutdown is a standard technique that provides excellent access and hemostasis, although reintroduction of the equipment in the event of abrupt closure may be limited by the need to perform a second procedure.

Percutaneous radial artery access has been demonstrated in Europe with the use of 6 French guiding catheters (Fig. 2-3), although this technique is still under evaluation in the United States. Radial artery sheath placement is considered less traumatic and potentially less risky if the artery is of sufficient size and arterial supply to the hand is not compromised. Before consideration of radial artery access, an Allen test should be performed by occluding both radial and ulnar arteries with pressure and releasing the ulnar artery to see if perfusion of the hand is rapid. Once the Allen test indicates a satisfactory ulnar supply to the hand, radial artery access is performed using a Seldinger technique with a 16- or 18-gauge short intravenous cannula through which a 0.025-in. guidewire is passed. Over the guidewire a 4F dilator is inserted. The 0.025-in. guidewire is exchanged for a 0.035-in. guidewire and a 6F arterial introducer sheath is positioned. The sheath is flushed and maintained with the same technique as for femoral artery puncture. Venous access should be obtained through an alternative route. Heparin is given after insertion of the arterial sheath. In patients who are anticoagulated, hemostasis upon removal of the radial artery sheath is easily obtained by direct pressure and has been used as a method of stent placement in some patients already anticoagulated before the procedure.

Arterial and Venous Access for High-Risk Interventions

For patients undergoing coronary interventions who are at high risk for complications requiring urgent placement of

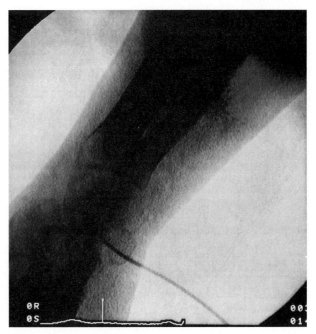

Radial artery catheter

Fig. 2-3.   Angiogram of radial arterial sheath placement for coronary angioplasty.

an intraaortic balloon pump or other hemodynamic support device, contralateral arterial and venous access is needed. In addition, continuous monitoring of pulmonary artery or wedge pressure for tolerance of ischemia may facilitate medical management during complex procedures. As a standby maneuver, small (5F) sheath introducers can be placed in the contralateral vessels at the beginning of the procedure. These sheaths will permit immediate vascular access should urgent hemodynamic support equipment be required. Cannulation of the contralateral artery or vein usually follows that of the primary access site. Two venous cannulae can be placed in a femoral vein if multiple venous catheters are anticipated.

For large (12-18F) cardiopulmonary support (CPS) cannulae, some operators use a surgical assistant for a cutdown. Most CPS systems can be placed percutaneously.

Difficult Vascular Access

Excessive vessel tortuosity. The most frequently encountered difficulty in advancing the guidewires or catheters into the aorta is tortuosity of the iliac or subclavian vessels, a condition often found in elderly patients. The steerable 0.035-in. Wholey guidewire has excellent characteristics for negotiating a tortuous vessel. Its flexible, relatively atraumatic curved tip is steerable and increases safety. In cases of extreme tortuosity, advancing a diagnostic catheter within several centimeters of the guidewire tip will increase torque control and pushability of the guidewire. A right Judkins coronary catheter can be used to change the direction of the guidewire tip. Once the wire is beyond the tortuous (or narrowed) segments, a long sheath can be positioned. Guidewire catheter exchanges will be needed.

Common equipment selection for tortuous vessels. Common equipment for tortuous vessels includes:
1. Wholey 0.035-in. wires, steerable
2. Long (300-cm) exchange wires, stiff shaft construction
3. Long sheaths (23 cm or, rarely, 90 cm)
4. Extra-stiff guidewires (0.018-0.038 in.)

In patients with tortuous iliac vessels, a long (23-cm) sheath may be used, recognizing the trade-off of multiple friction points for some straightening of the vessel. Catheter exchanges over a long (300-cm) exchange guidewire may be required to avoid undue procedure prolongation by repeated attempts to advance catheters across tortuous atherosclerotic segments. Extra stiff (Amplatz-type) guidewires may also be required.

Inguinal scarring. To insert an 8F sheath in a severely fibrotic groin or through a femoral bypass graft, successively dilate with 5, 6, 7, 8, and 9F dilators, then insert the 8F firm body sheath (Daig, Terumo, or Arrow).

Arterial Access in Patients with Peripheral Vascular Disease

Peripheral vascular disease complicating femoral arterial access can be managed by placement of vascular stents if required. This approach should be used if the peripheral vascular disease is an impediment to the positioning of the interventional equipment and no alternative routes exist. Before proceeding with intervention in the heart in patients with peripheral vascular disease, abdominal aortography and peripheral arteriography are necessary to evaluate the extent of disease. However, should an urgent coronary intervention be required; some operators advocate stent placement and proceeding to the coronary circulation directly.

CORONARY ARTERY ACCESS
Differences Between Coronary Access for Coronary Angiography and Coronary Interventions

Coronary access for coronary interventions is obtained using coronary guide catheters. For the purpose of coronary angiography, coronary access is required to deliver the contrast medium into the vessel selectively. For coronary interventions, on the other hand, the guide catheter is also expected to work as a platform for introduction of the balloon or device catheter into the coronary artery. Therefore, the guide catheter (1) should have a large lumen to allow introduction of treatment catheters yet enough stiffness to resist the backward motion and disengagement during the advancement of the balloon or device catheter into the coronary artery, and (2) should have a coaxial alignment with the proximal portion of the vessel. To meet these requirements, the guiding catheters are manufactured using relatively stiffer material with thinner walls. These are unique catheter types that require special placement techniques. The catheter tip is not tapered, increasing the chance of pressure damping. A softer plastic tip is usually attached to decrease the chance of tip trauma.

The unique characteristics of coronary guide catheter access may not be wholly appreciated by the beginner. The following points are useful to remember.

1. Catheter advancement and torquing should be gentle and gradual.
2. If the catheter is not engaged with minimal manipulation, a different size or shape must be tried instead of insisting on manipulating the catheter into the vessel.
3. Deep cannulation of the vessel should be avoided.
4. Catheter French size should be appropriate for the diameter of the proximal vessel.
5. Catheter size and shape are selected to be as minimally invasive as possible in accordance with the treatment plan. The majority of procedures can be accomplished with

Judkins-type (femoral) guide catheters. The size of the dilated vessel territory and the expected degree of difficulty in reaching the stenosis should be weighed against the possible proximal artery damage due to large or too invasive catheter shapes.

Coronary Guiding Catheter Types (Fig. 2-4)

Refer to *The Cardiac Catheterization Handbook* for a description of basic characteristics of these catheters.

A wide variety of shapes duplicating diagnostic catheter shapes and several novel curves comprise guide catheters. Tip shapes are listed in Table 2-1.

The arteries in which good backup guiding support is most difficult to achieve are, in order of difficulty, the right, circum-

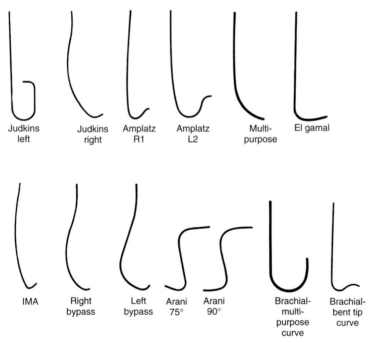

Fig. 2-4.   Tip configurations of guiding catheters for coronary angioplasty. (From Kulick DL, Rahimtoola SH, editors: *Techniques and applications in interventional cardiology,* St. Louis, 1991, Mosby, p 60.)

TABLE 2-1.   Types of guide catheters

Guide	Advantages	Disadvantages
For LAD lesions:		
JL4	Routine	Backs out
AL2	Easy to place	Good backup, but may dissect ostium
Nesto	Good support	Learning curve needed
For the right coronary artery:		
JR4	Easy use	Poor backup
Hockey stick	Deep seating	Deep seating
Multipurpose, El-Gamal	Deep seating	Deep seating
Arani	Excellent backup	Difficult to engage, deep seating
For highly tortuous RCAs— left Amplatz	Excellent backup	Difficult to engage, deep seating
For circumflex lesions:		
JL4	Routine placement	Backs out
AL2	Easy placement	Good backup, but may dissect ostium
Voda	Easy to seat, excellent backup	Deep engagement
Multipurpose	Good backup	Difficult to seat
Artery	*Alternative catheters*	
RCA	El-Gamal	
RCA, grafts	Hockey stick	
RCA	Arani	
CFX	Voda	
LAD, RCA	Nesto	

flex, and left anterior descending coronary arteries. Saphenous vein grafts and internal mammary artery (IMA) have
unique problems but are less frequent occurrences.

Femoral "Judkins"-type guide catheters.   The Judkins
left coronary catheter has a double curve. The length of the
segment between the primary and the secondary curve determines the size of the catheter (i.e., 3.5, 4.0, 5.0, or 6.0 cm). The
proper size of the left Judkins catheter is selected depending
on the length and width of the ascending aorta. In a small

person with a small aorta, a 3.5-cm catheter is appropriate, while in a large person or in one with an enlarged or dilated ascending aorta (e.g., as a result of aortic stenosis, regurgitation, or Marfan's syndrome), a 5.0- or 6.0-cm catheter may be required.

A left 4-cm Judkins catheter fits in most adult patients. When catheter size is adequate, the catheter tip is aligned with the long axis of the left main coronary trunk. A smaller (3.5-cm) catheter in the same patient will tip upward, and a larger (5.0-cm) catheter will tip downward into the coronary cusp. When the coronary orifice is not cannulated appropriately, the catheter should be replaced with a better-fitting catheter rather than manipulated into the coronary artery. Sometimes a slight counterclockwise rotation of the catheter may be necessary to improve alignment of the catheter tip with the left main trunk.

These catheters have shapes that are similar to the diagnostic Judkins catheter shapes. Various modifications, including short tips, smoother curves, half-sizes, or anterior or posterior tip directions, are available. The great majority of angioplasty procedures are performed using Judkins-type catheters. They are easy to manipulate. The depth of the cannulation usually can be adjusted well.

Amplatz guide catheters. In addition to similar curve sizes as diagnostic angiography catheters, there are size (half-sizes or 0.75 sizes) or shape modifications. The left Amplatz-type catheter is a preshaped half-circle with the tip extending perpendicular to the curve. Amplatz catheter sizes (left 1, 2, and 3; and right 1 and 2) indicate the diameter of the tip curve. In most normal-sized adults, 2 left and 1 right (modified) Amplatz catheters give satisfactory results. In the left anterior oblique (LAO) projection, the tip is advanced into the left aortic cusp. Further advancement of the catheter causes the tip to move upward into the left main trunk. It is necessary to push the Amplatz catheters slightly to disengage by backing the catheter tip upward and out of the left main ostium. If the catheter is pulled instead of first being advanced, the tip moves downward and into the left main or circumflex artery. Unwanted deep cannulation of the circumflex might tear this branch or the left main trunk. Amplatz catheters have a higher incidence of coronary dissection than

Judkins-type catheters. This is a very important safety issue. With this in mind, Amplatz catheters often provide excellent backup support. Sometimes it may be difficult to pass the tip angle with large-shaft catheters or devices. The right Amplatz (modified) catheter has a smaller but similar hook-shaped curve. The catheter is advanced into the right coronary cusp. As with Judkins right catheters, the catheter is rotated clockwise for 45° to 90°. The same maneuver is repeated at different levels until the right coronary artery is entered. After coronary injections, the catheter may be pulled, advanced, or rotated out of the coronary artery. Amplatz catheters could also be used from the brachial route.

Graft catheters.   There are right and left graft and internal mammary catheters with shapes similar to the diagnostic counterparts. They also may be useful in cannulating native vessels with unusual origins or proximal courses.

The right coronary vein graft catheter is similar to a right Judkins catheter with a wider, more open primary curve allowing cannulation of vertically oriented coronary artery vein graft.

The left vein graft catheter is similar to the right Judkins catheter with a smaller and sharper secondary curve allowing easy cannulation of left anterior descending and left circumflex vein grafts. Such grafts are usually placed higher and more anterior than the right coronary grafts with a relatively horizontal and upward takeoff from the aorta.

The internal mammary artery graft catheter has a short, hook-shaped tip configuration that facilitates the engagement of internal mammary artery grafts, especially in patients with very vertical origin of the internal mammary artery at the juncture of the subclavian and common carotid arteries.

Multipurpose and brachial guide catheters. Multipurpose guide catheter shapes (Fig. 2-4) are similar to multipurpose diagnostic catheters. These can be introduced from the femoral or brachial route. The catheter is somewhat difficult to manipulate but gives excellent support in situations such as vertically oriented right coronary artery grafts. Brachial guide catheters are marketed in various tip shapes, including Sones, Castillo, or multipurpose curves and have woven dacron or extruded walls. Brachial guide catheters are shorter. Shorter catheters allow regular-length balloon catheters to be used in the distal part of the long grafts.

The multipurpose or Sones-type catheter is introduced through a right brachial arteriotomy (or percutaneous sheath) and is advanced over a guidewire into the ascending aorta under fluoroscopic guidance. There may be a sharp caudal turn near the origin of the carotid artery, which usually requires careful J-tipped guidewire manipulation for passage. An inexperienced operator manipulating the catheter in this area may dissect or perforate the subclavian artery. To decrease the kinking and tortuosity of brachiocephalic vessels, the patient is instructed to turn his or her head to the left, with the chin extended (as if trying to see the ceiling corner), and to inspire deeply. The operator also may pull the arm straight and raise the arm toward the head at a 90° angle with the chest wall.

Cannulation of the left coronary artery using a multipurpose catheter is performed in the LAO projection. The catheter tip is advanced against the aortic valve and pushed to form a U-shaped loop with upward movement of the tip toward the left main trunk. The tip position is verified with small contrast injections. Once the catheter tip is near the left main coronary artery orifice, a slight counterclockwise rotation of the catheter brings the tip into the left main. Withdrawing the catheter slightly causes the tip to seat in the left main, achieving a more stable angiographic position. Because the catheter moves considerably with breathing, stability is assured by advancing or withdrawing the catheter slightly as needed.

Cannulation of the right coronary artery is also performed in the LAO projection. A smaller U-shaped curve can be formed in the right cusp with the tip directed to the left coronary orifice. Rotate the catheter clockwise into the right cusp, keeping the shortened U-shaped loop. Once the tip is engaged, the catheter has a tendency to go very deeply into the right coronary artery, requiring catheter adjustments during respiratory cycles. In patients with a vertically originating right coronary artery, the Sones catheter may go directly into the right coronary artery when it is first advanced through the right arm.

Preshaped Coronary Catheters for Brachial Use

Preshaped catheters should be introduced and advanced over the J-tipped guidewire. A preshaped brachial, or Castillo,

(Fig. 2-4) catheter (size 1, 2, or 3) with a curved tip configuration similar to the Amplatz catheter is used effectively from the right or left arm. This catheter is manipulated in a fashion similar to that described for the Amplatz catheter.

Specially curved catheters. Specially curved catheters have been designed by various interventionalists to provide increased backup support, such as Arani 75 and 90° catheters (for right coronary arteries) (Fig. 2-4), El-Gamal (for vein grafts), Noto (for right coronary arteries), Nesto (for left coronary arteries) (Fig. 2-5A shows different guide catheter backup positions. Fig. 2-5B shows Nesto guide catheter shape.), or Voda (right or left circumflex arteries), which are among the current ones. Deep cannulation of the vessels could occur, sometimes in a poorly controlled fashion. Relatively sharp angles may create difficulty in advancing large-bore balloon or device catheters. A hockey stick catheter has a 90° tip angle, which may be useful in engaging bypass grafts or right coronary arteries.

Reshaping the catheter. Sometimes slight heat modification of the catheter shape allows better access to the coronary artery. However, this should be done by an experienced operator. An introducer catheter or a large guidewire should be kept within the guide to prevent lumen collapse. The catheter should be checked for structural damage before reinsertion. It should be kept in mind that once it is heat modified, the catheter may perform differently from the nominal characteristics.

Small-size French guide catheters. Coronary angioplasty can be performed using 6 or 7 French large lumen guide catheters. Use of 5 or 6 French diagnostic catheters to introduce over-the-wire balloon catheters has also been reported. Small-size catheters allow early patient ambulation. They can be used from the brachial or radial (6 French) routes. Visualizing the coronary artery may be difficult with these catheters. In case of the need for larger-shaft catheters, the whole system must be removed from the coronary. However, small guide catheters may be exchanged over an 0.018-in. coronary guidewire if necessary. Another potential problem is relatively weak backup support. However, this may be overcome by deeply cannulating the proximal vessel, which can be accomplished more easily and with less trauma than with larger guiding catheters.

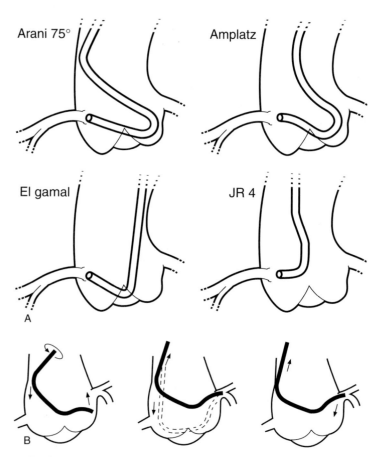

Fig. 2-5. **A,** Backup positions for guide catheter support for right coronary artery angioplasty using the four most common guide catheters. (From Freed M, Grines C, editors: *Manual of interventional cardiology,* Birmingham, Michigan, 1992, Physician's Press, p 20.) **B,** Unique Nesto configuration for guide catheter placement in left coronary artery. (From Nesto RW: Performance characteristics of a new shape of guiding catheter for PTCA of the left coronary artery, *Cathet Cardiovasc Diagn* 24:144-148, 1991.)

Side hole versus no side hole. With the exception of atherectomy guide catheters (9.5 to 10 French), left coronary catheters should be without side holes (perfusion ports) so that one can detect the pressure damping. The same is true for internal mammary catheters. On the other hand, side-hole catheters are very useful in safely cannulating small right coronary or graft vessels. Distal vessel visualization may be a problem. Undetected proximal pressure gradients may occur, complicating distal gradient evaluations.

Cannulating Coronary or Graft Ostia
Left coronary artery

Short left main, separate ostia left anterior descending, and circumflex arteries. Use of a left Judkins catheter that is one size smaller than that usually selected (i.e., 3.5-cm instead of 4.0-cm size; Figs. 2-6 and 2-7) permits selective cannulation of the left anterior descending artery in patients with a short left main artery. For cannulation of the circumflex ostium (Fig. 2-4), slight withdrawal and counter-clockwise rotation of the standard 4-cm left Judkins catheter or a left Judkins catheter that is one size larger is helpful. An Amplatz-type catheter is especially useful for cannulating the circumflex ostium separately, but it must be used with care to avoid dissection of the proximal or ostial location.

High left coronary artery takeoff. An unusually high origin of the left main coronary artery from the aorta usually can be cannulated using an Amplatz-type catheter. To cannulate the high-origin left main trunk through the brachial approach, a brachial guide catheter may be utilized.

Wide aortic root. In patients with a relatively horizontal and wide aortic root with upward takeoff of the left main coronary artery, a large-curve left Judkins (5 or 6 cm), an Amplatz-type left coronary catheter, or a "Voda"-shaped catheter may be required. In these cases brachial approach using multipurpose or brachial guide catheters works very well.

Posterior origin of left main. Slight counterclockwise rotation and advancement of the left Judkins catheter may bring the tip to the left main. Sometimes it may be necessary to heat-reshape the tip to give a posterior out-of-plane direction. Another option is a left Amplatz catheter.

Right coronary artery. The origin of the right coronary artery shows more variation than the left coronary artery. Extra backup support is difficult to obtain with standard JR4-type catheters. Directing the catheter tip to the right in the

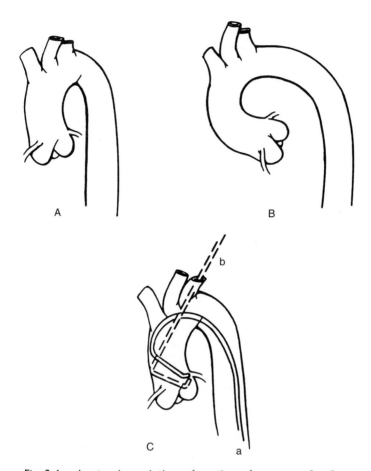

Fig. 2-6.   Anatomic variation of aortic arch, root, and valve plane: **A,** normotensive; **B,** hypertensive. **C,** Changes in secondary curves of left Judkins catheter when inserted via femoral approach (a) or from left brachial approach. (b) Right brachial approach can also be used. (From Topol EJ: *Textbook of interventional cardiology,* ed 2, Philadelphia, 1994, W. B. Saunders, p 553.)

usual fashion using the lateral view permits easy cannulation of the slightly anterior origin of the right coronary artery in the right cusp.

High and upward takeoff of a right coronary artery.   A relatively high origin of the right coronary artery may require a left or right (modified) Amplatz-type catheter (Fig. 2-5).

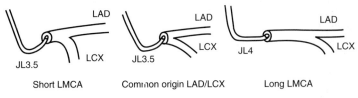

Fig. 2-7. Left anterior descending artery guide catheter positioning with different secondary curve sizes. (From Jang GD: *Angioplasty,* New York, 1987, McGraw-Hill, p 303.)

Wide aortic root. In a patient with a horizontal and wide aortic root, cannulation of the right coronary orifice may require an Amplatz or hockey stick catheter.

"Shepherd's crook" right coronary artery. In this situation, a right Judkins catheter provides poor support. A left Amplatz (0.75 to 1), hockey stick, or Arani catheter may provide better support, especially for relatively distal lesions. However, deep cannulation of the vessel is frequent with these catheters, and proximal vessel trauma can occur, especially in small aortic roots.

Anomalous coronary artery origin. The most frequent anomaly is a circumflex origin from a proximal right coronary artery, or a separate orifice just posterior to the right coronary

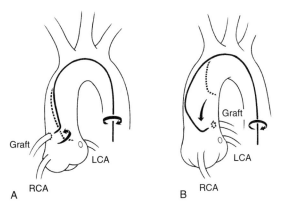

Fig. 2-8. Method of use for Judkins right catheter in cannulating saphenous venous bypass graft conduits. (From Tilkian AG, Daily EK: *Cardiovascular procedures: diagnostic techniques and therapeutic procedures,* St. Louis, 1986, Mosby.)

Superior directed vein graft

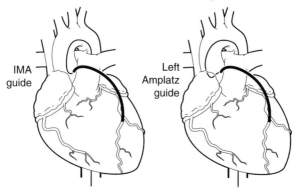

Transverse directed vein graft

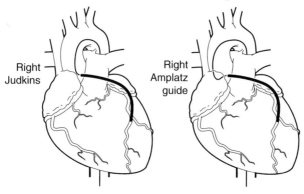

Inferior directed vein graft

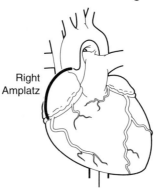

artery orifice. When there is a common trunk, a right Judkins catheter may be sufficient. A separate left circumflex orifice can be entered by rotating the right Judkins more posteriorly. Better engagement and support may be obtained (because of the downward course of the proximal circumflex) by a right Amplatz or a multipurpose guide catheter.

Extreme anterior or left coronary cusp origin of the right coronary artery can be engaged by using a left Amplatz catheter. More leftward origin of a right coronary artery (also tends to be higher) can be entered using a left bypass guide.

Saphenous vein bypass grafts (Figs. 2-8 and 2-9). To decrease the manipulation time and to select the best catheter shape, the diagnostic angiogram should be reviewed carefully for the location of the aortic anastomosis and proximal course of the vessel. Anatomic landmarks should be noted. Avoid unnecessary manipulation of catheters in vein grafts, especially in old grafts that may contain friable atherosclerotic material with potential risk of embolization.

Right coronary bypass vein graft catheterization (Fig. 2-9). The right coronary vein graft usually can be entered using a 4-cm right Judkins-type catheter. The right coronary catheter is placed in the ascending aorta at a level that is slightly higher than the expected level of the right coronary vein graft orifice, and the catheter is rotated clockwise from 45° to 90°. This will cause the catheter tip to move along the left border of the ascending aortic silhouette in the left anterior oblique position. When the right graft is anastomosed to the far right side of the aorta, a counterclockwise, rather than clockwise, rotation of the catheter may be necessary. In some cases the right Judkins or right bypass catheter may fall too short, in which case a multipurpose catheter may work very well. In

← _____

Fig. 2-9. Saphenous vein graft ostium orientations. Different guide catheters should be selected based on the angle of graft takeoff, superior, transverse, or inferior orientation. (From Pinkerton CA, Slack JD, Orr CM, Vantassel JW, Smith ML: Percutaneous transluminal coronary angioplasty in patients with prior myocardial revascularization surgery, *Am J Cardiol* 61:15G-22G, 1988.)

this situation, the catheter tip is pointed toward the left-hand side of the screen in the anteriopposterior (AP) or right anterior oblique (RAO) position. Advancement or withdrawal while rotating the catheter tip might be necessary for graft engagement. In case of right vein graft vertical takeoff, the right coronary Judkins catheter tip may be directed toward the wall rather than into the lumen, making adequate opacification of the vein graft difficult. In these cases, a right coronary bypass vein graft catheter should be used. Because of the wide primary curve, the right vein graft catheter tip usually points downward and more parallel to the axis of the graft. Sometimes this catheter may have a tendency to move deeply into the right coronary vein graft. A right modified Amplatz catheter can also be used for horizontal or vertical takeoff vein grafts.

Left anterior descending vein graft catheterization. The right Judkins catheter is placed at a level slightly higher than the expected level of the left anterior descending vein graft orifice, and 30°-45° clockwise rotation is applied. The catheter tip will appear foreshortened in the LAO view and will be pointing toward the right-hand side of the screen of the ascending aorta silhouette in the RAO view. In some patients, it may be necessary to use a left coronary vein graft catheter or left Amplatz catheter. A slight clockwise rotation of the catheter at the level of the expected aortic anastomosis site of the left anterior descending graft will engage the catheter into the ostium.

The left anterior descending graft may course horizontally or downward after the origin. In some cases, however, it makes an upward curve before it turns toward the apex. In these cases, the need for stronger backup support may require the use of a left Amplatz catheter or deep cannulation of the proximal vessel using a hockey stick or El-Gamal catheter.

Circumflex vein graft catheterization. Repeating the same maneuver described for left anterior descending vein graft cannulation using right Judkins or left vein graft catheters is usually a successful maneuver.

Internal mammary artery graft cannulation

Left internal mammary artery. The left internal mammary artery originates anteriorly from the caudal wall of the subclavian artery distal to the vertebral artery origin. There are many variations in the shape of the aortic arch and origin and direction of the subclavian artery (Fig. 2-10). The left subclavian artery can be entered using an IMA catheter. The catheter is advanced into the aortic arch up to the level of the left subclavian artery origin (Fig. 2-11). The guidewire is left in the catheter. Subsequently, the catheter is withdrawn slowly and rotated counterclockwise. The catheter tip is deflected cranially, usually engaging the left subclavian artery at the top of the aortic knob in the anteroposterior projection. The guidewire is advanced into the subclavian artery. The catheter is advanced. The guidewire is withdrawn. More than one attempt is often necessary to engage into the subclavian artery. Once the subclavian artery is engaged, the catheter is advanced slightly over a guidewire beyond the internal mammary orifice. A J-tipped or a Wholey wire is helpful to guide the catheter into the subclavian artery. Once the catheter has been advanced beyond the internal mammary artery take-off, the catheter is withdrawn slowly and small contrast injections are given to visualize the internal mammary artery

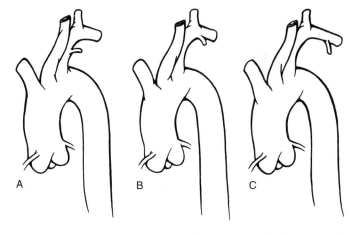

Fig. 2-10. Anatomic variation of the origin of the internal mammary artery from the subclavian artery: **A,** proximal; **B,** mid; **C,** distal. Although the femoral approach is easier for anatomy A, the ipsilateral brachial approach is more difficult than might appear initially. (From Topol EJ: *Textbook of interventional cardiology,* ed 2, Philadelphia, 1994, W. B. Saunders, p 560.)

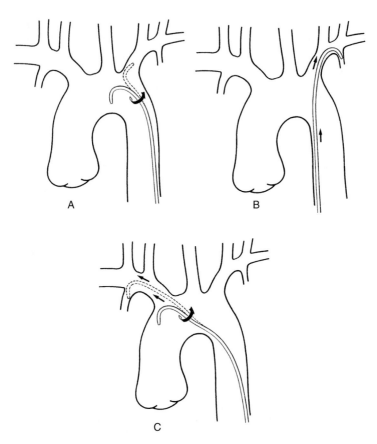

Fig. 2-11.   **A-C,** Technique of catheterization of the internal mammary arteries. Clockwise rotation is employed for both left and right IMA engagement. (From Tilkian AG, Daily EK: *Cardiovascular procedures: diagnostic techniques and therapeutic procedures,* St. Louis, 1986, Mosby.)

orifice. The catheter tip should be directed caudally and ante-riorly. At the level of the internal mammary orifice, a slight counterclockwise rotation and advancement may be neces-sary to cannulate the artery.

Vigorous manipulation of the catheter and deep intubation of the internal mammary artery should be avoided because of the hazard of dissection. Only catheters with no side holes should be used to be able to see the pressure damping, which indicates potentially dangerous deep cannulation. Moreover, side-hole catheters are not preferable in this location because of the poor opacification of the graft, especially after the balloon catheter is advanced. The patient should be informed about the sensations in the shoulder and anterior chest wall during nonionic contrast-media injection.

Right internal mammary artery catheterization. Right internal mammary artery cannulation is less common and more difficult than left internal mammary artery cannulation. The right brachiocephalic truncus is entered using a right Judkins catheter by rotating the tip with a counterclockwise rotation at the level of the brachiocephalic truncus (Fig. 2-11). The catheter is advanced into the subclavian artery over a guidewire. The rest of the cannulation procedure is similar to that described for left internal mammary artery graft cannulation.

In patients for whom cannulation of the subclavian artery is not possible because of excessive tortuosity or obstructive lesions, an internal mammary artery catheter can be introduced through a brachial (ipsilateral) artery, using either a percutaneous or cutdown approach, and advanced beyond the mammary artery orifice over a guidewire. The catheter is withdrawn slowly by making frequent, small contrast injections.

CORONARY GUIDING CATHETERS
Selection of Guiding Catheters Based on Angiographic Clues

Guide catheters differ from diagnostic catheters in two critical areas: a less open secondary curve tip and a potentially shorter nontapered ostial portion of the catheter. Although the majority of left coronary arteries are effectively cannulated with classic standard Judkins left 4-cm curves, guiding catheters may require the shorter Judkins left 3.5-cm or other configurations to engage adequately. A dilated aortic root may thus be satisfactorily engaged with the Judkins left 4-cm and, on rare occasion, Judkins left 5-cm guiding catheters.

With regard to right coronary arteries, the upward-angled high-takeoff or Shepherd's crook configuration represents a particularly difficult problem for angioplasty guide seating. For engagement of upgoing right coronary artery takeoffs, an Amplatz left coronary artery and Arani or hockey stick have been recommended. Although the internal mammary artery guide has been used, its support against the aortic cusp and posterior aorta is less than that provided by the just mentioned catheters.

Brachial Guiding Catheters

Brachial catheters usually are straight catheters with an end hole and two side holes placed close to the tip. The brachial catheter can be used for both left and right coronary interventions.

SHEATH CARE AND HEMOSTASIS AFTER CORONARY ANGIOPLASTY

Timely and safe removal of the arterial sheath with minimal patient discomfort is an integral part of a successful coronary angioplasty procedure. Percutaneous entry-site complications are a significant cause of morbidity and increased length of hospitalization. With the increased use of stents and other devices requiring large sheaths or continuous anticoagulation, sheath care and hemostasis after angioplasty have become more important. Therefore the coronary angioplasty plan should always include provision for time, personnel, and other resources that are necessary for this part of the procedure. The importance of appropriate sheath care and hemostasis should not be downplayed by concerns of time or resources.

Care of the In-Dwelling Sheath

The arterial and venous access sheaths are almost always left in place because of the high-dose heparin given during the procedure. Some institutions remove sheaths a few hours after the procedure, while some others prefer overnight heparinization with next-day sheath removal. In selected patients, same-day sheath removal is a safe alternative with obvious economical consequences. In case of coronary dissection, thrombus, or intraprocedure closure, heparin treatment is usually continued for 24 to 72 hours.

The presence of a sheath in a heavily anticoagulated patient predisposes perisheath hemorrhage and local or retroperitoneal hematoma. Important points in avoiding and treating these complications include the following:

1. Do it right the first time. Meticulous arterial puncture and sheath placement technique decrease future problems considerably.
2. Identify and remedy perisheath bleeding and hematoma that start during the procedure. Sometimes a one-French-size larger sheath may control the bleeding effectively.
3. Always place an appropriate-size obturator in the sheath to prevent kinking.
4. Use clear, transparent dressing to cover the puncture area.
5. The puncture site should be inspected and palpated at each check in addition to the detection of distal pulses. If the brachial artery is used, measure arm circumference periodically to detect hematoma.
6. Mark the hematoma borders and check frequently to see whether a rapid enlargement takes place.
7. Use closed sterile systems to monitor side arm pressures. Minimize blood drawing from the sheaths.
8. Be aware of a gradual but persistent downward trend in blood pressure and upward trend in heart rate. These may be the only clues to excessive bleeding (e.g., retroperitoneal hematoma).
9. Take necessary measures to ensure patient comfort.

Hemostasis

Since sheath removal takes place in the patient wards, appropriate measures should be taken to maintain sterility and decrease contamination.

1. Use sterile gloves and sterile technique.
2. Position the patient horizontally. Adjust bed height and your position to be able to exert maximum pressure with minimum fatigue.
3. Give local anesthetic (10 to 20 cc of 1% Lidocaine).
4. Give oral and/or IV analgesics before sheath removal.
5. Have atropine and IV fluids within reach.
6. Before removing the sheath, check that:
   a. Heparin is stopped for an appropriate time;
   b. If heparin is continued, PTT should be <50 sec;
   c. Vital signs are stable;
   d. No chest pain is present. No plans for recatheterization are made.
7. Remove the arterial sheath first. Avoid prolonged pressure on the femoral vein. Prolonged venous occlusion,

especially with pressure devices, may cause venous thrombosis. Check the leg and foot for cyanosis.

8. Duration of pressure holding (usually 20 to 45 min) depends on the sheath size, coagulation status, and ease of controlling the bleeding.

9. When longer pressure application is needed (such as continued heparinization, removal of large sheaths, intraaortic balloon pump catheters, or cardiopulmonary support cannulae), Fem-Stop (USCI-Bard, Inc.) is the preferred device. It provides stable position, relative patient comfort, and easy adjustment of the degree of pressure applied. C-clamps or other devices may also be used. Pressure devices are not intended for unsupervised application. The duration of the pressure application should be kept at a minimum to decrease the complications, such as skin necrosis, femoral nerve compression paralysis, or venous thrombosis.

10. Several types of plugging devices, including collagen plugs, pulley devices, and percutaneous arterial suture closures, have been invented in the recent years. These devices are aimed at immediate sheath removal in fully anticoagulated patients, thereby decreasing the duration of bed rest and overall hospitalization. Some authors found collagen plugs to be very safe and effective, while others emphasized the uncommon but serious complications, such as arterial occlusion or embolism, or periplug bleeding with extensive hematoma.

Care After Sheath Removal

Strict bed rest for 6 to 12 hours depending on the sheath size is required. Ambulation should be gradual. An important point is to extend the strict bed rest up to 24 hours after sheath removal in patients who are continued on heparin. This simple measure has decreased groin complications significantly, especially after stent implantation.

Continued anticoagulation after sheath removal, large (10 French) sheaths, and hematoma are risk factors for pseudoaneurysm development. Palpation for pulsatile mass and auscultation for bruits should be performed routinely until discharge. Femoral pseudoaneurysm may become prominent (mature) >24 hours after sheath removal.

SUGGESTED READINGS

Cragg AH, Nakagawa N, Smith TP, Berbaum KS: Hematoma formation after diagnostic angiography: effect of catheter size, *J Vascular Intervent Radio* 2(2):231-233, 1991.

Deligonul U, Roth R, Flynn M: Arterial and venous access. In Kern MJ, editor: *The cardiac catheterization handbook,* ed 2, St. Louis, 1995, Mosby, pp 45-107.

deSwart H, Dijkman L, van Ommen V, et al.: The hemostatic puncture closure device versus a conventional pressure bandage: preliminary results of a randomized study (abstr), *Circulation* 88: I-251, 1993.

Gardiner GA, Meyerovitz MF, Strokes KR, et al.: Complications of transluminal angioplasty, *Intervent Radiol* 159:201-208, 1986.

Oweida SW, Roubin GS, Smith RB, Salam AA: Postcatheterization vascular complications associated with percutaneous transluminal coronary angioplasty, *J Vasc Surg* 12:310-315, 1990.

Roberts SR, Main D, Pinkerton J: Surgical therapy of femoral artery pseudoaneurysm after angiography, *Am J Surg* 154:676-680, 1987.

3

ANGIOGRAPHY FOR INTERVENTIONAL PROCEDURES

Morton J. Kern, Ubeydullah Deligonul, Steven E. Nissen, and Alexander Khoury

ANGIOGRAPHY TECHNIQUES

In years before angioplasty was performed, definition of coronary artery narrowings sufficient for surgical revascularization required only identification of disease location without detailed characterization of plaque, associated branch points, or lesion morphology. Because interventional procedures require precise definition of lesion length and morphology, as well as location and relationship to side branches, angiography has taken on an even more critical role. The interventionist needs to assess several definitive aspects of the vessels and lesions under study.

Objectives for Angioplasty-Angiography
1. Identify relationship of coronary ostium to aorta for guide catheter selection
2. Identify target vessel, pathway, and angle of entry
3. Identify lesion morphology using angulated views eliminating vessel overlap
4. Separate and identify associated side branches and degree of atherosclerosis in branch ostia

5. Identify distal distribution of target vessel and collateral supply
6. Determine the diameter of the coronary artery at the target site

Optimal definition of proximal coronary anatomy is critical to guide and balloon catheter selection. Assessment of calcium from angiography is known to be less reliable than endovascular echocardiography, but still serves a useful purpose in assessing risks associated with the procedure. Classical terminology for defining angiographic projections with regard to left and right anterior oblique, cranial and caudal angulation, and lateral projections remains as defined in previous discussions for diagnostic coronary angiography (see *The Cardiac Catheterization Handbook*, Chapter 5).

For percutaneous transluminal coronary angioplasty, visualization of vessel bifurcations, origin of side branches, the portion of the vessel proximal to a significant lesion, and previously "unimportant" lesion characteristics (length, eccentricity, calcium, and the like) are critical. In the case of a total vessel occlusion, the distal vessel should be visualized as clearly as possible by injecting the coronary arteries that supply collaterals and taking cineangiograms with panning long enough to visualize late collateral vessel filling.

Optimizing the angiographic image is also critical to angiography for interventions. Excellent image quality enhances clinical studies and their accurate interpretation for decisions. Modification of catheterization technique to reduce motion artifact during imaging, optimal use of beam restrictors (collimation) to reduce scatter, improved image contrast, and meticulous supervision of film processing can enhance clinical results. In the coming era of filmless, all-digital cardiac imaging, data processing analysis and storage will remain critical issues for angiographers.

A working knowledge of the principles of radiographic imaging permits the interventionalist to improve diagnostic and therapeutic procedures. Awareness of the inverse square law of radiation propagation will dramatically reduce the exposure of the operator and the team. Obtaining quality images should not necessitate increasing the ordinary procedural radiation exposure to either the patient or catheterization personnel.

COMMON ANGIOGRAPHIC VIEWS FOR ANGIOPLASTY

The routine coronary angiographic views described below should include those that best visualize the origin and course of the major vessels and their branches in at least two different projections (preferably orthogonal). Naturally, there is a wide variation in coronary anatomy, and appropriately modified views will need to be individualized.

Nomenclature for Angiographic Views

For all catheterization laboratories, the x-ray source is under the table and the image intensifier (Figs. 3-1, 3-2; Tables 3-1, 3-2) is directly on top of the patient. They are moving in opposite directions in an imaginary circle in which the patient is positioned in the center. The body surface of the patient that faces the observer determines the specific view. This relationship holds true whether the patient is supine, standing, or rotated.

AP position.   The image intensifier is directly over the patient, with the beam perpendicular to the patient lying flat on the x-ray table. The AP view or shallow RAO displays the left main coronary artery in its entire perpendicular length. In this view, the left anterior descending and left circumflex artery branches are overlapped. Slight RAO or LAO angulation may be necessary to clear the density of the vertebrae and the catheter shaft in the thoracic descending aorta.

RAO position.   The image intensifier is to the right side of the patient. The RAO caudal view shows the left main coronary artery bifurcation from a view perpendicular to the LAO/cranial angle. The origin and course of the circumflex/ obtuse marginals, intermediate branch, and proximal left anterior descending segment are well seen. This view is one of the best two views for visualization of the circumflex artery. The left anterior descending beyond the proximal segment is obscured by overlapped diagonals.

The RAO or AP/cranial view is used to open the diagonal along the mid and distal left anterior descending. Diagonal branch bifurcations are well visualized. The diagonal branches are projected upward. The proximal left anterior descending and circumflex usually are overlapped. Marginals may overlap, and the circumflex is foreshortened.

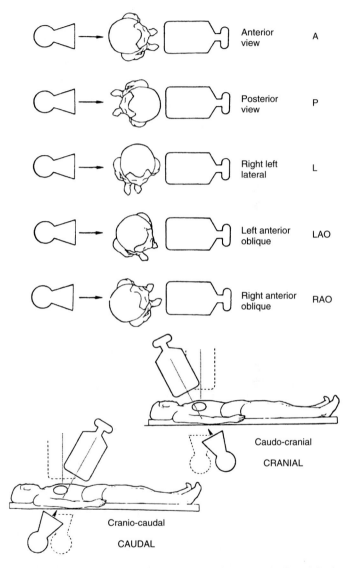

Anterior
view   A

Posterior
view   P

Right left
lateral   L

Left anterior
oblique   LAO

Right anterior
oblique   RAO

Caudo-cranial

CRANIAL

Cranio-caudal

CAUDAL

Fig. 3-1. Nomenclature for angiographic views. (Modified from Paulin S: Terminology for radiographic projections in cardiac angiography, *Cathet Cardiovasc Diagn* 7:341, 1981.)

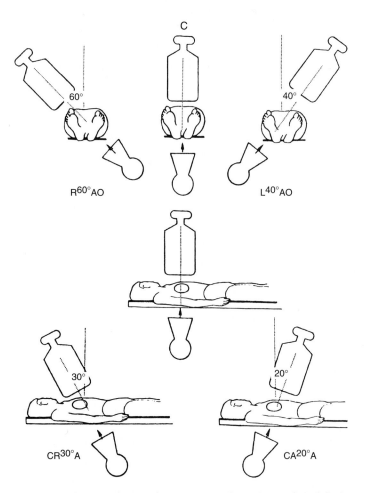

Fig. 3-2. Nomenclature for angiographic views. (Modified from Paulin S: Terminology for radiographic projections in cardiac angiography, *Cathet Cardiovasc Diagn* 7:341, 1981.)

LAO position. In the LAO position, the image intensifier is to the left side of the patient. The LAO/cranial view also shows the left main coronary artery (slightly foreshortened but perpendicular to the RAO view), left anterior descending, and diagonal branches. Septal and diagonal branches are separated clearly. The circumflex and marginals are foreshortened and overlapped. Deep inspiration, moving the density of the diaphragm out of the field, is essential for this view.

TABLE 3-1. Recommended "key" angiographic view for specific coronary artery segments

Coronary segment	Origin/bifurcation	Course/body
Left main	AP	AP
	LAO cranial	LAO cranial
	LAO caudal*	
Proximal LAD	LAO cranial	LAO cranial
	RAO caudal	RAO caudal
Mid LAD	LAD cranial	
	RAO cranial	
	Lateral	
Distal LAD	AP	
	RAO cranial	
	Lateral	
Diagonal	LAO cranial	RAO cranial, caudal, or straight
	RAO cranial	
Proximal circumflex	RAO caudal	LAO caudal
	LAO caudal	
Intermediate	RAO caudal	RAO caudal
	LAO caudal	Lateral
Obtuse marginal	RAO caudal	RAO caudal
	LAO caudal	
	RAO cranial (distal marginals)	
Proximal RCA	LAO	
	Lateral	
Mid RCA	LAO	LAO
	Lateral	Lateral
	RAO	RAO
Distal RCA	LAO cranial	LAO cranial
	Lateral	Lateral
PDA	LAO cranial	RAO
Posterolateral	LAO cranial	RAO
	RAO cranial	RAO cranial

* Horizontal hearts.
AP, Anterioposterior; *LAD,* left anterior descending artery; *LAO,* left anterior oblique; *PDA,* posterior descending artery (from RCA); *RAO,* right anterior oblique; *RCA,* right coronary artery.
From Kern MJ, editor: *The cardiac catheterization handbook,* St. Louis, 1995, Mosby, p 286.

The LAO angle should be set so that the left anterior descending course is parallel to the spine and stays in the "lucent wedge" bordered by the spine and the curve of the diaphragm. Cranial angulation tilts the left main coronary artery down and permits view of the left anterior descending/cir-

TABLE 3-2. Coronary angiographic projections

Artery	Routine*	Supplemental[†]
Projections for diagnostic coronary arteriography		
Left coronary	RAO (10-30)	RAO (15-30) CR (15)
	RAO (15) CA (15)	Spider [LAO 40-60, CA 20-30]
	LAO (45-60) CR (15-25)	
	LAT	AP ± CR (15-25)/CA (15-25)
Right coronary	LAO (30-60)	LAO (30-45) CR (10-15)[‡]
	RAO (30)	LAT
Angiographic projections for PTCA		
Left anterior descending	RAO (30)	Spider
	RAO (15-30) CR (15) vs. RAO (15) CA (15)[§]	RAO (0-10) CR (20-40) LAT CR (10-15) or CA (10-15)
	LAO (40-60) CR (15-25)	
	LAT	
Circumflex	RAO (15) CA (15-25)	RAO (30)
	LAO (60)	Spider
	LAT	LAO (60) CR (15)
Right coronary artery	LAO (30-60)	LAO (20-30) CR (10-15)[c]
	RAO (30)	RAO (10-30) CR (10-15)
	LAT	

* Degrees of angulation satisfactory for most patients are suggested in parentheses but may vary depending on anatomy.
† One or more supplemental views may be needed. Indications for these and possible additional views (not listed) are given in the text.
‡ LAO cranial view may replace nonangulated LAO as routine view in many patients.
§ For choice of RAO cranial versus caudal, see text and appended graphics section.
From Boucher RA, Myler RK, Clark DA, Stertzer SH: Coronary angiography and angioplasty, *Cathet Cardiovasc Diagn* 14:269-285, 1988.

cumflex bifurcation. Too steep an LAO/cranial angulation or shallow inspiration produces considerable overlapping with the diaphragm and liver, degrading the image.

The LAO/caudal view ("spider" view) (Fig. 3-3) shows the left main coronary artery (foreshortened) and bifurcation of the left main coronary artery into the circumflex and left anterior descending. Proximal and midportions of the circum-

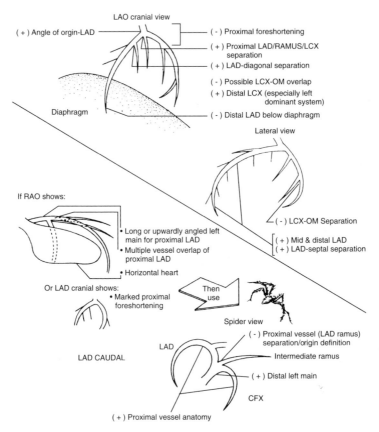

Fig. 3-3. Diagramatic view of left coronary artery demonstrating special positioning to best observe branch segments. (From Boucher RA, et al.: Coronary angiography and angioplasty, *Cathet Cardiovasc Diagn* 14:269-285, 1988.)

flex are usually seen excellently with the origins of obtuse marginal branches. Poor image quality may be due to overlapping of diaphragm and spine. The left anterior descending is considerably foreshortened in this view.

A lateral view shows the mid and distal left anterior descending best. The left anterior descending and circumflex are well separated. Diagonals usually are overlapped. The (ramus) intermediate branch course is well visualized.

Note: Think of the "oblique" view as turning the left/right shoulder forward (anterior) to the camera (image intensifier).

Cranial/caudal position.   For the cranial/caudal position, the nomenclature refers to image intensifier angles in relation to the patient's long axis.

Cranial.   In the cranial position, the image intensifier is tilted toward the head of the patient.

Caudal.   In the caudal position, the image intensifier is tilted toward the feet of the patient.

The cranial and caudal views are "open" overlapped coronary segments that are foreshortened in regular views (Fig. 3-3).

Remember: Cranial views for the left anterior descending artery; caudal views for the circumflex artery.

Angulation for the Right Coronary Artery

When considering which views to use, and because of the individual variations in anatomy, performing small (1- to 2-ml) test injections in inspiration is very helpful in obtaining the appropriate oblique and axial angulations and setup for panning.

The LAO/cranial view shows the origin of the right coronary artery, the entire length of the right coronary artery, and the posterior descending artery bifurcation (crux). Cranial angulation tilts the posterior descending artery down to show vessel contour and reduce foreshortening. Deep inspiration is necessary to clear the diaphragm. The posterior descending artery and posterolateral branches are foreshortened.

The RAO view shows the mid right coronary artery and the length of the posterior descending artery and posterolateral branches. Septals, supplying occluded left anterior descending via collaterals, may be clearly identified. The posterolateral branches are overlapped and may need the addition of the cranial view.

The lateral view also shows the right coronary artery origin (especially in those with more anteriorly oriented orifices) and mid right coronary artery well. The posterior descending artery and posterolateral branches are foreshortened.

Angulation for Saphenous Bypass Grafts

Coronary artery saphenous vein grafts are visualized in at least two views (LAO and RAO). It is important to show the aortic anastomosis, the body of the graft, and the distal anastomosis. The distal runoff and continued flow or collateral channels are also critical. The graft vessel anastomosis is best seen in the view that depicts the native vessel best. A general strategy for graft angiography is to perform the standard views while assessing the vessel key views for specific coronary artery segments (see Table 3-1) to determine the need for contingency views or an alteration/addition of special views. Therefore, the graft views can be summarized as follows:

1. Right coronary artery graft: LAO cranial, RAO, and lateral
2. Left anterior descending graft (or internal mammary artery): lateral, RAO cranial, LAO cranial, and AP (the lateral view is especially useful to visualize the anastomosis to the left anterior descending)
3. Circumflex (and obtuse marginals) grafts: LAO and RAO caudal

Techniques for Coronary Arteriography

Since deep inspiration may change the proximal course of the artery and the spatial relation of lesion to anatomic landmarks, guide angiograms should be taken in such a way that frequent inspiratory effort leading to patient fatigue during manipulation is not necessary. Select a view requiring minimal inspiratory hold while providing optimum presentation of the lesion.

Power injection versus hand injection for coronary arteriography. Power injection of the coronary arteries has been utilized in thousands of cases in many laboratories and is equal in safety to hand injection. However, hand injection of the coronary arteries offers advantages in ease of administration of intracoronary drugs and rapid successive injections with varying degrees of opacification for either severely diseased or high-flow coronary arteries. In the latter case, a power injector at a fixed setting might require several injections to find the optimal contrast delivery flow rate.

Typical settings for power injections are as follows:

1. Right coronary artery: 4-6 ml at 3-4 ml/sec, maximal psi 150
2. Left coronary artery: 8-10 ml at 4-5 ml/sec, maximal psi 150

Panning techniques. Many laboratories use x-ray image mode sizes of <7 in. diameter, which precludes having the entire coronary artery course visualized without panning over the heart to include late filling of the distal arterial or collateralized segments. In addition, in most views some degree of panning will be necessary to identify regions that are not seen from the initial setup positioning. Some branches may unexpectedly appear later from collateral filling or other unusual anatomic sources.

Angiographic thrombolysis in myocardial infarction (TIMI) classification of blood flow. TIMI flow grading has been used to assess, in a qualitative fashion, the degree of restored perfusion achieved after thrombolysis or angioplasty in patients with acute myocardial infarction. Table 3-3 provides descriptions used to assign TIMI flow grades.

TABLE 3-3.   Thrombolysis in Myocardial Infarction (TIMI) flow

TIMI flow grades	
Grade 3 (complete reperfusion)	Anterograde flow into the terminal coronary artery segment through a stenosis is as prompt as anterograde flow into a comparable segment proximal to the stenosis. Contrast material clears as rapidly from the distal segment as from an uninvolved, more proximal segment.
Grade 2 (partial reperfusion)	Contrast material flows through the stenosis to opacify the terminal artery segment. However, contrast enters the terminal segment perceptibly more slowly than more proximal segments. Alternatively, contrast material clears from a segment distal to a stenosis noticeably more slowly than from a comparable segment not preceded by a significant stenosis.
Grade 1 (penetration with minimal perfusion)	A small amount of contrast flows through the stenosis, but fails to fully opacify the artery beyond.
Grade 0 (no perfusion)	There is no contrast flow through the stenosis.

Modified from Sheehan F, Braunwald E, Canner P, et al.: The effect of intravenous thrombolytic therapy on left ventricular function: a report on tissue-type plasminogen activator and streptokinase from the Thrombolysis in Myocardial Infarction (TIMI) Phase I Trial, *Circulation* 72:817-829, 1987.

Angiographic classification of collateral flow.   Collateral flow can be seen and classified angiographically. The late opacification of a totally or subtotally (99%) occluded vessel through antegrade or retrograde collateral channels will assist in correct guidewire placement, lesion localization, and a successful procedure. The collateral circulation is graded angiographically as follows:

Grade	Collateral appearance
0	No collateral branches seen
1	Very weak (ghostlike) opacification
2	Opacified segment is less dense than the source vessel and filling slowly
3	Opacified segment is as dense as the source vessel and filling rapidly

Collateral visualization will help establish the size of the recipient vessel to select an appropriately sized balloon. Determination whether the collateral circulation is ipsilateral (e.g., proximal right coronary artery (RCA) to distal RCA collateral supply) or contralateral (e.g., CFX to distal RCA collateral supply) and exactly which region will be affected should collateral supply be disrupted is important to gauge procedural risk. The evaluation of collaterals must be included when making decisions on which vessels should be protected or lost during coronary angioplasty.

Assessment of coronary stenoses. Assessment of the degree of narrowing. The evaluation of the degree of a stenosis relates to the percentage reduction in the diameter of the vessel. This is calculated in the projection where the greatest narrowing can be observed. Exact evaluation is almost impossible and, in fact, the lesions are roughly classified. Six categories can be distinguished in this way:

0 = normal coronary artery
1 = irregularities of the vessel
2 = narrowing of less than 50%
3 = stenosis between 50% and 75%
4 = stenosis between 75% and 95%
5 = total occlusion

Coronary lesion descriptions for angioplasty. In 1988, the American College of Cardiology and the American Heart

Association Task Force characterized coronary lesions by specific characteristics, classifying lesions as type A, B, or C (Table 3-4).

Coronary artery descriptors. General characteristics of the artery proximal to the lesion dilated are as follows:

• *Tortuosity:* None/mild = straight proximal segment or only one ≥60° bend. Moderate = two ≥60° bends proximal to the lesion. Severe = three or more ≥60° bends proximal to the lesion.

• *Arterial calcification:* Light = proximal arterial wall calcification (not necessarily the lesion) seen as thin lines(s). Heavy = easily seen calcification.

Target lesion descriptors. Angiographic characteristics of the dilated lesion are as follows.

• *Arrangement of the lesion(s):* Tandem = two lesions located within one balloon length (i.e., both lesions can be covered

TABLE 3-4.   Characteristics of type A, B, and C lesions

Lesion-specific characteristics	
Type A lesions (high success, >85%; low risk)	
Discrete (<10 mm length)	Little or no calcification
Concentric	Less than totally occlusive
Readily accessible	Not ostial in location
Nonangulated segment, <45°	No major branch involvement
Smooth contour	Absence of thrombus
Type B lesions (moderate success, 60-85%; moderate risk)	
Tubular (10 to 20 mm length)	Moderate to heavy calcification
Eccentric	Total occlusions <3 months old
Moderate tortuosity of proximal segment	Ostial in location
Moderately angulated segment, >45°, <90°	Bifurcation lesions requiring double guidewires
Irregular contour	Some thrombus present
Type C lesions (low success, <60%; high risk)	
Diffuse (>2 cm length)	Total occlusion >3 months old
Excessive tortuosity of proximal segment	Inability to protect major side branches
Extremely angulated segment >90%	Degenerated vein grafts with friable lesions

From Ryan TJ, Raxon DP, Gunnar RM, et al.: Guidelines for percutaneous transluminal coronary angioplasty. *J Am Coll Cardiol* 12:529-545, 1988.

during single balloon inflation). Sequential = two lesions located at a distance longer than the balloon.

- *Length:* Discrete = ≥5 mm in length. Tubular = 5-10 mm in length. Diffuse = >10 mm in length.
- *Eccentricity:* Concentric = lumen axis is located along the long axis of the artery or on either side of it, but by no more than 25% of the normal arterial diameter.
- *Ostial:* Lesion is located at the aorto-ostial or at the bifurcation points.
- *Side branch:* Bypassable side branch (1.5 mm or larger).
- *Contour:* Smooth, irregular, or ulcerated.
- *Thrombus:* Definite = intraluminal, round filling defect, visible in two views, largely separated from the vessel wall and/or documentation of embolization of this material. Possible = other filling defects not associated with calcification, lesion haziness, irregularity with ill-defined borders, intraluminal staining at the total occlusion site.
- *Stenosis calcification:* Calcification at the actual lesion site.
- *Angulation:* None/mild = lesion located on a straight segment or <45° bend. Moderate = 45°-90° bend. Severe = >90° bend. Bend should be evaluated in end-diastolic frame.

Problems and Solutions in the Interpretation of Coronary Angiograms

Vessel overlap.   Because coronary angioplasty requires a clear view of the target vessel that may be overlapped, multiple angles are required to reveal locations of lesions not previously considered important.

Poor vessel opacification.   Poor contrast opacification of the vessel may lead to a false impression of an angiographically significant lesion or lucency that could be considered a clot. Inadequate mixing of contrast and blood presents as a luminal irregularity. A satisfactory bolus injection of contrast must be delivered if adequate opacification is to be achieved and the angiogram interpreted correctly. Enhanced contrast delivery can be best achieved by obtaining better coaxial engagement of the guiding catheter or using a larger-size catheter, injecting during Valsalva maneuver phase III, or using a power injector.

Total vessel occlusion.   Total occlusion of a vessel may be erroneously suspected if a catheter is subselective in its location or an anomalous origin and course of a vessel are not recognized. A short left main coronary artery may lead to opacification of only the left anterior descending, and a presumption of a circumflex occlusion or anomalous position may result. If this is thought to be the case, an aortic cusp "flush" injection of contrast may reveal the second vessel. Subselective injections into each vessel separately may be necessary if the left main artery is too short to opacify both vessels simultaneously. This problem may also occur for subselective injection into a large right coronary artery conus branch that does not visualize the main right coronary artery adequately.

Vasospasm.   Catheter-induced spasm may appear as a fixed stenotic lesion. This has been observed in both right and left (and left main) coronary arteries and must be considered when an organic lesion is the only suspected anomaly. Nitroglycerin will reverse coronary spasm and should be administered in such cases when a question of catheter-induced spasm exists. Catheter-induced spasm may occur not only at the tip of the catheter touching the artery, but also more distally. Repositioning of the catheter and administration of nitroglycerin (100-200 μg through the catheter) may clarify if the presumed lesion is structural and not spastic. Often a change to a smaller-diameter (6 or 5 French) catheter or catheters that do not seat deeply may help.

Special Problems

Defining left main coronary anatomy.   Since the engagement of the guide catheter into the left coronary ostium is critical to the successful performance of angioplasty, any disease within the left main coronary artery should be identified. Important left main coronary artery disease should be considered a contraindication to elective angioplasty for unprotected dilatation of proximal left coronary vessels. Optimal views to identify the left main coronary artery remain the same as for those during diagnostic studies, with a shallow right anterior oblique with cranial or caudal angulation often providing an excellent view. In addition, complementary left anterior oblique caudal view (spider view) will display the left main artery in an orthogonal projection.

Safe coronary angiography of patients having left main coronary artery stenosis remains one of the few critical situations in which the operator and the team may affect the life and death of the patient directly. In general, interventions are not performed through left main stenosis ≥40% diameter. However, some situations will warrant angioplasty, directional coronary atherectomy, or stenting despite some degree of left main stenosis. These interventions are high risk and should not be contemplated except by the most experienced interventionalist under exceptional circumstances.

Left circumflex coronary artery takeoff.   The angle of departure of the circumflex artery represents the most difficult aspects of angioplasty in this vessel. Since the circumflex may be up-going and then immediate down-going, a right-angle bend of the circumflex is best appreciated from the left anterior oblique caudal view. Horizontal takeoffs in the left anterior oblique cranial of the circumflex artery permit easy passage of the system in the proximal portion of the coronary artery. A transfer to the right anterior oblique caudal projection will facilitate movement down the coronary artery. Guide catheter selection for the circumflex artery often requires longer (i.e., 4.0 JL4 guides, left Amplatz, or Voda) guides with special tips.

Diagonal branch origin. Visualization of diagonal branches from the left anterior descending artery is often best performed using right anterior oblique with cranial projections or AP with cranial projections adequately identifying the takeoff from the left anterior descending artery path. Lateral projections are often excellent, but fail to reveal diagonal origins unless significant cranial angulation can be established. The mid and distal left anterior descending artery segments are best seen with the lateral projection.

ANGIOGRAPHIC AND VIDEO IMAGING SYSTEMS
Video Systems and Fluoroscopy (Fig. 3-4)

In modern interventional practice, video systems and fluoroscopy have an increasingly important role in safe and effective procedures. Video and fluoroscopy systems have evolved more rapidly than any other component in the x-ray system. A typical video camera used for fluoroscopy has a lens which focuses light from the output phosphor of the image intensifier. The incident light strikes a target in the video camera composed of small globules of photoconductive material.

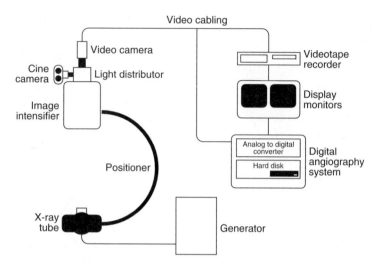

Fig. 3-4. Angiographic imaging chain. Both cinefilm and digital angiographic data are produced from the same x-ray-generated images.

Each small globule of material is insulated from surrounding areas. In general, the larger the target area, the better the image quality.

Video signal generation. The light-sensitive material emits electrons in quantities proportional to the intensity of the incident light. The free electrons are attracted to an anode in the video camera and each globule of photoconductive material thus becomes positively charged, acting as a small capacitor. An electron beam subsequently scans the photoconductive material progressively discharging each tiny globule of material. The resulting current flows through a conductive signal plate and, following appropriate amplification, constitutes the video signal emerging from the camera. The voltage of the video output signal is proportional to the intensity of light that struck each point in the target.

A television monitor works in an opposite but analogous fashion. An electron beam scans a fluorescent screen that emits light in proportion to the number of electrons striking the phosphor. A control grid modulates the current of the scanning beam based on the voltage of the incoming video signal. The resulting television image varies in brightness at each point in the image proportional to the amount of light that originally illuminated the video camera. The accuracy of video reproduction is determined by the precision with which the video camera converts light into an electrical signal and the accuracy with which the monitor converts the video signal into a fluorescent image.

Scanning modes.   Television monitors and video cameras use two different scanning methods. Traditional television monitors scan 525 lines in an interlaced fashion such that one half of the lines are scanned each 1/60th sec. (Fig. 3-5). This interlaced approach results in two fields and one frame each 1/30th of a second (30 frames/sec). Interlacing is employed to accommodate the flicker fusion frequency of the human eye. If a full frame were reproduced every 1/30th sec, the image would exhibit annoying flicker. Because part of each frame is updated each 1/60th sec, the image is perceived without noticeable flicker.

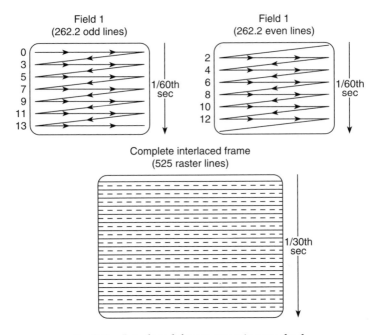

Fig. 3-5.   Interlaced frame-scanning method.

Most (but not all) video systems in modern catheterization laboratories include video cameras and monitors with 1024 high-line-rate video. Advanced systems use progressive-scan video cameras rather than the interlaced approach. The progressive-scan systems use a video camera that scans all 1024 lines of the image each 1/60th sec, avoiding flicker. Because there are 1024 scan lines, not 525, raster-line effects are reduced. Despite improvements, the 1024-line video does not produce images with twice the resolution of 525-line systems, because the low x-ray dose image used for fluoroscopy has interference from quantum mottle. High-line-rate video cameras also generate more electronic noise than 525-line systems. Despite these limitations, a high-line-rate fluoroscopic image and such systems should be the standard in interventional laboratories.

Another advance in interventional radiology is pulsed fluoroscopy. These fluoroscopic systems are short pulses of x-ray similar to that of cineangiography, reducing or eliminating motion artifact (blur) and improving image quality, particularly for rapidly moving coronaries. A reduction in x-ray dose, though more efficient exposure, may be noted. However, pulsed fluoroscopy systems generally require a grid-control x-ray tube, an expensive addition.

Image lag.   Image lag is defined as the degree of persistence of the image on the target of the video camera. During fluoroscopy, because low radiation exposure is employed, images contain considerable quantum noise. Video cameras take advantage of lag time to smooth the image appearance during fluoroscopy. Excess lag time will result in objectionable motion blur, a problem following acquisition of digital imaging systems.

Sophisticated television systems in catheterization suites control camera lag according to the application. During fluoroscopy, moderate lag smooths the noise, but when recording video images during digital angiography, the camera is electronically altered to yield low lag characteristics. Such techniques utilize an electronic edge-enhancing filter to increase the apparent sharpness of the image. A different technique, known as unsharp masking, improves image sharpness and contrast. Sophisticated image filters used for fluoroscopy are adaptive, changing their characteristics according to the requirements of the image.

Video recording systems. In modern laboratories, video tape recorders have assumed a secondary role, because digital angiographic systems have replaced video recorders as the principal means used to review images during interventional procedures. Cassette decks, including $\frac{3}{4}$-in. and $\frac{1}{2}$-in. VHS, rarely offer more than 300 lines of resolution. A few laboratories have adopted the improved $\frac{1}{2}$-in. super-VHS format to store images in a "cine-less" laboratory. At the moment, this practice results in suboptimal image quality and poor archival properties, and it cannot be recommended.

Digital Angiography

Digital imaging uses the voltage of analog video signal produced during image acquisition, which is proportional to the brightness in the original image. An analog-to-digital converter samples the video signal and converts the voltage levels into a series of discrete numbers. The number of possible gray levels for each pixel is determined by the number of bits available for analog-to-digital conversion. In cardiac digital angiography, this is typically 8 bits (1 byte), which in binary numbers corresponds to 256 possible gray levels. No matter how many discrete levels are assigned, the digital representation does not exactly reproduce the original signal and contains a series of discrete steps known as quantization error. For coronary angiography, the typical 256 gray levels have a quantization error that is clinically negligible.

The horizontal and vertical sampling rate of the digital-to-analog converter determines the matrix size of the digital image. Most current systems generate 512 horizontal and 512 vertical samples, each referred to as a picture element, or pixel. Cardiac digital angiography, thus, consists of a 512 × 512 pixel acquisition with 8 bits of gray scale per pixel. With a 512 × 512 matrix, the digital system will generate 3.4 pixels/mm for a 15-mm (6-in.) image intensifier. A top-quality image intensifier will resolve 4 to 5 line pairs per millimeter. At least 2 pixels are required to reproduce each line pair. Thus, a 512 × 512 digital image undersamples the available information. An 8-bit gray scale (256 levels) should be adequate for minimizing quantum noise at exposures of 20-25 μR per frame. Higher doses, such as might be used for peripheral vascular imaging, may require 10-12 bits under certain circumstances.

Cardiac digital angiography requires large data storage capacity. A single 512 × 512-pixel, 8-bit image represents 262,144 bytes of data. A 30-frame/sec digital coronary angiography generates 30 × 262,144 bytes per second, or about 7.5 million bytes of data per second (7.5 megabytes). An 8-sec coronary injection requires about 60 megabytes, and a full angiographic study may require up to 1 billion bytes of data (1 gigabyte). For 1000 cases, the storage requirements for complete archiving of these studies are approximately 1000 gigabytes (1 terabyte). In current interventional practice, images are stored temporarily on a computer hard disk for immediate replay and review. The size of the hard disk determines the capacity of the digital imaging system, typically 2500 to 25,000 images (2 to 14 complete patient studies).

Advantages.   It is possible to acquire useful arterial images with much smaller amounts of contrast than with film angiography and to store and analyze images in a more quantitative fashion. In addition, the digital approach allows the performance of a number of manipulations on the stored images. The contrast image can be amplified or enhanced. One image can be subtracted from another and then that image can be subtracted from a third image. Digital image manipulations allow many views that are not possible with film radiograms.

Disadvantages.   Digital angiography systems may not provide the exquisite detail found in radiographic films. Moreover, the digital subtraction procedure is very sensitive to motion. It often requires a patient who is alert and aware of what is going on and who can cooperate during the procedure.

Digital (subtraction) angiography system.   There are two types of digital subtraction angiography systems, pulsed systems and fluoroscopy (real-time systems).

Pulsed system. The pulsed system acquires images relatively infrequently. One image per second with a 512 × 512 digital matrix is a typical acquisition rate. Some systems may indicate that 5-10 images per second can be acquired. (Cineangiographic filming acquisition rates are >30 frames/sec.)

Pulsed systems require special TV cameras. Pulsing requires high-powered, three-phase, 12-pulse x-ray generators. They operate by pulsing the generator at high milliamperage currents, which provide a heavy burst of x-ray energy to the image intensifier in an attempt to obtain sharp images. A single image is scanned by the TV camera, which overcomes the blurring of the x-ray image. Images are stored until after the run is complete.

Once the run is complete, the operator retrieves these images and subtracts them from each other. Image acquisition runs must begin several seconds before the contrast media are due to arrive at the anatomical region of interest and must continue long enough so that the operator can be certain that a person with slow circulation has passed all the contrast media through the region of interest. The unopacified image (mask) is subtracted from the images with the contrast in the vessels with a restraint image remaining of only the opacified vessel without interference from other structures such as bones.

Fluoroscopic (real-time) system. The second type of system is called a real-time system. These systems operate at fluoroscopic x-ray levels and normal TV frame rates (30 frames/sec). They normally do not require a special TV camera, and fluoroscopic milliamperage levels from 5 to 20 mA produce quite satisfactory imaging. The milliamperage required will depend on the age and performance of the image intensifier and the TV camera. A three-phase x-ray generator is not required. Because of the fluoroscopic x-ray requirements, and unlike pulsed systems, special heavy-duty x-ray tubes are not required. A 300,000-heat-unit tube is quite satisfactory.

The image processing in real-time systems occurs as the acquisition run (and the examination) progresses. The subtracted image can be observed on the TV monitor as the examination is proceeding. This ability to see the contrast agent passing through the region of interest allows the operator to terminate image acquisition and fluoroscopy as soon as the contrast media have passed. There is no need to run on past contrast media passage as with pulsed systems.

Real-time systems are designed to be added to most fluoroscopic x-ray generators. Real-time systems have the ability to do subtraction angiography with IV injection for primary and secondary arteries (peripheral vessels only). To visualize tertiary and very small vessels, intraarterial catheterization often is required.

Digital archiving: Cine replacement. Digital angiography is attractive as a long-term storage medium for archiving cardiac catheterization studies. Digital information allows production of multiple copies with no image degradation. Digital data can be transmitted electronically for remote examination and consultation. The economic cost of storing patient studies may be reduced relative to current film technology with a cost of approximately $100.00 per patient for film and development. Digital studies may cost less than $10.00 per patient.

At the time of this publication, a committee from the American College of Cardiology and the National Electrical Manufacturers Association (NEMA) has been formed to address the issue of standardization. Until the development of a standard is accepted, most laboratories should defer conversion to digital archiving.

Vascular tracing. A procedure called vascular tracing, or road mapping, often is provided in digital angiographic systems. After arterial injection of small amounts of contrast material, the vascular tracing function will "remember" the path of the contrast media as they travel through the arteries. As the contrast media travel down the artery, it traces out the path of the entire arterial system in that area. Once the digital trace is complete, a "hard copy" (photograph or print) can be made, or it can be subtracted from an image with no contrast media in it. The major value of this technique for relatively stationary vascular anatomy is in "runoff" studies for detecting blood clots or blockages in the legs or arms.

Digital fluoroscopy aids. Many digital angiographic systems utilize functions of the image processor during fluoroscopy, when subtraction angiography is not being performed. One of these functions is image noise reduction during fluoroscopy by integrating several successive frames. Another is "last image hold," which allows the operator to retain the last image displayed on the monitor each time the fluoroscopic foot switch is released.

Another capability is electronic radiography. This turns the x-rays on just long enough for the system to acquire and freeze an image and then automatically turns the x-ray off again. This is similar to spot filming with the fluoroscope. One other function that can be provided during normal fluoroscopy is contrast enhancement.

Quantitative coronary angiography. The degree of coronary stenosis is quantitated from the cineangiogram and, in clinical practice, is usually a visual estimation of the percentage of diameter narrowing using the presumed proximal normal arterial segment and the ratio of normal diameters to stenosis diameters. This technique is widely applicable in clinical practice but is inadequate for the quantitative methodology done in most research studies. The intraobserver variability may range between 40% and 80%, and there is frequently as wide as a 20% range on interobserver differences. Quantitative methodology uses digital calipers or automated or manual edge detection systems. Densitometric analysis with digital angiography also provides quantitative lesion measurements.

MEDICATIONS USED IN CORONARY ANGIOGRAPHY

Recording medications on cinefilm during angiography will help assess events during procedural reviews.

If drugs are given during the course of the catheterization that may affect the angiograms in any way, the film can be marked with a cineangiographic exposure of a radioopaque drug marker to identify the drug and indicate that a change in the subsequent arteriograms may be present. Examples of such drugs are sublingual or intracoronary nitroglycerin, ergonovine, and drugs used during thrombolytic therapy (e.g., streptokinase). A radiographic clock marker may also be used to indicate the time of such events.

Radiographic Contrast Media

The contrast material is selected from commercially available liquid solutions appropriate for the specific examination to be conducted. All contrast materials are x-ray "dense" (as a result of iodine), as compared to anatomical structures that are x-ray "lucent," and absorb x-rays in order to provide different gray shades in x-ray images. The quantity and concentration of contrast materials used are specific medical decisions. Factors included in these decisions are the patient's age, size, general health, and allergies.

All contrast agents contain iodine, an effective absorber of x-rays. Although all agents are derivatives of benzoic acid, the number of iodine molecules and ionic and osmolar composition will vary. Osmolarity, viscosity, sodium content, and other additives and properties are different among these agents. Table 3-5 provides a summary of commonly used contrast agents for coronary and left ventricular angiographic studies. Selection of a contrast agent for the particular laboratory is, to a large extent, a matter of personal preference. Major differences among the contrast agents include cost, induction of bradycardia and hypotension, and impairment of left ventricular function. Thousands of studies have been performed safely with conventional high-osmolar/ionic agents and pose no major risks. However, considerable data exist to suggest that the newer, low-osmolar/nonionic agents may be safer and provide satisfactory diagnostic quality, especially for high-risk patients. Indications for low-osmolar/nonionic contrast agents include unstable ischemic syndromes, congestive heart failure, diabetes, renal insufficiency, hypotension, severe bradycardia, history of contrast allergy, severe valvular heart disease, and use of internal mammary artery injection.

Ionic contrast media produce hypotension by peripheral arterial vasodilation, transient myocardial dysfunction, and decreasing circulating volume and blood pressure after osmotic diuresis (initially contrast media increased circulating fluid volume by osmotically shifting fluid into vascular space).

TABLE 3-5. Angiographic contrast agents

	Iodine (mg/ml)	Osmolality (mosm/kg)	Additives
A. Ionic, high osmolality			
Renografin-76	370	1940	NaEDTA, NaCitrate
Hypaque-76	370	2016	NaCaEDTA
MD-76	370	2140	NaEDTA, NaCitrate
Angiovist	370	1076	NaCaEDTA
Vascoray	400	2400	NaH_2Po_4, NaCaEDTA
B. Nonionic			
Omnipaque	350	844	$Na_2CaEDTA$
Isovue	370	796	$Na_2CaEDTA$
Optiray	350	600	$Na_2CaEDTA$
C. Ionic, low osmolality			
Hexabrix	320	600	$Na_2CaEDTA$

Table 3-6 lists medications commonly used during cardiac catheterization.

Coronary Vasodilators

Nitroglycerin.   Nitroglycerin is the most commonly used drug during coronary arteriography and ventriculography. Nitroglycerin dilates peripheral arteries, venous beds, and coronary arteries. Nitroglycerin is a very safe and short-acting drug. It can be given through the sublingual, intravenous, intracoronary, or intraventricular route. Sublingual (or oral spray) nitroglycerin (0.4 mg) is almost always given before coronary arteriography. Exceptions include patients in whom coronary spasm may be suspected and those with hypotension (<90 mmHg systolic pressure). In patients with documented coronary spasm, sublingual or intracoronary nitroglycerin is given to eliminate coronary spasm. In patients with unstable angina, IV infusions of nitroglycerin of up to 250 μg/min with a systolic blood pressure of 90 mm Hg are permissible. In patients with elevated left ventricular end-diastolic pressure in the catheterization laboratory from ischemia or from congestive heart failure, intraventricular or IV boluses of 200 μg of nitroglycerin will reduce left ventricular end-diastolic pressure and is appropriate if not required before or after ventriculography. Nitroglycerin increases coronary blood flow without a marked reduction in pressure in doses of 50, 100, and 200 μg (intracoronary). In doses of more than 250 μg, hypotension without further increases in coronary blood flow may be evident.

Calcium channel blockers.   Calcium channel blockers dilate vascular smooth muscle and reduce heart muscle contractility, and some agents block atrioventricular (AV) nodal conduction. Calcium channel blockers are used to reduce peripheral vascular resistance, reduce blood pressure, and increase coronary blood flow. These agents are given orally before the performance of angioplasty and are in use chronically by patients with ischemic heart disease. Acute use in the cardiac catheterization laboratory is indicated for hypertension and ongoing myocardial ischemia with increased blood pressure or sudden recurrent supraventricular tachycardia (verapamil, diltiazem). Doses for calcium channel blockers are as follows:

TABLE 3-6.   Medications used in the cardiac catheterization laboratory*

Inotropics

    Digitalis, 0.125-0.25 mg IV >4 hr apart
    Dobutamine, 2-10 μg/kg/min IV drip
    Dopamine, 2-10 μg/kg/min IV drip
    Epinephrine, 1:10,000 IV
    Isoproterenol, 1 mg/min IV drip

Antiarrhythmics, anticholinergics, beta blockers, calcium blockers

    Adenosine, 5-12 mg IV bolus
    Atropine, 0.5-1.2 mg IV
    Bretylium, 100-300 mg IV bolus
    Diltiazem, 10 mg IV
    Esmolol, 4-24 mg/kg IV drip (beta blocker)
    Lidocaine, 50-100 mg IV bolus; 2-4 mg/min IV drip
    Procainamide, 50-100 mg IV
    Propranolol, 1 mg bolus; 0.1 mg/kg in 3 divided doses (beta blocker)
    Verapamil, 2-5 mg IV, may repeat dose to 10 mg (calcium channel
      blocker)

Analgesics, sedatives

    Diazepam, 2-5 mg IV
    Diphenhydramine, 25-50 mg IV
    Meperidine, 12.5-50 mg IV
    Morphine sulfate, 2.5 mg IV
    Naloxone, 0.5 mg IV

Anticoagulants

    Heparin, 2000-5000 units IV; 1000 units/hr IV drip; 10,000-unit bolus
      for PTCA

Vasodilators

    Nitroglycerin, 1/150 sublingual; 100-300 μg IV or IC
    Nitroprusside, 5-50 μg/kg/min IV

Vasoconstrictors

    Aramine, 10 mg in 100 ml saline, 1 ml IV
    Ergonovine, 0.4 mg IV in divided doses
    Norepinephrine, 1:10,000 IV; 1 ml doses IV

Diuretic

    Furosemide, 20-100 mg IV

Metabolic buffers

    Calcium chloride and/or gluconate, 10 mEq
    Sodium bicarbonate, 50 mEq

Miscellaneous

    Protamine, 15-50 mg IV
    Succinylcholine, 1-4 mg IV

---

* The list is meant to be neither all-inclusive nor exclusive of emergency life-support techniques or standards.

1. Nifedipine, 10-20 mg PO
2. Diltiazem, 30-60 mg PO; 10 mg IV
3. Verapamil, 120 mg PO; 2.5-5 mg IV

Papaverine.   Papaverine is a potent arterial vasodilator used in the investigation of coronary vasodilatory reserve. Intracoronary papaverine causes a marked increase in blood flow in the right coronary artery in doses from 4 to 8 mg and in the left coronary artery in doses from 8 to 12 mg. Doses exceeding these recommended levels do not appear to provide an increase over the maximal blood flow. Rare cases of papaverine-induced *torsade de pointe* (Ventricular Tachycardia) have been reported, and antiarrhythmic preparations for this unusual event should be in place before administration of intracoronary papaverine.

Adenosine.   Adenosine is used for breaking supraventricular tachycardia (SVT) and is the drug of choice for intracoronary induction of maximal hyperemia for coronary vasodilator reserve. For the right coronary artery, intracoronary adenosine of 6-8 μg and for the left coronary artery 12-18 μg produces optimal results. Adenosine (0.14 μg/kg/min IV) infusions produce sustained and equivalent hyperemia. Adenosine hyperemia lasts <60 sec after drug administration is ended.

Acetylcholine.   Acetylcholine dilates normal coronary arteries and constricts diseased vessels. Intracoronary doses of 20, 50, and 100 μg have been used to induce coronary spasm in patients in Japan. The drug is very short-acting and rapidly reversed, making it excellent for catheterization laboratory use. Marked bradycardia and heart block have been reported with the use of acetylcholine. Temporary pacing is required during its administration. Continuous infusions of 0.02 to 2.2 μg/kg/min (10^{-8}, 10^{-7}, 10^{-6} M) have been used to identify normal endothelial function of coronary vessels.

Anticholinergics for Vagal Reactions

Atropine.   Atropine is used to block vagally induced slowing of the heart rate and hypotension. Doses of 0.6 to 1.2 mg IV given immediately will reverse bradycardia and hypotension within 2 min. It is important to remember that in elderly patients, heart rate may not slow during vagal episodes in which the only manifestation is low blood pressure. This low blood pressure can be alleviated by the administration of IV atropine and normal saline. In the rare patient in whom IV access is not immediately available, intraarterial atropine (in the aorta) can be administered.

Antiarrhythmic Drugs

Lidocaine.   Lidocaine is an antiarrhythmic drug used to block or reduce the number of ventricular extra-systoles. Lidocaine can be administered as a bolus of 50 to 100 mg intravenously before ventriculography if a stable and quiet catheter position within the left ventricle cannot be obtained. In patients in whom myocardial ischemia is developing during cardiac catheterization or angioplasty, lidocaine for frequent ventricular ectopy is indicated. A bolus of 50 to 100 mg intravenously followed by 1 to 2 mg/min infusion is usually satisfactory.

Cardiac Agonists

Isoproterenol.   Isoproterenol (Isuprel) is a pure beta agonist that increases heart rate and causes peripheral vasodilatation. It is indicated during cardiac arrest with refractory bradycardia. Isuprel has been used for provocation of heart stress (increased heart rate) in patients with valvular heart disease or hypertrophic cardiomyopathy.

Dopamine.   Dopamine is a potent vasoconstrictor. In low doses, it causes renal vasodilatation. In high doses, it causes peripheral vasoconstriction, elevating the blood pressure and increasing myocardial contractility. Dopamine from 2 to 15 µg/min will cause vasoconstriction, elevating the blood pressure.

Dobutamine.   Dobutamine is a potent inotropic agent with no peripheral vasoconstrictor effects. It increases cardiac contractility (inotropy) and is especially useful in patients with congestive heart failure. It may be used in conjunction with a potent vasodilator such as nitroprusside in those patients with markedly elevated LV filling pressures and poor cardiac output.

Epinephrine.   Epinephrine (1:10,000) is a naturally occurring catecholamine that stimulates cardiac function. It is administered only during cardiac emergencies. This medicine will increase heart rate and blood pressure immediately, sometimes to excessive levels. This should be reserved for cases in which cardiac resuscitation is required or in which refractory hypotension is present and not responding to peripheral vasoconstrictors. Transthoracic administration of epinephrine through a long needle is not required during cardiac catheterization in which IV or intraarterial access already is obtained. One milliliter of 1:10,000 dilution given intravenously can increase systemic pressure during hypotension to a safe level until IV vasopressors have been prepared. This dose has a duration of action between 5 and 10 min.

Arterial Vasodilators

Nitroprusside.   Nitroprusside is a potent short-acting intravenous arterial vasodilator used in the treatment of aortic insufficiency, mitral regurgitation, hypertensive crisis, and congestive heart failure. Doses administered range from 10 to 100 μg/min and must be monitored by direct arterial pressure measurement.

RADIATION EXPOSURE DURING CORONARY ANGIOPLASTY

Cardiac angiography with combined fluoroscopy and cineradiography carries the highest patient x-ray doses in diagnostic radiology. Coronary angioplasty will deliver greater x-ray exposure because of the more complicated and time-consuming nature of this procedure. Previous studies have demonstrated that operator exposure is 93% greater for angioplasty than for routine diagnostic coronary angiography. This increase is due to longer fluoroscopy times in angioplasty without corresponding longer cineradiography times. Because of the angled projections used in coronary angioplasty, increased x-ray exposure may be present. The scattered x-ray dose has been reported to be four times higher with angioplasty than with diagnostic cardiac catheterization (Fig. 3-6).

Fluoroscopy Times

A study of radiation risk to patients from coronary angioplasty by Pattee et al. indicated that radiation doses varied considerably during the procedure due to large differences in exposure times. Fluoroscopy time per angioplasty case averaged 19 min, but in some procedures exceeded 60 min. Average patient skin entrance exposure per angioplasty pro-

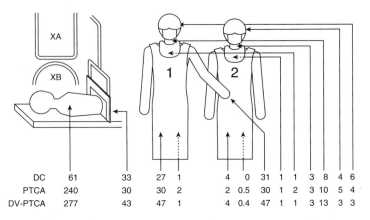

DC	61	33	27	1	4	0	31	1	1	3	8	4 6
PTCA	240	30	30	2	2	0.5	30	1	2	3	10	5 4
DV-PTCA	277	43	47	1	4	0.4	47	1	1	3	13	3 3

Fig. 3-6. Radiation exposure rates for two operators during coronary angioplasty. DC, Diagnostic catheterization; DV-PTCA, double-vessel PTCA; XA, x-ray amplifier in plane A; XB, x-ray amplifier in plane B. (Modified from Finci L, et al.: Radiation exposure during diagnostic catheterization and single- and double-vessel percutaneous transluminal coronary angioplasty, *Am J Cardiol* 60:1401-1403, 1987.)

cedure was 32 μC/kg (124 R), of which 70% was from cineradiography. Cancer mortality risk per angioplasty procedure was 8×10^{-4}. The study indicated that skin exposures estimated for angioplasty are, on average, higher than for other x-ray procedures, and that the cancer mortality risk does not exceed the mortality risk of bypass surgery (Table 3-7). Good professional practice requires maximal benefit-to-risk ratio for angioplasty procedures employing high-dose fluoroscopy or cineradiography.

New Device Procedure Times (Table 3-8)

New intracoronary interventional devices increase radiation exposure. Federman et al., of the Mayo Clinic, found that in 900 patients, two-thirds undergoing balloon angioplasty and one-third undergoing directional atherectomy or other new procedures including 37 with intracoronary stent placement, the duration of fluoroscopy for angioplasty was 24 ± 18 min, which was greater than for directional atherectomy (18 ±

TABLE 3-7. Organ doses and risks of cancer mortality for average coronary angioplasty procedure

Organ	Organ dose (cGy)*	Cancer mortality risk ($\times 10^{-6}$)
Red bone marrow	2.29	92
Bone (surfaces)	2.29	9.2
Lung	9.35	636
Thyroid	0.99	5.9
Breast (women)	4.89	157
Total risk		
Men		743
Women		899

* 1 Gy = 1 J/kg = 100 rads: 1 cGy = 1 rad.
From Pattee PL, Johns PC, Chambers RJ: Radiation risk to patients from percutaneous transluminal coronary angioplasty, *J Am Coll Cardiol* 22:1044-1051, 1993.

8 min). Fluoro times were similar, at 25 and 29 min. When atherectomy or laser angioplasty was performed with balloon angioplasty, or if emergency intracoronary stent placement was performed, the duration of fluoroscopy was significantly prolonged compared to angioplasty alone. Increased radiation exposure should be expected when emergency procedures are required.

TABLE 3-8. Estimated radiation entrance exposure to patients using phantom model data

Procedure*	Entrance exposure	
	Fluoroscopy (R)	Cine (R)
Isolated BA	43	25
Isolated DCA	32	23
DCA + BA	66	29
Isolated laser	45	18
Laser + BA	57	27
Elective stenting	52	27
Emergency stenting	96	41

* BA, Balloon angioplasty; DCA, directional coronary atherectomy; *laser*, laser coronary angioplasty.
From Federman J, Bell MR, Wondrow MA, Grill DE, Holmes DR Jr: Does the use of new intracoronary interventional devices prolong radiation exposure in the cardiac catheterization laboratory?, *J Am Coll Cardiol* 23:347-351, 1994.

TABLE 3-9.   Radiation dose and angulation

View	Dose (relative increase)
Image intensifier position	
RAO 30-60°	1
LAO 30-60°	2.6-6.1
Increasing angulation	
LAO 30°	1
LAO 60°	3
LAO 90°	9

Angulated views and radiation exposure (Table 3-9)

LAO views produce 2.6 to 6.1 times the operator dose as equivalently angled RAO views.* Steeper LAO views also increased operator dose. LAO 90° produces 8 times the dose of LAO 60° and 3 times the dose of LAO 30°.

Fluoroscopy produced more radiation than cine during angioplasty by 6:1. Reducing the steepness of angulation will reduce operator radiation dosage.

PERIPHERAL VASCULAR ANGIOGRAPHY

Digital subtraction angiography is the method of choice for identifying peripheral vascular disease. Cineangiography also provides satisfactory information if the filming time, frame rates, and contrast dosages are properly established.

Renal arteriography (see Chapter 11)

Selective renal arteriography or arteriography obtained from aortic flush is used to evaluate the renal artery origins and vasculature. *Remember:* For renal artery identification during aortography, the artery origins usually arise at L_1 vertebrate (just below the T_{12} ribs). Selective renal arterial injections provide the most detail. The left anterior oblique projection often provides the best view of the renal artery ostia in a majority of patients. Acutely angled takeoffs of the renal artery may require specially shaped catheters or a brachial arterial approach from above. Atherosclerotic disease of the renal artery usually involves the proximal one-third of the renal artery

* Pitney MR, et al.: Modifying fluoroscopic views reduces operator radiation exposure during coronary angioplasty, *J Am Coll Cardiol* 24:1660-1663, 1994.

and is seldom present without abdominal atherosclerotic plaques. A renal artery stenosis alone is rarely the sole determinant for surgery or angioplasty. Refractory hypertension and determination of the renin-angiotensin levels are usually the indicators for an interventional (angioplasty or stent) procedure. Renal artery fibromuscular dysplasia may occur and appear as atherosclerotic disease. This finding is often present in middle-aged women with other vessels involved, most commonly cerebral or visceral arteries. Unlike that of atherosclerotic narrowing, the proximal one-third of the main renal artery is usually free of disease.

Angiography of the Thoracic and Abdominal Aorta

Aortography is indicated for suspected aneurysms or dissections by clinical, historical, or procedural signs. Injection techniques are the same as for ascending aortography. Evaluation of peripheral lower extremity disease requires identification of iliac bifurcation and common femoral artery patency before subselective injections.

Angiography of Lower Extremities

Based on clinical signs and symptoms of arterial insufficiency to the legs, suspected obstructions of vessel are screened with echo-Doppler before angiography is performed. Small-diameter (5 French) catheters are satisfactory. Reduced volumes of contrast (10 to 20 ml over 1 to 2 sec) are injected during filming with panning down the artery, following the course to the most distal locations. Angulated views may be necessary to open bifurcations and overlying vessels that obscure the vessel origin. When possible, angiographic filming should extend at least to the ankle. Long cut-films that cover the entire lower extremity on a moving table are available in radiologic suites. In cardiac catheterization laboratories, cineangiographic filming with prolonged filming and panning down to the ankle must be tested before obtaining final views. Digital subtraction techniques are available commonly in many modern laboratories. Nonionic contrast agents are less painful for peripheral vascular angiography as compared to ionic contrast agents.

The area most frequently involved in peripheral atherosclerotic disease involves the distal superficial femoral artery at

the abductor canal (Fig. 3-7). One major challenge encountered with femoral-iliac angiography is the contralateral (opposite leg) approach over the aortic bifurcation of the iliac
vessels. To enter the opposite iliac artery, often a right Judkins
or internal mammary artery graft catheter is selected and
advanced with a guidewire over the bifurcation and down
into the opposite femoral artery. The wire is passed down
into the selected artery. The catheter may be advanced and
exchanged (over a long, 300-cm wire) for an appropriate angiographic or balloon dilatation catheter, as required. The calf,
tibial, and knee (popliteal) arteries are the next most commonly involved vessels after the superficial femoral artery.
Disease in the deep femoral artery (femoral profunda) is rare.
Pathways of collateralization are often rich and varied in

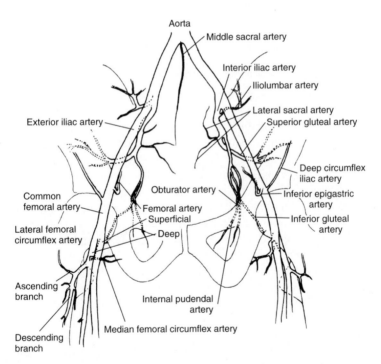

Fig. 3-7.   Pelvic and proximal femoral arterial branches. (From
Johnsrude IS, et al.: *A practical approach to angiography*, ed. 2,
Boston, 1987, Little, Brown.)

patients with chronic distal femoral artery disease, especially in total occlusions of the superficial femoral artery that reconstitutes at or below the knee, close to the branching trifurcation of the tibial and deep peroneal arteries.

SUGGESTED READINGS

Arvidson H: Angiographic observations in mitral valve disease, with special reference to the volume variations in the left atrium, *Acta Radiol* (suppl 158):1-40, 1958.

Balter S, Sones M Jr, Brancato RL: Radiation exposure to the operator performing cardiac angiography with U-arm systems, *Circulation* 58:925-932, 1978.

Boucher RA, Myler RK, Clark DA, Stertzer SH: Coronary angiography and angioplasty, *Cathet Cardiovasc Diagn* 14:269-285, 1988.

Dillon JC: Inexpensive radiation protective glasses, *Cathet Cardiovasc Diagn* 5:203-208, 1979.

Dodge HT, Sandler H, Ballew DW, Lord JD Jr: The use of biplane angiocardiography for the measurement of left ventricular volume in man, *Am Heart J* 60:762-776, 1960.

Federman J, Bell MR, Wondrow MA, Grill DE, Holmes DR Jr: Does the use of new intracoronary interventional devices prolong radiation exposure in the cardiac catheterization laboratory?, *J Am Coll Cardiol* 23:347-351, 1994.

Finci L, Meier B, Steffenino G, Roy P, Rutishauser W: Radiation exposure during diagnostic transluminal coronary angioplasty, *Am J Cardiol* 60:1401-1403, 1987.

Gertz EW, Wisneski JA, Gould RG, Akin JR: Improved radiation protection for physicians performing cardiac catheterization, *Am J Cardiol* 50:1283-1286, 1982.

James TN, Bruschke AVG, Bothig S, et al.: Report of WHO/ISFC task force on nomenclature of coronary arteriograms, *Circulation* 74:451A-455A, 1986.

Judkins MP: Guidelines for radiation protection in the cardiac catheterization laboratory. *Cathet Cardiovasc Diagn* 10:87-92, 1984.

Levin DC, Dunham LR, Stueve R: Causes of cine image quality deterioration in cardiac catheterization laboratories, *Am J Cardiol* 52:881-886, 1983.

Miller SW, Castronovo FP Jr: Radiation exposure and protection in cardiac catheterization laboratories, *Am J Cardiol* 55:171-176, 1985.

Pattee PL, Johns PC, Chambers RJ: Radiation risk to patients from percutaneous transluminal coronary angioplasty, *J Am Coll Cardiol* 22:1044-1051, 1993.

Rackley CE, Dodge HT, Coble YD Jr, et al.: A method of determining left ventricular mass in man, *Circulation* 29:666-671, 1964.

Sandler H, Dodge HT: The use of single plane angiocardiograms for the calculation of left ventricular volume in man, *Am Heart J* 75:325-334, 1968.

Wynne J, Green LH, Mann T, et al.: Estimation of left ventricular volumes in man for biplane cineangiograms filmed in oblique projections, *Am J Cardiol* 41:726-732, 1978.

4

CORONARY ANGIOPLASTY COMPLICATIONS AND ANTITHROMBOTIC THERAPY

Richard G. Bach, Ubeydullah Deligonul, Thomas M. Hyers, and Morton J. Kern

SECTION I. CORONARY ANGIOPLASTY COMPLICATIONS

Complications of coronary angioplasty include major ischemic events related to vessel closure that result in myocardial infarction and death, and minor complications predominantly involving vascular access (Table 4-1). More unusual complications, potentially more frequent with newer devices, include coronary ostial trauma and coronary perforation.

INCIDENCE OF MAJOR COMPLICATIONS

The incidence of complications is related to both patient and lesion characteristics, as well as operator skill and procedural factors.

TABLE 4-1. Potential complications following PTCA

Acute vessel closure (dissection, thrombus, spasm)
  Acute myocardial infarction
  Emergent coronary bypass surgery
  Death
Coronary artery emboli or perforation
Right ventricular perforation (with pacing catheter)
Coronary ostial dissection with guiding catheter
Fracture of guidewire within coronary circulation
Ventricular tachyarrhythmias
Severe angina
Transient hypotension
Transient bradyarrhythmias
Small coronary artery side-branch occlusion
Allergic reaction to radiographic contrast medium
Contrast nephropathy
Local vascular access-site complications: bleeding, arterial damage,
  thrombosis

From Kulick DL, Kawaniski DT: Percutaneous transluminal coronary angioplasty. In Kulick DL, Rahimtoola SH, editors: *Techniques and applications in interventional cardiology,* St. Louis, 1991, Mosby, p 76.

Early coronary angioplasty experience (National Heart, Lung, and Blood Institute [NHLBI] PTCA Registry 1977-1981) reported myocardial infarction occurring in 5% of patients, urgent coronary artery bypass graft surgery required in 7%, and death in 1%. The incidence of major complications has improved despite angioplasty currently being performed in more difficult patient subsets with multivessel disease, poor left ventricular function, and advanced age. The more recent NHLBI Registry (1985-1986) complication rates indicate that myocardial infarction occurs in 3.4%, emergency coronary artery bypass graft surgery in 4.3%, and death in 1% of patients. On average, success for coronary angioplasty has been maintained at a nearly constant favorable rate of >90%, with major complications occurring in <4% of patients. These rates will vary among patient subsets with various risk factors.

Clinical Risk Factors

Higher risk of adverse angioplasty outcome has been associated with a clinical presentation of unstable ischemia, likely due to the presence of intracoronary thrombus, impaired left ventricular function, and certain anatomic characteristics indicating increasing lesion complexity (Tables 4-2, 4-3).

Technical Risk Factors

Procedural factors, such as a failure to administer aspirin and adequate doses of heparin, balloon-to-artery ratio of >1.3, and a severe degree of angiographically apparent intimal dissection, also confer an increase in the risk of vessel closure.

The incidence of myocardial infarction varies depending on the interventional technique employed. Reported rates of myocardial infarction for the following devices have been established.

TABLE 4-2. Characteristics associated with increased mortality from cardiac catheterization

Age

Infants (<1 year old) and the elderly (>65 years old). Elderly women appear to be at higher risk than elderly men.

Functional class

Mortality in class IV patients is more than 10 times greater than in class I and II patients.

Severity of coronary obstruction

Mortality for patients with left main disease is more than 10 times greater than for patients with one- or two-vessel disease.

Valvular heart disease

Especially when combined with coronary disease, this condition is associated with a higher risk of death at cardiac catheterization than coronary artery disease alone.

Left ventricular dysfunction

Mortality for patients with left ventricular ejection <30% is more than 10 times greater than in patients with ejection fraction ≥50%.

Severe noncardiac disease

Patients with:
    Renal insufficiency
    Insulin-requiring diabetes
    Advanced cerebrovascular and/or peripheral vascular disease
    Severe pulmonary insufficiency

Modified from Grossman W: Complications of cardiac catheterization: incidence, causes and prevention. In Grossman W, editor: *Cardiac catheterization and angiography,* ed 3, Philadelphia, 1986, Lea & Febiger.

TABLE 4-3.   Factors associated with abrupt vessel closure during elective coronary angioplasty

1. Angiographic factors
    Intraluminal thrombus
    Type B and C lesions
    Multivessel disease
    Ostial right coronary artery disease
    Saphenous vein grafts
    Subtotal coronary occlusion
2. Clinical conditions predisposing to acute vessel closure
    Unstable angina
    Diabetes
    Female gender
    Advanced age (>80 years)
3. Conditions associated with increased mortality after major complication of coronary angioplasty
    Unstable angina
    Left ventricular ejection fraction <30%
    Congestive heart failure
    Multivessel disease
    Proximal right coronary artery stenosis
    Unstable angina
    Age >65 years
    Female gender

1. PTCA: <3%
2. Rotational atherectomy (rotablator)
    Q-wave myocardial infarction: 2%-3%
    Non-Q-wave myocardial infarction: 5%-6%
    [Predisposing factors: lesion length >4 mm, right coronary stenosis, acute angle of >60° bend, and female gender]
3. Coronary stenting
    From the Gianturco-Roubin stent multicenter registry, 5% for acute closure
    0.5% for stent elective placement
    [Risk factors for myocardial infarction included stenting vessels <3.0 mm diameter and presence of thrombus]
4. DCA: 10%-15% for elective procedures in native vessels; 5%-10% in saphenous vein grafts.
5. TEC catheter.
    For saphenous vein grafts, myocardial infarction occurred in 5.5% due to graft closure within 24 hours.

ACUTE MYOCARDIAL ISCHEMIA DUE TO ABRUPT CLOSURE

Prolonged ischemia due to impaired blood flow through the target vessel may cause complications by inducing arrhythmias, hypotension, infarction, and death if the ischemia is not treated in a timely manner. Acute ischemia is manifested by either one or any combination of the following: chest pain, ST-T wave changes, arrhythmias, or hypotension. A hypertensive response may sometimes be seen. Hypotension may be manifested by mental changes (e.g., yawning, confusion, or frank loss of consciousness). Management of acute ischemia induced by acute vessel closure must address the underlying causes. Treatment of dissection, thrombus, or a combination of these two mechanisms should be undertaken immediately.

Although many patients have features suggesting an increased potential for acute vessel closure, preventive techniques should help to limit the incidence of this occurrence.

1. All patients receive antiplatelet therapy (aspirin), and ischemic complications are increased if aspirin is omitted. Alternatives to aspirin include dipyridamole, ticlopidine, and potentially nonsteroidal antiinflammatory drugs.
2. A satisfactorily anticoagulated state with intravenous heparin should elevate the activated clotting time to >300 sec, and this can be easily monitored in the laboratory. A bolus of 10,000 U with a 1000-U/hr intravenous drip is the most common regimen employed for angioplasty. However, some patients empirically require more heparin. In the setting of acute vessel closure, an immediate assessment of the activated clotting time or activated partial thromboplastin time plus repeated administration of heparin and an increased infusion rate (as needed) is warranted.

While working on vessel reopening, the systemic consequences of acute myocardial ischemia are also treated. Maintenance of systemic hemodynamics should be addressed with fluid resuscitation, intraaortic balloon pumping, and intravenous vasopressors (Aramine or Dopamine) when necessary. Temporary transvenous pacemaking may also be required for heart block.

If repeated standard balloon inflations fail to restore adequate blood flow and are limited by continued severe isch-

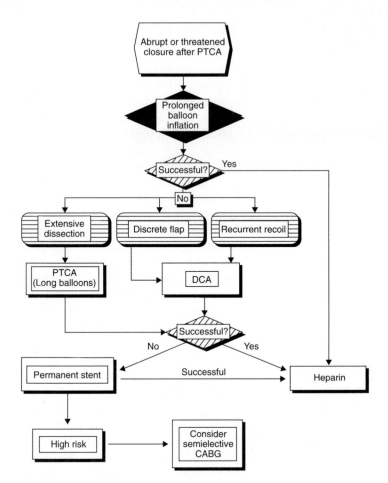

Fig. 4-1. Algorithm for treatment strategy for abrupt vessel closure. DCA, Directional coronary atherectomy; CABG, coronary artery bypass graft surgery. (From Popma JJ, Leon MB: Developing an integrated approach to the use of new devices for coronary intervention. In Topol EJ, editor: *Textbook of interventional cardiology,* vol 2, ed 2, Philadelphia, 1994, W. B. Saunders, p 980.)

emia, perfusion balloons (passive or active, if available) or stenting is indicated. Augmentation of coronary blood flow with intraaortic balloon pumping through perfusion balloons may be helpful. A flow chart for management of acute or threatened coronary occlusion after coronary angioplasty is shown in Fig. 4-1.

Coronary dissection. The most common cause of prolonged ischemia during angioplasty is coronary dissection. Although coronary dissection may be detected by characteristic angiographic imaging, at times, the dissection cannot be differentiated from thrombus formation, with lucent and linear streaking of contrast in and around the site of angioplasty. Coronary dissection is generally treated with prolonged balloon inflations or intracoronary stent placement.

Classification of coronary artery dissections followed the National Heart, Lung, and Blood Institute system A-F, where type A is minor radiolucencies within the coronary lumen due to contrast injection with no persistence of dye; type B is parallel tracks or double lumen impression of radiolucent area during contrast injection with no persistence; type C is

Dissection type	Description	Angiographic appearance
A	Minor radiolucencies within the coronary lumen during contrast injection with minimal or no persistence after dye clearance.	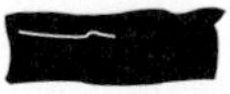
B	Parallel tracts or double lumen separated by a radiolucent area during contrast injection with minimal or no persistence after dye clearance.	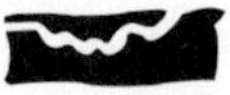
C	Extraluminal cap with persistence of contrast after dye clearance from the coronary lumen.	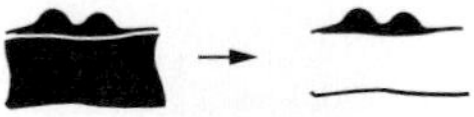
D	Spiral luminal filling defects.	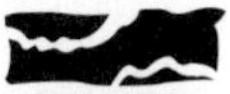
E+	New persistent filling defects.	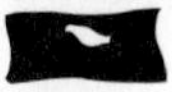
F+	Those non–A-E types that lead to impaired flow or total occlusion.	

+ May represent thrombus.

Fig. 4-2. Types of coronary artery dissections: NHLBI classification system. (Modified from Freed M, Grines C, editors: *Manual of interventional cardiology,* Birmingham, Michigan, 1992, Physician's Press, p 204.)

J.M., 67-year-old man

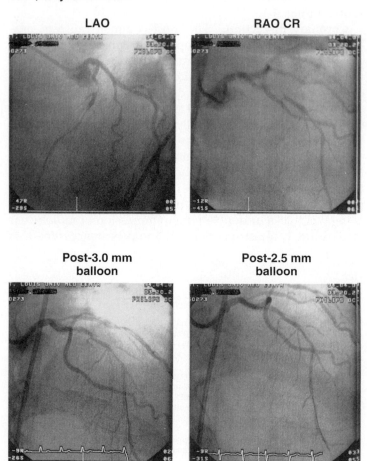

Fig. 4-3.   Case example of coronary dissection during PTCA.
(**A,** left panels) Proximal left anterior descending artery stenosis (95%) is eccentric and precedes diffuse distal disease. PTCA
with 2.5-mm and 3.0-mm PTCA balloons results in a dissection
(type C). (Right panel) A coiled perfusion balloon is placed
in dissection. Flow is maintained and ischemia reduced.
B, Dissection persisted despite prolonged balloon inflations.
Vessel was stabilized after placement of 3.5-mm Palmaz-
Schatz stent.

J.M., 67-year-old man

**Dispatch
perfusion
balloon inflated**

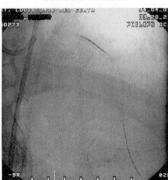

**Contrast in
drug lumen**

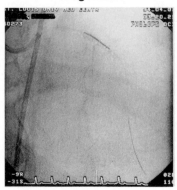

**Flow through
D₃ balloon**

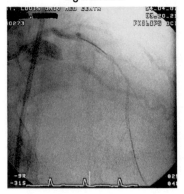

A

Fig. 4-3.   (*Continued*).

extra luminal cap with persistence of contrast after coronary
angiography; type D is spiral luminal filling defects in multiple areas of the vessel that persist; type E is new intraluminal
filling defects that persist; and type $\bar{r}$ is type A-E dissections
that lead to impaired flow or abrupt closure (Fig. 4-2).

J.M., 67-year-old man

Post-LAO

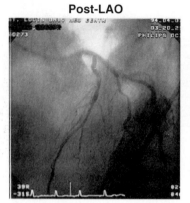

Post-RAO

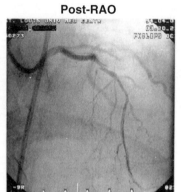

Poststent 3.5 mm

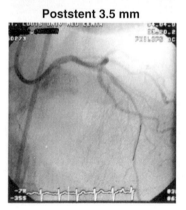

B

Fig. 4-3.   (*Continued*).

Prolonged balloon inflations, if tolerated, have recently been shown to successfully restore patency and reduce flow-limiting dissections in a majority of cases. Extensive spiral dissections are less likely to respond to prolonged balloon inflations than are focal ones. Total cessation of distal flow with the occurrence of dissection also decreases the chance of achieving a stable patency with prolonged inflations. Figure 4-3 illustrates management of a dissection during coronary angioplasty.

Autoperfusion Balloon Catheters

Prolonged balloon inflation can be maintained by autoperfusion balloons, provided systemic blood pressure exceeds 80 mm Hg. In most patients, a reduced incidence of myocardial necrosis and ischemia, and improved tolerance to balloon inflation, has been demonstrated with this technique. Elective autoperfusion balloon angioplasty can permit prolonged inflations without significant electrocardiographic evidence of ischemia. However, if a coronary-artery side branch is occluded during balloon inflation, myocardial ischemia will occur despite satisfactory flow through the major coronary lumen. Perfusion balloon catheters are larger and stiffer than standard angioplasty balloons and require better guide catheter support; in some cases, they may not negotiate tortuous coronary segments, although recently developed lower-profile autoperfusion balloons have made most coronary sites accessible. In assessing whether stent placement is feasible, we consider whether a reperfusion balloon catheter system can be advanced to the lesion. If this is not possible, then intracoronary stenting will be difficult.

Once the perfusion catheter is in place and the balloon is inflated, the guidewire is removed proximal to the proximal perfusion ports to enhance flow. Figure 4-4 illustrates use of a perfusion balloon for coronary angioplasty after acute myocardial infarction and shows the effect of wire pull-back from the reperfusion balloon on distal coronary blood flow. Care should be taken not to leave the monorail channel completely. Small-caliber guidewires may come out of the side holes during readvancement, requiring replacement with a larger or a straight-tip guidewire. The external hub of the over-the-wire balloons should be closed with a Y connector to allow periodic heparin saline flushing. The rotating adapter should be tightly closed around the guidewire. This will not be necessary with monorail catheters when periodic guide catheter flushing is given. The perfusion balloon position should be monitored frequently on the fluoroscope to detect balloon displacement. If transfer of the patient to surgery becomes necessary while the perfusion catheter is in place, deflate the balloon. Pull back the guide catheter to a safe distance from the ostium and secure the external end with

R.W., Acute ant MI

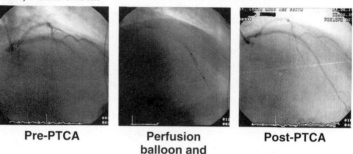

| Pre-PTCA | Perfusion balloon and flowire | Post-PTCA |

R.W., Distal LAD flow during removal of perfusion balloon guidewire

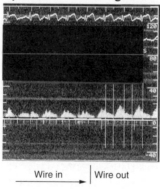

Wire in ⟶ | Wire out

Fig. 4-4.   Case example of PTCA for acute myocardial infarction using a reperfusion balloon catheter. (Top panels, left) Total occlusion of proximal left anterior descending artery during anterior infarction. (Middle panel) Flowtrack 40s perfusion balloon catheter. A Doppler flow velocity guidewire is positioned along side to record flow through the balloon. Final result is shown on right panel. (Lower panel) Flow velocity spectra with a guidewire inside the balloon and flow after guidewire is withdrawn. Flow velocity increases from 10 to 15 cm/sec. Velocity scale is 0 to 160 cm/sec.

sutures. The surgical team should be notified to remove the guide and perfusion catheter as a unit once the bypass is established.

Active hemoperfusion systems are available but have not proven superior to passive perfusion, provided systemic hemodynamics are stable. In high-risk patients, an active hemoperfusion system may provide benefit because systemic blood pressure may be insufficient to provide adequate perfusion pressure.

Stent placement (also see Chapter 5) should be considered for vessels in which other repeated attempts to maintain patency have failed. Factors that limit stent placement include thrombus, vessel size (>2.5 mm diameter), tortuosity, tolerance for anticoagulation, and ability to exchange guide catheters. Stent implantation after too many prolonged balloon inflations to "tack up" the dissection may not prevent myocardial infarction. The incidence of myocardial infarction increases with the time to stent placement. Table 4-4 lists conditions that preclude stent placement.

Systemic Hemodynamic Support Techniques

Intraaortic balloon counterpulsation, percutaneous cardiopulmonary bypass, and coronary sinus retroperfusion are the three major techniques for providing adjunctive hemodynamic support. These have been discussed under high-risk coronary angioplasty.

TABLE 4-4.   Indications that preclude bailout stent implantation

---

Anatomy
   Very small vessels (<2.0 mm)
   Severe angulation point
   Severe tortuosity
   Very long dissection
   Very proximal left anterior descending or circumflex dissection
      necessitating stent implantation in left main stem
   Thrombosis main component of acute occlusion
Clinical situation
   Refractory unstable angina (Braunwald class IIIB and IIIC)
   Acute myocardial infarction
   Contraindication for intensive anticoagulant or antiplatelet treatment

---

From de Feyter PJ, de Jaegere PPT, Serruys PW: Incidence, predictors, and management of acute coronary occlusion after coronary angioplasty, *Am Heart J* 127:643-651, 1994.

Intracoronary thrombus. Intracoronary thrombus has characteristic angiographic features (Fig. 4-5). Presumed intracoronary thrombus is also treated with prolonged balloon inflations and frequently intracoronary thrombolytics (urokinase, Chapter 8, "Difficult Angioplasty Situations"). It should be noted, however, that routine use of intracoronary thrombolytics has not been found to reduce, and may potentially increase, the risk of ischemic events. Should thrombus be present, intracoronary urokinase (100,000-750,000 U over 10-

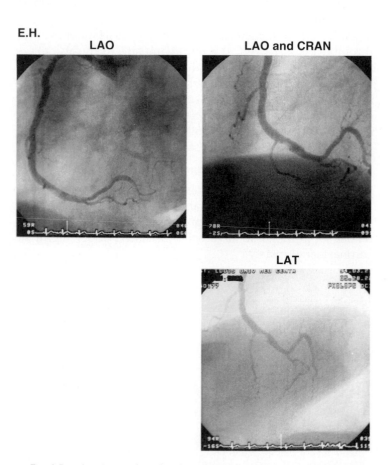

E.H.

LAO   LAO and CRAN

LAT

Fig. 4-5. Angiography of right coronary artery with thrombus before PTCA. Note the difficulty in visualizing the outline of thrombus in the left anterior oblique (LAO) view.

60 min) may be required. Additional intravenous heparin is used to reduce propagation of thrombus. A slow intracoronary infusion of 1000 U of heparin may also be useful. Prolonged low-pressure inflations using a slightly oversized balloon may work very well.

Coronary artery embolism. Occasionally, coronary air embolism will occur in the performance of procedure catheter exchange, balloon extraction, and reinsertion. Air embolism may occur under the following conditions:

1. Incomplete aspiration of guiding catheter upon introduction into the circulation
2. Balloon leakage or rupture
3. Prolonged negative suction of self-venting balloon catheters when exposed to room air
4. Introduction of balloon catheters into the guide
5. Removal of balloon catheters from deeply seated guiding catheters
6. Structural failure of catheter
7. Injection of air due to bubble in contrast injection line and/or syringe
8. Vacuum air accumulation on use of tracker exchange system

Management of coronary air embolus includes stabilization of hemodynamics and ischemia, analgesics, treatment of arrhythmias, circulatory support with pressors, intraaortic balloon pumping as needed, and inhalation of 100% fraction of inspired oxygen (FIO_2) by mask.

Air embolism is usually a self-limited condition that generally results in no serious compromise; however, acute myocardial infarction has been attributed to air embolus despite successful coronary angioplasty.

Clot embolism may follow guidewire penetration or balloon inflation in a proximal lesion containing thrombus or intracoronary thrombolytic administration. On rare occasions, some thrombus may be transported proximally via the deflated balloon catheter and may embolize in an uninvolved territory. Limitation of the balloon catheter movement until achieving a stable lumen is recommended. Embolus in a relatively large segment or branch of the artery may respond to balloon catheter passage and/or low-pressure balloon inflation. Thrombolytic infusions may be useful.

The *no-reflow phenomenon* is rarely encountered except in graft angioplasty. It is seen more often with the rotablator technique (see Chapter 6). Although frequently reversible, in the case of rotablator, the no-reflow phenomenon can last long enough to cause severe complications, such as myocardial infarction or death in other subsets of patients. There has been no specific treatment for no-reflow. Intracoronary vasodilators (nitroglycerin and verapamil) are routinely used. Other antiischemic measures, including intraaortic balloon pump support, should also be considered early in the course. Coronary bypass surgery fails to correct this problem.

Guide catheter obstruction.   Ischemia due to guide catheter ostial occlusion is treated by removal of the guide catheter or use of a catheter with side holes. Balloon catheters with relatively larger shaft sizes may create ischemia when they are inserted into relatively smaller arteries. The ischemia persists despite the balloon deflation. The solution is to remove the balloon into the guiding catheter after each inflation.

Coronary spasm.   Coronary vasospasm occurs frequently during angioplasty, and intracoronary nitroglycerin can readily reverse vasospastic tendencies. Some patients may require continuous intravenous nitroglycerin to remove this potentially complicating factor. Coronary vasospasm should be suspected in every case of reduced flow and excluded by the administration of intracoronary nitroglycerin.

Out-of-laboratory abrupt closure after coronary angioplasty.   Abrupt vessel closure can occur within the first 24 hr after angioplasty. The mechanism of abrupt closure usually involves dissection and/or thrombus with or without concomitant coronary vasospasm. Symptoms with ischemic electrocardiographic findings demand investigation. Nitroglycerin should be given. If there is no immediate response, decisions should be made for repeat angioplasty.

In the laboratory, prolonged balloon inflations to tack up a dissection flap against the lumen are performed. After obtaining a satisfactory angiographic result, the patient is continued on heparin for a minimum of 48 hr and returned to a monitoring area. Since closure can be related to heparin discontinuation, it has been our experience to stop heparin in such patients in the morning rather than in the early evening, so that if abrupt closure occurs, patient management can be achieved during full-service hours. If prolonged balloon inflations are not successful, a longer balloon (>30 mm) and/or stent should be considered. If the dissection flap is discrete and nonspiral, directional atherectomy excision of the flap may be performed. If these maneuvers are successful, intravenous heparinization is maintained and the patient treated in the same manner as after prolonged balloon inflation.

Bypass surgery for acute vessel closure. The need for emergency coronary bypass surgery after acute or threatened artery closure depends on various factors, including the amount of myocardium in jeopardy and the suitability of the anatomy to salvage techniques (autoperfusion balloons, stents). Mortality rates for emergency bypass after failed angioplasty range from 1% to 4%, with Q-wave myocardial infarction rates of 28% to 43%. Emergency bypass surgery limits the likelihood of the surgeons utilizing an internal mammary artery conduit. Intracoronary stenting has reduced significantly the need for emergency bypass surgery to <1% at experienced centers. However, unexpected events (abrupt out-of-lab closure) after stent placement still occur and may complicate this efficacious approach to a major coronary dissection. Elective bypass surgery even after stent placement, especially in vessels <2.5 mm in diameter, should be considered. Table 4-5 summarizes indications for *not* performing percutaneous reintervention.

Considerations for coronary angioplasty without on-site surgical backup should be limited. The ACC-AHA Task Force

TABLE 4-5. Various indications for not performing percutaneous reintervention

Expected problems in recrossing the lesion
  Tortuosity/calcification/angulation
  Unstable guiding catheter
Expected unfavorable redilation outcome
  Diffuse disease
  Long, spiral dissection
  Small caliber vessel
  Severe angulation
High risk of damage to left main (stem)
Severe hemodynamic instability
Additional significant (nondilatable) lesions

From de Feyter PJ, de Jaegere PPT, Serruys PW: Incidence, predictors, and management of acute coronary occlusion after coronary angioplasty, *Am Heart J* 127:643-651, 1994.

reporting guidelines for angioplasty in 1988 indicate that "an experienced cardiovascular surgical team should be available within the institution for emergency surgery for all angioplasty procedures." Given the commonly available surgical facilities in the country and the proximity of major medical centers to the population at large, it has not appeared warranted that angioplasty be performed in a center without on-site surgical backup, or at least surgical backup within 5-10 min of the facility that can be easily reached by ambulance transport. Although several European countries report coronary angioplasty performed in large numbers without surgical coverage, these centers have highly experienced operators with on-site air ambulance backup. The economic necessity of performing angioplasty without surgical backup does not appear warranted in the United States, where cardiovascular surgical facilities are widely available.

HYPOTENSION

Hypotension during angioplasty that is unrelated to myocardial ischemia may be the result of vasovagal stimulation, hypovolemia, retroperitoneal bleeding, or prolonged bed rest without appropriate hydration. These conditions are easily treated with fluid administration before or during the procedure.

Transient hypotension due to myocardial dysfunction may lead to a downward spiral of progressive ischemia and shock. Stabilization of blood pressure may occur with small intravenous doses of epinephrine or aramine. The epinephrine is in a 1/10,000 dilution, and 1 cc of this 10-cc syringe can be used to maintain pressure. The effect is dramatic and relatively short-lived (<5 min).

ARRHYTHMIAS
Severe Bradyarrhythmias

During coronary angioplasty, especially of the right coronary artery, bradycardia may require immediate temporary pacing. Most operators insert a prophylactic transvenous pacemaker into the right ventricle in anticipation of angioplasty involving sites in the vicinity of the sinus node artery or arteriovenous (AV) nodal artery. Caution must be exercised, even under urgent circumstances, to avoid perforation of the right ventricle and resultant tamponade. Transcoronary cardiac pacing using the angioplasty guidewire has been successfully reported and may serve as a reliable backup during interventional procedures complicated by bradyarrhythmias.

The angioplasty guidewire is hooked to a coronary pacing system with clips, and ventricular pacing through the transcoronary route is performed. The transcoronary pacing method can be performed successfully and may be a reliable backup system until a more definitive transvenous pacemaker can be inserted. Meier et al. report the use of coronary pacing during coronary angioplasty through guidewires and left ventricular pacing. This technique can be a satisfactory temporary pacemaker.

Ventricular Arrhythmias

During diagnostic and interventional studies, ventricular arrhythmias may result from transient myocardial ischemia, during contrast coronary injection, or catheter-induced ventricular stimulation (temporary pacemakers, Swan-Ganz catheter, deep guidewire manipulation). Ventricular arrhythmias can be managed with mechanical means (catheter repositioning), antiarrhythmics (Lidocaine), maintenance of left ventricular filling with fluids, and electrolyte replacement, as needed.

CARDIAC TAMPONADE

Cardiac tamponade may occur after temporary pacemaker placement with an unsuspected perforation of the right ventricle in an anticoagulated patient, or may occur rapidly if there is coronary perforation from guidewire, balloon catheter, or new device manipulation. Tamponade must be identified in patients undergoing coronary angioplasty as an unsuspected cause of hypotension.

Management of Pericardial Effusion after Guidewire or Catheter Perforation

Reversal of heparin and pericardial drainage using standard subxyphoid techniques may proceed depending on the degree of hemodynamic compromise. Heparin reversal may complicate an otherwise successful angioplasty and must be carefully considered. Expeditious placement and inflation of an autoperfusion balloon at the site of coronary perforation may be essential to control pericardial leakage from a ruptured or perforated artery.

Guidewire perforation, although rare, may cause cardiac tamponade, acute myocardial infarction, or require emergency coronary artery bypass surgery. The penetration of a guidewire through a coronary artery is not always associated with significant complications, but should be monitored closely and steps taken to ensure that tamponade and/or continued bleeding are controlled. Depending on the clinical situation, management of coronary guidewire perforation has included nonoperative management with prolonged coronary balloon compression to tamponade the puncture site, or emergency pericardiocentesis with urgent surgical repair and coronary artery bypass surgery. Intraaortic balloon counterpulsation for hemodynamic stabilization with control of pericardial hemodynamics has been recommended. Early recognition and monitoring of pericardial effusion permit selection of an aggressive or conservative management mode for arterial perforation during angioplasty. Further treatment is based on hemodynamic responses and does not always require intervention.

THE UNDILATABLE LESION

Some lesions may not respond to balloon angioplasty despite high-pressure inflations. In these cases, the lesions may be either rigid and severely calcified, or they may be elastic and have severe recoil.

Relatively acute vessel renarrowing following angioplasty without obvious dissection has been attributed to vessel recoil, possibly due to severe fibrous composition of the plaque and artery. In these cases, directional coronary atherectomy or stent is recommended over rotablator, since rotablator may inadvertently encounter a dissection not angiographic apparent and thus produce a further complication.

In some cases the elastic component can be very fibrous and firm and may also respond to rotablator. In rigid calcified lesions, rotablator has a significant advantage and can manage these adequately. Residual stenosis after rotablator procedure requires further balloon angioplasty, DCA, or stent, depending on the size of the vessel and residual angiographic appearance.

PERIPHERAL VASCULAR COMPLICATIONS AFTER CORONARY INTERVENTIONS

Routine coronary angioplasty may be associated with problems related to the vascular access site that include:

1. Femoral artery pseudoaneurysm
2. Large hematoma requiring transfusion
3. Persistent bleeding requiring vascular surgical closure
4. Thromboembolism

The incidence of local vascular complications during diagnostic coronary angiography is 0.46% in the Society for Cardiac Angiography and Interventions Registry. The incidence of vascular access site complications following percutaneous coronary revascularization is higher than with diagnostic procedures. Recent studies of new device technologies of percutaneous revascularization (i.e., stent, atherectomy, and laser) have reported vascular access site complications in 5.9% to 29% of procedures. Vascular complications occurred more frequently following intracoronary stenting (14%) and extractional atherectomy (12.5%) than with conventional balloon angioplasty (3.2%). Hemorrhagic (i.e., femoral or retroperitoneal hematoma) and arterial traumatic (i.e., A-V fistula and pseudoaneurysm formation) complications are more common following percutaneous transluminal coronary revascularization. Major hematomas and pseudoaneurysm formation are the most frequent complications, accounting for up to 80% of access-site complications. Pseudoaneurysms are often due to inappropriately low or lateral femoral artery puncture site, inadequate arterial compression, or excessive anticoagulation at the time of sheath removal.

Clinical and procedural risk factors of vascular access site that are associated with complications have been reported. Various clinical and procedural factors, including performance of more complex procedures (i.e., use of larger arterial sheath sizes, longer procedural duration), patient comorbidity (i.e., older age), and the co-administration of pharmacologic therapies (aspirin, intravenous heparin, and fibrinolytic therapy), have been identified as contributing to an increased risk of vascular access-site complications. Vascular access-site complications occur more frequently among females, older patients ($\geq$65 years old), and those patients with peripheral vascular disease and small body surface areas. Higher rates of postprocedural access-site hemorrhagic complications occur with concomitant use of fibrinolytic agents and with the duration and extent of heparin anticoagulation.

In addition, multivariate analysis indicated that age >70 years, stenting, multiple procedures, and low platelet count were also independent predictors of major vascular complications. In stent patients, increased anticoagulation, low platelet count, hypertension, and same-day sheath removal protocol with activated clotting time guidance were independent predictors of vascular complications. These factors should be kept in mind when expressing the risk of vascular complications to patients undergoing new devices. Procedures with the highest rate of surgical repair after interventional procedures include balloon valvuloplasty, intraaortic balloon pumping, and procedures involving 10F or larger sheaths.

Risk factors for vascular complications after stenting and atherectomy also included use of thrombolytic agents and long postprocedural periods of anticoagulation (>6 hours).

Postprocedural management of patients undergoing percutaneous transluminal coronary revascularization requires close clinical observation and meticulous care of the vascular-access wound site, especially when receiving novel dosing regimens of antiplatelet and antithrombin agents.

Important steps that can limit vascular access-site hemorrhagic complications are listed in Table 4-6 and include the following:

1. Preprocedural identification of variables associated with higher risk for bleeding complications
2. Limiting the degree of systemic anticoagulation during (i.e., maintain an activated clotting test [ACT] of 300 to 350 sec) and following (i.e., maintain an activated partial thromboplastin time of 1.5 to 2.0 times baseline control) the percutaneous transluminal coronary revascularization
3. Meticulous care in obtaining arterial and venous vascular access
4. Bed rest following the procedure, ensuring patient comfort with appropriate analgesia
5. Determination of the ACT (i.e., <150 to 160 sec) before sheath removal

TABLE 4-6.   Management strategies to limit bleeding complications following PTCA

Preprocedural risk assessment
  Clinical variables
    Age
    Gender
    Weight
  Angioplasty procedure
    Heparin dosing (weight-adjusted, ACT: 300-350)
    Arterial puncture
  Postprocedural
    Meticulous clinical care
    Sheath removal (target ACT, bed rest)
    Blood-product transfusion protocol

ACT, Activated clotting time.

6. Bed rest for a minimum of 8 hr following sheath removal to facilitate hemostasis

7. Limitation of blood-product transfusions by the institution of specific transfusion guidelines

Vascular access-site complications require early identification and diagnosis. Sanguinous oozing around the access site usually requires either a dressing change, temporary manual compression, or, at times, an "upsizing" of the vascular sheath (e.g., from 8 French to 9 French). A large or continually expanding femoral or brachial vascular access-site wound necessitates the differentiation of a hematoma, A-V fistula, or pseudoaneurysm by use of vascular duplex color flow ultrasonography.

Femoral Pseudoaneurysm

Femoral artery pseudoaneurysm is a well-recognized complication of cardiac catheterization and coronary angioplasty. Its incidence is higher with larger-diameter vascular access sheaths and catheters. Secondary complications of pseudoaneurysm that may involve the femoral artery include infection, distal embolization, and hemorrhage. In general, pseudoaneurysms <2 cm in diameter are at lower risk for rupture than larger aneurysms. Nonsurgical management and observation for small pseudoaneurysms, especially with intraluminal clot, have been successful. Infrequently, hemorrhage may occur during the administration of prolonged anticoagulation in the postinterventional period. Superficial femoral pseudoaneurysms may be a risk factor for rupture. The incidence of pseudoaneurysms is 0.3% to 0.7%. Duplex Doppler-guided pseudoaneurysm compression is a technique that is an effective nonsurgical management of this condition.

1. After locating the pseudoaneurysm cavity and communicating track, the surface of the Doppler imaging probe is pressed downward over the imaged track using continuous color flow Doppler monitoring.
2. The compression angle should be sufficient to obliterate the arterial inflow into the pseudoaneurysm cavity.
3. A registered vascular technologist or skilled technician may apply the compression.
4. The positioning of the probe should avoid compression of the femoral nerve and artery.
5. Manual compression is then maintained for 10-min intervals, after which pressure is slowly released and inflow into the pseudoaneurysm reassessed.
6. Compression can be continued for 45 min.
7. If compression longer than 2 hours is performed with nonclosure of the communicating track, surgical intervention may be required. Duplex Doppler ultrasound-guided compression of the femoral artery pseudoaneurysm is successful in more than 80% of patients in whom the technique is applied.

Other hemostasis systems involve the anchor, the vasoseal, and the surgical needle placement technique.

Limb Ischemia

Management of limb ischemia depends on the probable cause, which includes the following.

1. *Acute probable thromboembolism:* For thromboembolism, thrombectomy via catheter can be performed. Intraarterial nitroglycerin for vasospasm may be helpful. Vascular surgical consultation should be obtained with Doppler assessment of pulses.
2. *Sheath-induced ischemia:* For sheath-induced ischemia, remove the sheath. Consult vascular surgery for pulse loss or persistent bleeding.

Expanding Hematoma

For expanding hematoma, stop anticoagulation. Apply firm pressure for 20-30 min. Consult vascular surgery as above.

Venous Occlusion

After prolonged clamp or other pressure-device application, femoral venous thrombosis may develop, with swelling, pain, and cyanosis in the extremity. Resume heparinization. Consult vascular surgery.

Retroperitoneal Bleeding

Bleeding into the retroperitoneal space may occur due to a high femoral arterial puncture. Anticoagulation worsens the situation. Various signs and symptoms due to retroperitoneal bleeding have been reported, including back pain, flank pain, lower abdominal quadrant pain, urgency, peritoneal irritation signs, and so on. A high index of suspicion should be kept, with emergency computerized tomographic (CT) scan for the diagnosis. Hypotension or clinical signs of hypovolemia with or without a major drop in hemoglobin should alert one to the possibility of retroperitoneal hemorrhage. Treatment consists of discontinuation of anticoagulation, IV volume replacement, transfusions, and vascular surgery.

Blood Product Transfusions

New interventional angioplasty devices may produce superior results, but introduce greater expense, new complications, and increase the incidence of local vascular complications and requirement for blood transfusion. Prototypic guidelines for blood product transfusions adapted from Welch et al. are listed in Table 4-7. Asymptomatic patients with evidence of clinical bleeding should receive crystalloid infusion to correct hypovolemia. Transfusion "thresholds" should be avoided at all costs. For example, many clinicians utilize a hemoglobin concentration of <10 g/dl as a threshold to initiate transfusion therapy. Normovolemic anemia (i.e., hemoglobin concentration of 7 to 10 g/dl) is often clinically well tolerated. Packed red blood cell transfusion should be administered only if signs or symptoms of anemia or acute blood loss occur. In addition, hemoglobin concentrations of <7 g/dl or a hematocrit of <21% is usually not well clinically tolerated, often necessitating blood-product transfusion. Administration of packed red blood cells should be performed on a "unit-by-unit" basis with a goal of obtaining symptom relief. The guidelines for other blood-product transfusions including platelets are listed in Table 4-7.

TABLE 4-7.   Transfusion guidelines

Packed red blood cell transfusions:
  Correct hypovolemia (crystalloid infusion)
  Avoid transfusion "thresholds"
  Transfuse only if
    Signs/symptoms occur
    Hematocrit falls <21%
    "Unit-by-unit" basis: relief of symptoms
Other transfusions:
  Severe/acute bleeding/emergency surgery
  Administer random donor platelets for:
    Emergency measure
    Severe asymptomatic thrombocytopenia (i.e., <50,000/mm^3)
    Thrombocytopenia (<100,000/mm^3) associated with bleeding
    Bleeding time >9 min
  Reserve cryoprecipitate and fresh frozen plasma for true coagulation
    abnormalities

From Welch HG, Meehan KR, Goodnough LT: Prudent strategies for elective red blood cell transfusion, *Ann Intern Med* 116:393-402, 1992.

COMPLICATIONS RELATED TO RADIOGRAPHIC CONTRAST MEDIA
Anaphylactoid Reactions

Contrast-mediated anaphylactoid reactions to contrast often occur upon first exposure to contrast media and recur with the same severity on subsequent exposures. Direct complement activation is postulated to be the mechanism. Clinical manifestations of anaphylactoid reaction include urticaria in approximately 1% of patients, angio edema or bronchospasm in 0.03%, and circulatory shock in 0.01% of patients. Patients with history of anaphylactoid reactions are at high risk of recurrence, ranging from 15% to 35%. Recurrence is reduced to 5% to 10% for minor reactions and <1% for severe reactions upon pretreatment with prednisone, diphenhydramine, and cimetidine (H1 and H2 blockers).

Contrast Nephropathy

Contrast nephropathy may occur in patients with compromized renal function who receive doses of radiographic contrast media in quantities >100 ml. The incidence for a detectable change in renal function of >1 mg/dl rise in creatinine is <1% for hospitalized patients. In patients with baseline creatinine >1.5 mg/dl, the risk increases by two to three times. In diabetic renal insufficiency, the risk may occur in 30% to 50% of patients. Kidney-transplant recipients are also at high risk for contrast-induced nephropathy when the volume exceeds 125 ml per exposure. Mechanisms to reduce contrast nephropathy include limiting the amount and frequency of contrast administration and preprocedural hydration. It is unknown whether mannitol, calcium channel blockers, angiotensin converting enzyme (ACE) inhibitors, or renal-dose dobutamine infusions provide benefit to indicate their general use for renal dysfunction in patients.

CHOLESTEROL EMBOLI

Cholesterol embolization is a rare event, with an incidence of <0.2%. Cholesterol emboli originate from plaques in the abdominal aorta, but have been reported to occur with interventions involving popliteal arteries, descending thoracic aorta, and internal carotid arteries. Clinical features of cholesterol emboli include blue toe syndrome, restless leg syndrome, livedo reticularis (blue/red mottling of the skin in a netlike pattern along the buttocks, legs, and feet). Peripheral pulses are intact with this syndrome. Renal insufficiency is common, but differentiated from contrast nephropathy in that the renal dysfunction is delayed for several weeks following the procedure. Diagnosis is made by clinical examination, increased sedimentation rate, transient hematoma, skin mottling, and skin biopsy. Management is conservative. Anticoagulation has not proven to be beneficial and may prevent epithelization of the atherosclerotic debris, thus prolonging the syndrome. Corticosteroids have no beneficial effect despite the vasculitis-type response.

CEREBRAL VASCULAR ACCIDENTS

The incidence of cerebral vascular accidents during diagnostic catheterization reported in the Society for Cardiac Angiography and Interventions Registry was 0.7%. Risk factors were patients with low ejection fraction (<30%) and patients who have percutaneous balloon valvotomy at 1%. Cerebrovascular accident (CVA) is associated with embolic events related to atheromatous or thrombotic particles being dislodged from arterial surfaces, guidewires, or catheters. Verte-

TABLE 4-8. Overview of the management of complications during coronary angioplasty

Complications/precautions	Treatment
Myocardial infarction (0.2%)	Intracoronary nitroglycerin (rule out spasm)
	Consider intracoronary thrombolysis or possible coronary aspiration embolectomy
	Emergency aorto-coronary bypass
Cerebrovascular accident (0.1%)	Observation
Systemic heparinization	Stabilization
Cleaning of guidewires	Neurologic consultation
Aspirate/flush catheters as frequently as safe	
Remove air bubbles in any of the tubing, solution, or injection syringe	
Caution when changing bottles of contrast media	
Maintain all tubing and catheter connections tight	
Large vessel dissection (0.1%)	No further coronary injections
Never advance guidewire or catheter against resistance, catheter tip location confirmed by gentle contrast injection	If ischemia produced, emergency aorto-coronary bypass
Do not manipulate catheter in coronary ostium, monitoring pressure of catheter tip	If dissection associated with thrombus but no ischemia, use heparin (controversial)
Do not inject with damped pressure	
Acute pulmonary edema	Oxygen, morphine (2 to 5 mg IV), nitrates (100 to 200 μg IV), furosemide (20 to 200 mg IV)
Treat preexisting CHF optimally	
Limit contrast medium, avoid LV angiography	Nitroprusside for afterload reduction with dopamine or dobutamine
Use nonionic or low-osmolar contrast-media agent	Intraaortic balloon pumping
Avoid further hypotension	Endotracheal intubation, sedation, monitoring PCWP
Limit flush solution volume	
Check oxygen saturation	

Cardiogenic shock	
Careful patient selection	If shock caused by coronary occlusion, treat with emergency PTCA or CABG
Prophylactic IABP for high risk	Manage as high risk with hemodynamic support
Atropine (0.125 to 0.25 mg Aramine (metaraminol))	
Rule out pericardial tamponade with RA and RV pressures (also urgent echocardiogram)	
Ventricular tachycardia, asystole, or fibrillation (0.6%)	Cough to maintain blood pressure
Use nonionic contrast agents in high-risk patients	Remove catheter from coronary ostium
ECG and blood pressure should be normal before proceeding	CPR followed by prompt defibrillation
Do not inject when catheter tip pressure is damped	Defibrillation (200 J)
Use atropine, volume expansion, or Aramine (metaraminol)	Lidocaine (50-mg bolus, 2 to 4 mg/min IV)
Hypotension	Refractory VF usually as a result of extensive CAD; emergency percutaneous cardiopulmonary bypass should be considered
Air embolism	Same as cerebrovascular accident
For prevention and treatment, see *The Cardiac Catheterization Handbook*	
Hematoma of femoral artery (0.1% major, 1% to 2% minor)	Evacuation rarely required
Puncture below inguinal ligament	Surgical consult for enlarging hematoma, compartment syndrome or cool extremity
Attention to compression	Discontinue anticoagulation (weigh risk or coronary vessel occlusion)
	Prolonged compression if patient coughing, has aortic insufficiency, hypertension, or if heparin is not reversed
Retroperitoneal bleeding	Reverse anticoagulants
Low hematocrit, tachycardia (if not receiving beta blockers)	Volume replacement
Avoid high (above inguinal ligament) femoral artery puncture	Transfusion if Hct <25
Hypotension, low abdominal or flank pain, within 2 to 12 hr of procedure early warning signs	CT scan

Continued on page 144.

TABLE 4-8. Overview of the management of complications during coronary angioplasty—cont'd

Complications/precautions	Treatment
Cardiac tamponade	
Avoid stiff catheters in RA or RV; pacing catheters handled gently	Reverse anticoagulation
	Prompt pericardiocentesis with catheter drainage
Avoid posterior LA wall during transseptal catheterization	Cardiovascular surgery consultation
	Surgical exploration and closure for persistent bleeding
Contrast-agent nephrotoxicity	Generally self-limited; dialysis rarely needed
See *The Cardiac Catheterization Handbook*	
Hydration, mannitol, furosemide, and nonionic contrast agents	
Contrast-agent reaction	
See *The Cardiac Catheterization Handbook*	
Vasovagal reaction	
See *The Cardiac Catheterization Handbook*	

CAD, Coronary artery disease; *CHF*, congestive heart failure; *CPR*, cardiopulmonary resuscitation; *CT*, computerized tomography; *Hct*, hematocrit; *IABP*, intraaortic balloon pump; *LA*, left atrium; *LV*, left ventricle; *PCWP*, pulmonary capillary wedge pressure; *RA*, right atrium; *RV*, right ventricle; *VF*, ventricular fibrillation.

Modified from Tilkian AG, Daily EK: *Cardiovascular procedures: diagnostic techniques and therapeutic procedures*, St. Louis, 1986, Mosby.

bral basilar insufficiency may be associated with brachial procedures. Carotid embolic events are more commonly associated with femoral procedures. Contrast injection alone during routine diagnostic angiography may cause transient neurologic deficits including seizure, confusion, and bilateral cortical blindness. All events generally resolve spontaneously with a highly favorable prognosis.

An overview and summary of the complications and their management during coronary angioplasty are provided in Table 4-8.

SECTION II. ANTITHROMBOTIC THERAPY

Familiarity with commonly used antithrombotic agents is required in the management of interventional cardiology patients. This section outlines how various antithrombotic agents should be used. The authors thank Dr. Thomas Hyers for permitting us to use his material as published in the *Handbook of Antithrombotic Therapy* (published by Dr. Thomas Hyers, Department of Internal Medicine, St. Louis University, St. Louis, Missouri, 1994). Table 4-9 lists available thrombolytic and acute thrombotic agents.

HEPARIN

1. Route of administration: intravenous or subcutaneous, *not intramuscular*

TABLE 4-9. Available thrombolytic or antithrombolytic agents

Generic drug	Brand name	Company
Heparin		
Warfarin	Coumadin™	DuPont Pharma
Aspirin		
Ticlopidine	Ticlid™	Syntex
Thrombolytic agents		
Anistreplase	Eminase™	SmithKline Beecham
Streptokinase	Kabikinase™	Kabi
	Streptase™	Astra
Tissue plasminogen activator	Activase™	Genentech
Urokinase	Abbokinase™	Abbott
Low-molecular-weight heparin	Lovenox™	Rhone-Poulenc
(Enoxaparin)		Rorer

2. Absorption and clearance
   a. Plasma half-life of 60 to 90 min when given intravenously
   b. Slower absorption and clearance when given subcutaneously
3. Mode of action
   a. Heparin is a mixture of glycosaminoglycans (mucopolysaccharides) that combine with a plasma protein called antithrombin III (AT III) to make the AT III a highly effective inhibitor of thrombin and several other clotting factors.
   b. Heparin requires the presence of AT III to be effective.
4. Duration of action: minutes to hours when given intravenously, several hours when given subcutaneously
5. Frequency of dosing
   a. Constant infusion intravenously
   b. Every 8 to 12 hours subcutaneously
6. Monitoring (Table 4-10)
   a. Heparin therapy is usually monitored by the activated partial thromboplastin time (aPTT) or the activated clotting test (ACT).
   b. When blood levels of heparin have been measured directly, antithrombotic efficacy occurs between 0.2 unit 0.4 unit/ml.
7. Indications (Table 4-11)
   a. Following percutaneous coronary angioplasty (4 to 48 hours)
   b. Treatment of unstable angina
   c. Following anterior wall myocardial infarction (7 to 10 days)
   d. Prevention of deep venous thrombosis
   e. Treatment of pulmonary embolism and deep venous thrombosis
8. Precautions
   a. Bleeding
      (1) Keep aPTT between 1.5 and 2.5 times the laboratory's mean normal value.
      (2) Avoid concurrent use of other antithrombotics unless indicated.
   b. Thrombocytopenia
      (1) Heparin can cause an immune-mediated thrombocytopenia which can lead to a platelet thrombus with stroke, loss of limb, or other ischemic events.

TABLE 4-10. Heparin dosing algorithm (1300 U/hr maintenance dose)
Intravenous heparin: monitoring and adjusting dosage*

aPTT[†]	Rate change (ml/hr)	Dose change (U/24 hr)	Additional action	Next aPTT
≤45	+6	+5.760	Rebolus with 5000 U	4-6 hr
46-54	+3	+2.880	None	4-6 hr
55-85[‡]	0	0	None	Next morning[§]
86-110	−3	−2.880	Stop infusion 1 hr	4-6 hr after restart
>110	−6	−5.760	Stop infusion 1 hr	4-6 hr after restart

D5W, Dextrose 5% solution.

* A starting bolus of 5000-10,000 U is given IV followed by IV infusion of 1300 U/hr (heparin 20,000 U in 500 ml D5W at approximately 33 ml/hr). The concentration of heparin is 40 U/ml. When aPTT is checked at 6 hr or longer, steady-state kinetics can be assumed. Dosage adjustments are made according to the protocol.

[†] Normal aPTT range with Dade-Actin FS reagent of 27 to 35 sec.

[‡] The therapeutic range of 55-85 sec is roughly equivalent to a plasma heparin concentration range of 0.2-0.4 U/ml by protamine titration or by inhibition of factor Xa. The therapeutic range will vary with different aPTT reagents and coagulation machines.

[§] During the first 24 hr, repeat aPTT in 4-6 hr. Thereafter, monitor aPTT daily unless it is subtherapeutic.

Modified from Hyers TM, Hull RD, Weg JG: Antithrombotic therapy for venous thromboembolis disease. Chest 102:408S-425S, 1992.

TABLE 4-11. Heparin administration

Indication	Dosing	Therapeutic range
Coronary angioplasty	10,000 U IV loading, 1000 U/hr IV	aPTT 1.5-2.5 times mean normal for laboratory
Acute myocardial infarction	5000 U IV loading, 1300 U/hr IV	aPTT 1.5-2.5 times mean normal for laboratory
	Subcutaneous therapy:	
	12,500-17,500 U subcutaneous q 12 hr	aPTT 1.5-2.5 times mean normal for laboratory
Unstable angina	5000 U IV loading, 1300 U/hr IV	aPTT 1.5-2.5 times mean normal for laboratory
Pulmonary embolus and deep venous thrombosis	5000 U IV loading, 1300-1700 U/hr IV	aPTT 1.5-2.5 times mean normal for laboratory
	Subcutaneous therapy:	
	2000 U IV loading, 17,500 U subcutaneous q 12 hr	aPTT 1.5-2.5 times mean normal for laboratory

(2) During acute treatment, monitor platelet count *daily*. If platelet count falls below 100,000/μl or otherwise falls precipitously or in a sustained fashion, *discontinue heparin*.

c. Osteopenia
   (1) Daily use of heparin in doses above 15,000 units for more than 6 months can lead to severe axial osteopenia.

Overlapping Heparin and Warfarin During Acute Anticoagulation

1. Heparin 5000-10,000 units IV bolus followed by 1000 to 1700* units/hour IV infusion
2. Obtain aPTT at 4 to 6 hours and keep aPTT between 1.5 and 2.5 times laboratory mean normal aPTT value
3. Start warfarin on day 1 at no more than 10 mg a day
4. Obtain platelet count daily
5. Give heparin and warfarin jointly for 5 to 7 days; stop heparin when PT gives an international normalized ratio (INR) of 2.0 to 3.0
6. Continue warfarin at an international normalized ratio (INR) of 2.0 to 3.0

Managing Bleeding in Patients Receiving Heparin

1. Minor bleeding
   a. Discontinue heparin
   b. Monitor vital signs, aPTT, hemoglobin (Hgb), hematocrit (HCT), platelet count
2. Major bleeding
   a. After intermittent dosing
      (1) Discontinue heparin
      (2) Monitor vital signs, aPTT, Hgb, HCT, platelet count
      (3) Give blood transfusions as necessary
      (4) Consider protamine reversal of heparin
   b. For patients receiving constant intravenous heparin:
      (1) Give protamine sulfate (1% solution) at 25 mg slow IV infusion over 10 min
      (2) Repeat aPTT in 20 min
   c. For patients receiving large doses (>5000 U) of subcutaneous heparin:
      (1) Give protamine sulfate (1% solution) 15 mg slow IV infusion over 10 min

* Current recommendations are 1700 U/hr for patients with low bleeding risk and 1300 U/hr for patients with higher bleeding risk.

(2) Repeat aPTT in 20 min and 1 hour
(3) It may be necessary to repeat the protamine SO_4 infusion after 1 hour because of the slow absorption of subcutaneous heparin

d. Protamine response
(1) Protamine SO_4 can cause *severe anaphylactoid reactions.* Use this agent only when severe bleeding warrants it. Have resuscitation equipment nearby.

Low-Molecular-Weight Heparin

Low-molecular-weight heparins are fractionated to have molecular weights between 3000 and 7000 (mean 3000 to 4500), in contrast to standard heparin (3000 to 30,000; mean 10,000 to 15,000). Low-molecular-weight heparins have a very predictable antithrombotic effect, which makes monitoring and dose adjustment unnecessary. When given subcutaneously, low-molecular-weight heparin has a longer plasma half-life than standard heparin. Each low-molecular-weight heparin behaves somewhat differently. Clinical results cannot be extrapolated from one preparation to another.

Only one low-molecular-weight heparin is currently available for clinical use. Enoxaparin is approved for deep venous thrombosis prophylaxis in patients undergoing hip replacement.

1. Dose: 30 mg subcutaneously q or every 12 hours starting the evening after surgery. Continue for 7 to 14 days or until patient is fully ambulatory.
2. Monitoring and dose adjustment: none required.

WARFARIN

1. Route of administration: oral
2. Absorption and clearance
   a. Absorption is rapid and nearly complete.
   b. Warfarin cleared from the blood and taken up by the liver over several hours.
3. Mode of action
   a. Racemic sodium warfarin is a coumarin derivative.
   b. The agent acts by inhibiting the gamma carboxylation of glutamic acid residues in the clotting proteins II (prothrombin), VII, IX, X.

4. Duration of action
   a. Daily warfarin takes 4 to 7 days to have its optimum effect.
   b. Large loading doses do not markedly shorten the time to achieve a full therapeutic effect.
   c. The following general recommendations for warfarin use are made:
      (1) Initiate therapy with either the estimated daily maintenance dose (2 to 5 mg) or, if a larger initial dose is chosen, start with no more than 10 mg.
      (2) Elderly or debilitated patients often require low daily doses of warfarin (2 to 3 mg).
      (3) Four to five days are required after any dose change or any new diet or drug interaction to reach the new antithrombotic steady state.
5. Frequency of dosing: daily
6. Monitoring (Table 4-12)
   a. Warfarin is monitored by the one-stage prothrombin time test.
   b. Prothrombin times are reported in seconds, as a ratio of the prothrombin time in seconds to the mean normal prothrombin time of the laboratory, or an INR.
   c. The INR is the most reliable way to monitor the prothrombin time.
7. Indications
   a. Stent placement
   b. Long-term secondary prevention of myocardial infarction (lifetime in enteric-coated aspirin failures)
   c. Stroke prophylaxis in atrial fibrillation (lifetime)
   d. Stroke prophylaxis in mechanical heart valves (lifetime)
   e. Stroke prophylaxis in tissue heart valves (4 to 6 weeks, then start enteric-coated aspirin)
   f. Long-term treatment of pulmonary embolus/deep venous thrombosis (PE/DVT) (3 to 6 months)
8. Contraindications and precautions
   a. Pregnancy
      (1) Warfarin is *contraindicated* during any stage of pregnancy because of its teratogenic and fetopathic effects.
      (2) Obtain *pregnancy test* before starting women of child-bearing potential on warfarin.

TABLE 4-12. INR comparisons

Thromboplastin reagent	Patient's PT in seconds / Mean normal PT in seconds = ratio	ISI	[ratio][ISI]	=	INR
A	18 sec/12 sec = 1.5	2.4	$1.5^{2.4}$	=	2.6
B	21 sec/13 sec = 1.6	2.0	$1.6^{2.0}$	=	2.6
C	24 sec/11 sec = 2.2	1.2	$2.2^{1.2}$	=	2.6
D	17 sec/12 sec = 1.4	2.8	$1.4^{2.8}$	=	2.6
E	38 sec/14.5 sec = 2.6	1.0	$2.6^{1.0}$	=	2.6

The intensity of anticoagulation is the same when reported as an INR, despite widely different prothrombin times in seconds and ratios.

b. Bleeding
   (1) Minimize risk by keeping therapy in the prescribed INR range
c. Purpura
   (1) This rare skin and subcutaneous necrosis has been seen in a few individuals during the first few weeks of therapy with warfarin.
   (2) The condition seems to be linked to protein C deficiency.
9. Dietary and other interactions with warfarin
   a. Patients taking warfarin should eat a diet that is constant in vitamin K.
      (1) Minimize changes in intake of green leafy vegetables (spinach, greens, and broccoli), green peas, and oriental green tea.
   b. Conditions that interfere with vitamin K uptake or interfere with liver function will increase the warfarin effect.
      (1) Expect a longer prothrombin time in patients with CHF, jaundice, hepatitis, liver failure, diarrhea, or extensive cancer or connective tissue disease.
      (2) Expect a longer prothrombin time when patients receiving warfarin are hospitalized for any reason.
   c. Metabolic alterations can affect the prothrombin time.
      (1) Expect a longer prothrombin time in patients with hyperthyroidism or high fever.
      (2) Expect a shorter prothrombin time in patients with hypothyroidism.

INR Considerations

Definition. The INR is the prothrombin time ratio that would have been obtained had the World Health Organization international reference thromboplastin been used.

The INR is important for chronically anticoagulated patients because commercially available thromboplastin reagents give quite different prothrombin times when a patient is taking warfarin. The international sensitivity index (ISI) of a thromboplastin relates it to an international reference thromboplastin. The use of a thromboplastin reagent with an ISI as close to 1.0 as possible, as recommended by the World Health Organization, will further reduce the variability of the

INR results. The INR is the most reliable way to compare prothrombin time measurements performed in different laboratories:

$$INR = \left(\frac{\text{patient's PT in seconds}}{\text{mean normal PT in seconds}}\right)^{ISI}$$

Table 4-12 shows the variability in prothrombin times when a single blood sample from an anticoagulated patient is split and sent to five different laboratories, each using a different commercially available thromboplastin.

Notes for INR use

1. The INR is the most reliable way to measure the anticoagulant effect of warfarin in stable patients on long-term therapy.
2. The INR was not designed to interpret prothrombin times that are used for evaluation of liver function or a bleeding abnormality.

Warfarin dosing algorithm to achieve INR of 2.0 to 3.0

Warfarin*: monitoring and dosage adjustment in stable anticoagulated patients

INR	Action
<1.5	Increase dose by 1 mg/day for 5 days of next week (5 mg total); repeat PT in 1 week
1.5-2.0	Increase dosage by 1 mg/day for 3 days of next week (3 mg total); repeat PT in 1 week
2.0-3.0	No change
3.0-4.5	Decrease dosage by 1 mg/day for 3 days of next week (3 mg total); repeat PT in 1 week
4.5-7.0	Decrease dosage by 1 mg/day for 5 days of next week (5 mg total); repeat PT in 1 week
7.0-10.0	Stop warfarin for 2 days; decrease dosage 1 mg/day for next week (7 mg total); repeat PT in 1 week
>10.0	Stop warfarin; contact patient for examination

* Coumadin,™ 1-mg tablet.

ASPIRIN

1. Route of administration: oral
2. Absorption and clearance: rapid absorption, peak plasma levels in 20 min, rapid clearance

TABLE 4-13.   Effective doses of aspirin

Before and after coronary angioplasty	325 mg qd
Acute myocardial infarction	160 mg qd (chewed)
Unstable angina	75 mg qd
Stable angina	325 mg qod
Primary prevention of MI	325 mg qod
Secondary prevention of MI	160 mg qd
Peripheral vascular disease	325 mg qd
Stroke prevention (after TIA)	30 mg qd
Mechanical heart valves (adjunctive therapy to warfarin)	100 mg qd

MI, Myocardial infarction; TIA, transient ischemic attack.

3. Mode of action: acetylates and inactivates platelet cyclooxygenase, inhibiting production of thromboxanes which are potent inducers of platelet aggregation and vasoconstrictors
4. Duration of action: days (for the lifetime of the platelet)
5. Frequency of dosing: daily or every other day
6. Monitoring
   a. None is routinely used.
   b. The template bleeding time can be used to gauge aspirin's effect on platelet function.
7. Indications (Table 4-13)
   a. Stable angina
   b. Unstable angina
   c. Acute myocardial infarction
   d. Coronary angioplasty
   e. Primary and secondary prevention of myocardial infarction
   f. Carotid or primary cerebrovascular disease (stroke prevention)
   g. Peripheral vascular disease
   h. Atrial fibrillation*
   i. Prosthetic heart valves†
8. Precautions
   a. Aspirin allergies (asthma)
   b. Active peptic ulcer disease or other bleeding predispositions

* Not as effective as warfarin; use when warfarin is contraindicated.
† Adjunctive therapy with warfarin.

9. Aspirin dosing regimens
   a. Effective doses of aspirin in clinical trials (see Table 4-13)
   b. Cautionary notes:
      (1) In general when used alone the dose is 325 mg qd
      (2) Aspirin dosing recommendations for specific indications can be found in Table 4-13.

TICLOPIDINE

1. Route of administration: oral
2. Absorption and clearance: rapid absorption, peak plasma level in 2 hours, plasma half-life of 12 hours, steady-state drug levels in 14 to 21 days
3. Mechanism of action: unidentified metabolite interferes with platelet membrane function by inhibiting adenosine diphosphate (ADP)-induced platelet-fibrinogen binding and platelet-to-platelet interactions.
4. Duration of action: days (for the lifetime of the platelet)
5. Dose and interval: 250 mg every 12 hours
6. Monitoring
   a. No direct monitoring
   b. Because of neutropenia, obtain CBC and WBC differential every 2 weeks for the first 3 months of therapy
7. Indications: ticlopidine is indicated for stroke prevention in patients who cannot take aspirin or fail aspirin therapy.
   a. Stroke prevention in patients with stroke precursors
   b. Secondary stroke prevention after completed stroke
8. Precautions
   a. Neutropenia—occurs in 1% to 3% of patients in the first 3 months of therapy. Monitor CBC and WBC differential every 2 weeks for the first 3 months.
   b. Not recommended in patients with severe liver disease.
   c. Dosage reduction may be necessary in patients with renal insufficiency. Monitor template bleeding time.

THROMBOLYTIC AGENTS

Thrombolytic agents are proteins that activate a plasma pro-enzyme, plasminogen, to the active enzyme plasmin. Plasmin then solubilizes fibrin and degrades a number of other plasma proteins, most notably fibrinogen.

1. Common agents
   a. Streptokinase (SK): derived for group C, β-hemolytic streptococci. Not fibrin specific. Activates adjacent plasminogen by forming a noncovalent SK-plasminogen activator complex. Plasma half-life 30 min. Stimulates antibody production making retreatment difficult.
   b. Urokinase (UK): derived from cultured human cells. Not fibrin specific. Activates plasminogen directly by enzymatic action. Plasma half-life 20 min.
   c. Tissue plasminogen activator (t-PA): derived by recombinant genetics from human DNA. Fibrin specific. Activates plasminogen associated with fibrin directly by enzymatic action. Plasma half-life 5 min.
   d. Anisoylated plasminogen-SK activator complex (Anistreplase): Derived by anisoylating human plasminogen to standard SK. Weakly fibrin specific. Complex activates adjacent plasminogen. Plasma half-life of 90 min.
2. Indications
   a. Acute myocardial infarction (SK, t-PA, Anistreplase)
   b. Acute pulmonary embolism (SK, UK, t-PA)
   c. Acute deep venous thrombosis (SK)
   d. Clotted AV fistula and shunts (UK)
3. Precautions
   a. Bleeding is the major complication of thrombolytic therapy. Consequently, absolute contraindications include dissecting aortic aneurysm, pericarditis, stroke, or neurosurgical procedures within 6 months of known intracranial neoplasm.
   b. Relative contraindications include major surgery or bleeding within 6 weeks, known bleeding diathesis, and severe uncontrolled hypertension.
   c. Allergic reactions: SK and antirelapse are potentially allergenic. Patients are usually pretreated with 100 mg of intravenous hydrocortisone.
   d. Antibody production: SK and anistreplase induce antibody production, which makes treatment with either of these agents less effective.

Other regimens for thrombolytic agents include the following:

1. Peripheral intraarterial infusion
   SK: 20,000 IU bolus followed by 2000 IU/min for 60 min
   UK: 6000 IU/min for 1 to 2 hours
   (both SK and UK should be given with concurrent systemic heparin)
2. Clotted IV catheter clearance with UK
   a. Inject UK 5000 IU in 1 ml into catheter.
   b. For central venous catheter, inject 5000 IU/ml in volume equal to volume of the catheter. Allow 30 to 60 min for thrombolysis.
3. Clotted AV cannula clearance with SK
   a. Inject SK 250,000 IU in 2 ml in each end of cannula.
   b. Clamp ends and allow 30 to 60 min for thrombolysis.

SUGGESTED READINGS

Abraham P, Harkonen S, Kjellstrand C: Contrast nephropathy. In Massry SG, Glasscock RJ, editors. *Textbook in nephrology,* Baltimore, 1983, Williams & Wilkins, 6:206.

Agrawal SK, Pinheiro L, Roubin GS, et al.: Nonsurgical closure of femoral pseudoaneurysms complicating cardiac catheterization and percutaneous transluminal coronary angioplasty, *J Am Coll Cardiol* 20:610-615, 1992.

Anderson HV, Willerson JT: Current concepts: thrombolysis in acute myocardial infarction, *N Engl J Med* 329:703-709, 1993.

Antithrombotic Therapy: The Third ACCP Consensus Conference, *Chest* 102:303S-549S, 1992.

Detre K, Holubkov R, Kelsey S, and the investigators of the National Heart, Lung, and Blood Institute: Percutaneous transluminal coronary angioplasty in 1985-86 and 1977-81: the National Heart, Lung, and Blood Institute Registry, *N Engl J Med* 318:265-270, 1988.

Dorros G, Cowley MJ, Simpson J, et al.: Percutaneous transluminal coronary angioplasty: report of complications from the National Heart, Lung, and Blood Institute PTCA Registry, *Circulation* 67:723-729, 1983.

Flynn MS, Aguirre FV, Donohue TJ, Bach RG, Caracciolo EA, Kern MJ: Conservative management of guidewire coronary artery perforation with pericardial effusion during angioplasty for acute inferior myocardial infarction, *Cathet Cardiovasc Diagn* 29:285-288, 1993.

Fuster V: Coronary thrombolysis—a perspective for the practicing physician, *N Engl J Med* 329:723-725, 1993.

Grines CL, Glazier S, Bakalyar D, et al.: Predictors of bleeding complications following coronary angioplasty (abstr), *Circulation* 84:II-591, 1991.

Hildner FJ, Javier FP, Tolentino A, Samet P: Pseudo complications of cardiac catheterization: update, *Cathet Cardiovasc Diagn* 8:43-47, 1982.

Johnson LW, Lozner EC, Johnson S, et al.: Coronary arteriography 1984-1987. A report of the Registry of the Society for Cardiac Angiography and Interventions, *Cathet Cardiovasc Diagn* 17:5-10, 1989.

Kahn JK, Hartzler GO: The spectrum of symptomatic coronary air embolism during balloon angioplasty: causes, consequences, and management, *Am Heart J* 119:1374-1377, 1990.

Lincoff AM, Popma JJ, Ellis SG, Hacker JA, Topol EJ: Abrupt vessel closure complicating coronary angioplasty: clinical, angiographic and therapeutic profile, *J Am Coll Cardiol* 19:926-935, 1992.

Lozner EC, Johnson LW, Johnson S, et al.: Coronary arteriography 1984-1987. A report of the Society for Cardiac Angiography and Interventions. II. An analysis of 218 deaths related to coronary arteriography, *Cathet Cardiovasc Diagn* 17:11-14, 1989.

Moscucci M, Mansour KA, Kent C, et al.: Peripheral vascular complications of directional coronary atherectomy and stenting: predictors, management, and outcome, *Am J Cardiol* 74:448-453, 1994.

Muller DWM, Shamir KJ, Ellis SG, Topol EJ: Peripheral vascular complications after conventional and complex percutaneous coronary interventional procedures, *Am J Cardiol* 69:63-68, 1992.

Oweida SW, Roubin GS, Smith RB, Salam AA: Postcatheterization vascular complications associated with percutaneous transluminal coronary angioplasty, *J Vasc Surg* 12:310-315, 1990.

Popma JJ, Satler LF, Pichard AD, et al.: Vascular complications after balloon and new device angioplasty, *Circulation* 88:1569-1578, 1993.

Sheikh KH, Adams DB, McCann R, et al.: Utility of Doppler color flow imaging for identification of femoral arterial complications of cardiac catheterization, *Am Heart J* 117:623-628, 1989.

Smith MC, Ghose MK, Henry AR: The clinical spectrum of renal cholesterol embolization, *Am J Med* 71:174-180, 1981.

Sorrell KA, Feinberg RL, Wheeler JR, et al.: Color-flow duplex-directed manual occlusion of femoral false aneurysms, *J Vasc Surg* 17:571-577, 1993.

Sutton JM, Ellis SG, Roubin GS, et al.: Major clinical events after coronary stenting: the multicenter registry of acute and elective Gianturco-Roubin stent placement, *Circulation* 89:1126-1137, 1994.

The GUSTO Investigators: An international randomized trial comparing four thrombolytic strategies for acute myocardial infarction, *N Engl J Med* 329:673-682, 1993.

Turpie AGG, Gent M, Laupacis A, et al.: A comparison of aspirin with placebo in patients treated with warfarin after heart valve replacement, *N Engl J Med* 329:524-529, 1993.

Welch HG, Meehan KR, Goodnough LT: Prudent strategies for elective red blood cell transfusion, *Ann Intern Med* 116:393-402, 1992.

Wyman RM, Safian RD, Portway V, et al.: Current complications of diagnostic and therapeutic cardiac catheterization, *J Am Coll Cardiol* 12:1400-1406, 1988.

5

STENTS

Antonio Colombo, Patrick Hall, Luigi Maiello, Shigeru Nakamura, Antonio Gaglione, Frank Aguirre, and Morton J. Kern

INTRACORONARY STENT IMPLANTATION
Introduction

Stents scaffold the artery wall from inside. Metallic stents are available configured as coil, mesh, or cage types. The three most common stents are shown in Fig. 5-1. Table 5-1 lists and compares features of several commercially available stents.

Proper stent implantation technique is integrally associated with a successful procedural outcome. When a procedure is performed with good stent implantation technique, procedural and postprocedural complications, including acute and subacute stent thrombosis, can be dramatically minimized if not avoided, and long-term results can be optimized. With intracoronary stent implantation it is important to create the most ideal conditions, producing improved stent outcomes even in the most challenging situations, such as emergency stent implantation, stent deployment in the presence of thrombus, and stent insertion in small or diffusely diseased vessels.

Elective and Emergency Stent Implantation

Elective stent placement is performed as a planned primary revascularization strategy. Stent implantation is performed in a controlled environment with sufficient time for optimizing the result without distraction. Elective stent implantation

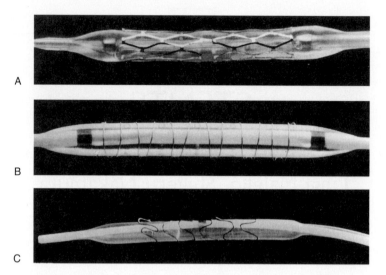

Fig. 5-1. Three common intracoronary stents. A, Palmaz-Schatz tubular slotted stent with center articulation. B, Gianturco-Roubin coiled wire stent. C, Wiktor coiled wire stent. (From MacIsacc AI, et al.: Comparison of three coronary stents: clinical and angiographic outcome after elective placement in 134 consecutive patients, *Cathet Cardiovasc Diagn* 33:199-204, 1994.)

also appears to improve long-term results as reflected by the reduced restenosis rates in the BENESTENT and STRESS trials.

Early application of stent after the occurrence of angioplasty-induced dissection decreases the need for emergency bypass surgery and the risk for myocardial infarction. Emergency stent implantation (also known as bailout) is performed for acute or threatened vessel closure. Stent implantation requires working during significant ischemia, which may limit optimization of stent expansion and precipitate subtle changes in technique, such as incomplete stent coverage of the entire lesion and a willingness to accept a less than optimal angiographic result. These features may make the difference between a successful and an unsuccessful procedure. Delays between the time of acute or threatened closure and stent implantation may also affect the clinical outcome. In particular, thrombus may form during the delay in stent implantation

TABLE 5-1. Comparison of some commercially available stents

	Wallstent	Gianturco-Roubin	Palmaz-Schatz	Wiktor
Diameter limitations	None	4.0 mm	None	Yes
Material	Stainless steel	Stainless steel	Stainless steel	Tantalum
Flexibility	+++	+++	+	++
Balloon—expandable	Postplacement	++	++	++
Ease of placement	+	+++	+	++
Needs predilatation	No	Yes	Yes	Yes
Visibility	+	+ (tantalum ↑)	++	+++
Shortens as expands	++++	No	+	No
Thrombogenicity	++	++ (tantalum ↓)	+	++ (tantalum ↓)
Used for dissection	++	+++	? Trackability	?
Amount of metal	+++	+	++	+
coatings	Yes	Yes	?	Yes

?, Precise effect is unknown.

and contribute to slow flow and an increased likelihood of stent thrombosis.

Indications

A primary elective stent is indicated for use in selected patients
1. Eligible for balloon angioplasty
2. With symptomatic ischemic heart disease due to discrete (length <15 mm)
3. With *de novo* native coronary artery lesions with a reference vessel diameter in the range of 3 to 4 mm

In this patient population, stenting the coronary artery produces a larger luminal diameter, maintains arterial patency, and reduces the incidence of restenosis at 6 months as compared with balloon angioplasty. The stent, however, represents a permanent implant into the coronary artery. One-year and longer follow-up is not well characterized.

Contraindications

Contraindications can be divided based on patient and anatomic factors.

Patient factors.   When anticoagulation is not used, patient contraindications are similar to those for coronary angioplasty. When anticoagulation is used, contraindications include:
1. Gastrointestinal bleeding that prevents 4 to 5 hours of anticoagulation during or following the stent procedure
2. Inability to take antiplatelet therapy
3. Conditions limiting use of long-term coumadin, intracranial hemorrhage, recent surgery, or bleeding diathesis

Anatomic factors

1. Small vessels, less than 2.5 mm
2. Vessels with poor distal runoff
3. Vessels supplying poorly functional or nonfunctional myocardium
4. Heavily calcified vessels

Special Patient Populations

Current data have not established the safety and effectiveness of the stent for patients with any of the following characteristics:

1. Patients whose lesions would require the placement of more than one stent per lesion
2. Patients with coronary artery reference vessel diameters of <3 mm
3. Patients with significant thrombus at the lesion site
4. Patients with lesions located in saphenous vein grafts, the left main coronary artery, ostial lesions, or lesions located at a bifurcation
5. Patients with restenotic lesions
6. Patients with diffuse disease or poor outflow distal to the identified lesion
7. Patients with tortuous vessels in the region of the obstruction or proximal to the lesion
8. Patients within 7 days of an acute myocardial infarction
9. Patients with significant impairment of left ventricular function. Clinical studies suggest that patients with impaired left ventricular function may be at increased risk of complications associated with interventional techniques.

STENT IMPLANTATION

Part of the preprocedural considerations involves choosing the correct equipment to optimize stent delivery to the appropriate site. Operators should anticipate the potential need for stent implantation even if there is no commitment to stent insertion before an angioplasty procedure. Generally, stent implantation is performed from the femoral approach with 8 French sheaths and guide catheters.

Equipment needed includes:
1. Stent—coiled, tubular, woven, or self-expanding
2. 6F-9F guide
3. 6F-9F sheath
4. 0.014- to 0.018-in. extra-support guidewire

Guiding Catheter Selection for Stents

Coaxial guiding catheter support is essential for effective stent delivery. Guide catheter selection is especially important when stent implantation is performed in an angulated circumflex or Shepherd's crook right coronary artery, tortuous vessels, or vessels with long dissections. In these anatomic conditions, Amplatz guiding catheters (usually with an AL2 curve) or Voda guiding catheters provide good support for stent deployment. Stent delivery into saphenous vein graft conduits to the circumflex or left anterior descending artery sometimes requires Amplatz guiding catheter support.

Starting a stent procedure with a guiding catheter that provides good support is especially important when stent implantation is performed with a bare stent, as is the case with the Gianturco-Roubin stent or the Palmaz-Schatz stent, which is hand crimped on a delivery balloon. However, the use of an extra support guidewire or short stent may compensate to some degree for a lack of ideal guiding catheter support.

The internal lumen of the guiding catheter is also important with certain types of stents, particularly, the Gianturco-Roubin stent. The 3.5- or 4.0-mm Gianturco-Roubin stent requires large-lumen 8 French (0.86-in. internal diameter) guiding catheters or 9 French guiding catheters. Guiding catheters with side holes are of limited use during intracoronary stent implantation. The profiles of all stent delivery systems are larger than balloon catheters and, in general, contribute to excessive loss of contrast through the side holes. This may limit precise stent positioning during delivery. The use of intravascular ultrasound also requires 8 French guiding catheters.

Guidewires for Stent Implantation

For the straightforward stent implantation procedures, a 0.014-in. guidewire provides sufficient support. Extra-support guidewires (0.014 or 0.018 in.) provide a good "rail" when stent implantation is undertaken in lesions with extreme proximal angulation or tortuosity and lesions with long dissections. The extra-support guidewires are particularly helpful for interventional cardiologists who are learning stent implantation techniques. The extra guidewire support assists both guiding catheter support and stent delivery. The extra-support 0.014-in. wires are helpful when using the Palmaz-Schatz delivery system and the 0.018-in. extra-support guidewires for Gianturco-Roubin stent delivery. Though helpful in stent delivery, extra-support guidewires (particularly 0.018-in. guidewires) can sometimes damage the distal vessel or precipitate vessel spasm. A strategy of exchanging back to a floppy-tipped wire after stent delivery may prevent distal vessel trauma or distal vasospasm.

Stent Types (Fig. 5-1)

There are now over 24 stent configurations undergoing evaluation. The following describes several of the most commonly used stents.

Palmaz-Schatz. The Palmaz-Schatz stent (Johnson & Johnson Interventional Systems, Warren, N.J.) is a balloon-expandable, stainless-steel stent with a tubular slotted design. The standard length is a 15-mm stent consisting of 7-mm tubular slotted segments with a 1-mm central articulation. The stent is available with a spiral central articulation and also in variable lengths (8-, 10-, 15-, and 20-mm lengths).

The stent provides good radial support and lesion coverage and is a first choice for vein grafts, ostial lesions, and many types of native coronary artery lesions. The biliary stent is also used in vein grafts and is helpful in more precise stent placement in ostial lesions because of its visibility. The stent has more limited flexibility in comparison to other types of stents. This drawback can be overcome by using the short or disarticulated Palmaz-Schatz stent. A short stent is very useful when stenting distal to a previously deployed stent. The use of the sheath delivery system prevents the stent from dislodging during delivery and withdrawal. However, the compromise is less flexibility, increased profile, and decreased visibility with contrast injections.

Gianturco-Roubin. The Gianturco-Roubin stent (Cook Cardiology, Bloomington, Ind.) is a balloon-expandable, stainless-steel, flexible, coiled stent that is available in 12-mm and 20-mm lengths. The flexibility allows for relatively good trackability in tortuous vessels or lesions with long dissection and can be delivered quickly in the bailout situation. The 20-mm stent provides longer lesion coverage than other stents. The 12-mm length is useful in focal lesions and for delivery to lesions distal to deployed stents, provided the deployed stent is well expanded. The 3.5- or 4.0-mm stent requires large-lumen 8 French or 9 French guiding catheters.

Wiktor. The Wiktor stent (Medtronic International Vascular, Inc., Danvers, Mass.) is a balloon-expandable tantalum stent wrapped in a helical coil structure and available in a 17-mm length. The stent is visible, with relatively good trackability. There appears to be good radial support by intravascular ultrasound. The stent is good in bend lesions and long lesions. Care should be taken when performing intravascular ultrasound, as the stent struts can be modified by the ultrasound catheter and when recrossing the stent with noncompliant balloon catheters.

Micro.   The Micro stent (Arterial Vascular Engineering, Santa Rosa, Calif.) is a balloon-expandable, stainless-steel stent. This stent is premounted on a balloon in nonarticulated multiples of 4 mm, with the available lengths being 4, 8, and 12 mm. The short stent unit length allows it to be used in short lesions, tortuous anatomy, and for complex situations such as stent delivery through a deployed stent. The short stent units and low-profile delivery balloon provide excellent trackability. Sometimes stent migration or gaps between stent units are identified upon intravascular ultrasound evaluation.

Cordis.   The Cordis stent (Cordis Corporation, Miami, Fla.) is a balloon-expandable tantalum coil stent. Stent has good visibility, flexibility, and trackability in tortuous vessels and for distal lesions. The stent provides good rail support although, when stents are placed on bends, small gaps appear between the stent struts. This does not appear to compromise the lumen but may prevent full stent site optimization during post-stent balloon dilation. The dense tantalum structure may make it difficult to appreciate the lumen at the time of the follow-up angiography.

Stent Implantation Technique

Predilation.   Prior to elective stent implantation, predilation is generally essential. Predilation with a balloon that is slightly undersized relative to the reference vessel diameter is a safe strategy. Full balloon expansion with the predilation balloon will facilitate subsequent stent delivery. Using a balloon that is sized correctly to the angiographic vessel diameter for both the predilation and final optimization dilation is another strategy that has been used and may be more cost-effective. Predilatation with a markedly undersized balloon may not be effective and can have an impact on stent delivery success or initial stent expansion.

Stent delivery and implantation.   Implantation is similar to the balloon angioplasty technique. Guiding catheters used must have lumen sizes which are suitable to accommodate the introduction of the stent delivery system. When catheters are in the body, manipulation should be performed only under fluoroscopy with radiographic equipment that provides high-quality images.

Utilizing standard procedures for balloon angioplasty, an introducer sheath with a side-arm adapter is placed in the femoral or brachial artery and flushed with saline. Under fluoroscopic control, the stenotic lesion is gently probed with a 0.014-in. vascular guidewire. Once the lesion is traversed, a standard balloon angioplasty procedure is performed. Care should be taken not to overdilate the lesion. In order to minimize the potential for balloon angioplasty-related complications, the lesion may be intentionally underdilated. Following a wire exchange (if necessary), the balloon angioplasty catheter is withdrawn, leaving the guidewire positioned across the lesion.

Verify the position of the stent. For delivery systems with a sheath, inject saline through the sheath to purge the system and to facilitate sheath withdrawal. Then advance the sheathed stent/balloon assembly over the 0.014-in. exchange wire to the site of the previously dilated lesion. After advancement of the stent delivery system, remove the lockout device from the back end of the stent delivery system and loosen the Tuohy-Bourst valve.

Under fluoroscopic observation, the sheath is pulled back, exposing the stent at the lesion site. The radioopaque markers of the balloon catheter should bracket the previously dilated lesion to assure proper positioning of the stent. Attach the inflation device and inflate the balloon to at least 5 atm pressure, but do not exceed the labeled maximum inflation recommendation (Table 5-2).

TABLE 5-2.   Maximum recommended inflation pressure for Palmaz-Schatz stent

Balloon diameter (mm)	Maximum recommended inflation pressure (atm)	Stent length at nominal diameter (mm)
3.0	8	15.1
3.5	6	14.7
4.0	6	14.3

Fluoroscopic visualization during stent expansion should be used in order to judge the optimum expanded stent diameter as compared to the proximal and distal native coronary artery diameter(s). Optimal expansion requires that the stent be in full contact with the arterial wall. If the stent is not optimally expanded by the stent delivery balloon, a larger balloon (up to 4 mm) or high inflation pressures (>14 ATM) may be used to expand the stent to its optimal size. The final stent internal diameter should match the size of the referenced vessel diameter. All efforts should be taken to assure that the stent is not underdilated.

It is important that the stent cover the entire length of the dissection or lesion without leaving any inflow and outflow obstruction. Excessive manipulation may cause dislodgement of the stent from the carrier balloon. Figure 5-2 shows an

J.W., 62-year-old man

RCA Stent

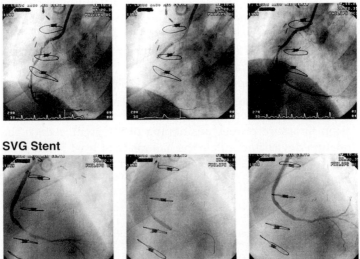

SVG Stent

Fig. 5-2. Angiograms of primary Palmaz-Schatz stent placement in right coronary artery (RCA) (top panels), and in the same patient in a saphenous vein graft conduit to the distal RCA (bottom panels).

example of stent deployment in native and saphenous vein graft locations.

Technical Notes for Stent Preparation and Delivery

1. For the Palmaz-Schatz stent, do not preinflate the balloon catheter. This could cause premature expansion and dislodgement of the stent from the balloon. If any resistance is encountered while advancing the sheath or stent/balloon assembly to the site of the previously dilated lesion, the assembly may be withdrawn through the introducer sheath and guide catheter and the procedure aborted.

2. The Palmaz-Schatz sheath should not be withdrawn until the operator is ready to expand the stent. In the event of inadvertent advancement of the sheath, the entire system should be removed from the patient and another system should be utilized for treatment. "Snagging" of the stent on atherosclerotic plaque in the arterial lumen may occur if the stent is advanced without the protective sheath, leading to an inability to place the stent at the intended treatment site.

3. Do not apply negative pressure to the Palmaz-Schatz catheter before placement of the stent across the lesion and retraction of the sheath. This may cause premature dislodgement of the stent from the carrier balloon.

4. Do not exceed recommended balloon inflation pressure. Stents should be sized to assure full contact with the vessel wall. Stent-vessel wall contact should be verified through angiography and/or intravascular ultrasound.

5. Although most stent delivery balloon catheters are strong enough to expand the stent without rupture, circumferential tear of the carrier balloon distal to the stent and before complete expansion of the stent could cause the balloon to become tethered to the stent, requiring surgical removal. In case of rupture of the balloon, it should be withdrawn and, if necessary, a new balloon catheter exchanged over the guidewire to complete expansion of the stent.

6. When treating multiple lesions, the distal lesion should be stented initially, followed by stenting of the proximal lesion. Stenting in this order obviates the need to cross the proximal stent in placement of the distal stent and reduces the chances of dislodging the proximal stent.

7. When recrossing a recently implanted stent, care should be taken to assure that the guidewire is placed within the lumen and not between the stent and the vessel wall. Otherwise, inadvertent dislodgement of the stent may occur, leading to inappropriate positioning of the stent.

8. If there is inflow or outflow obstruction or residual vessel narrowing, a freshly prepared balloon catheter should be advanced into and through the stented area for further dilatations. If there is thrombus, urokinase may be infused into the coronary artery. An appropriately sized balloon will ensure complete compression of the stent structure against the wall without leaving space between the vessel wall and the stent, which may be a source for thrombus formation and cause abrupt closure.

9. Coronary artery stent implantation is associated with the risk of immediate and/or long-term occlusion of lesion-associated side branches. Serial quantitative data obtained from 66 cases that included side branches with a diameter >1 mm indicated that coronary stenting minimally increased the risk of acute side-branch occlusion over that associated with conventional balloon angioplasty. When side-branch occlusion occurred, it was usually in the presence of underlying branch ostial disease. The patency of side-branch ostia was maintained at 6-month follow-up. Nevertheless, should the side branch become occluded, future crossing of the ostium to gain access to the side branch is extremely difficult. Artery site branches usually will not be affected by stent.

STENT OPTIMIZATION STRATEGY

Once the stent has been deployed, the process of stent optimization (postdilation) begins. The five essential features of the stent optimization technique are as follows:

1. Selection of an appropriately sized, noncompliant balloon based on angiographic reference vessel diameter

2. High-pressure balloon dilatation of the stent (usually *above* 15 atm inflation pressure)

3. Elimination of any inflow or outflow lesions by additional stent implantation, especially if the stent margin has a dissection

4. Full lesion coverage, a process that involves having no fear of multiple and/or overlapping stent implantation
5. Achievement of an optimal angiographic result with a <10% stenosis by visual estimates

High-Pressure Balloons

Stent optimization complications have been reduced significantly by using balloons for final dilations that are not angiographically oversized relative to the angiographic vessel size and by the use of balloons that are more dependable at high pressures. These balloons should have the most favorable characteristics at high pressures of 18 to 20 atm. The use of pressures above 15 atm is associated with additional improvement in stent expansion in 30% of stent implantation procedures. Noncompliant balloons allow direct expansile force to the most resistant part of the lesion without causing overexpansion in other parts of the balloon. Quarter-diameter sizes are particularly beneficial in small vessels but have the disadvantage of being available only in 20-mm balloon lengths. Short (10-mm) balloon lengths, at present, come only in half-diameter sizes. A short balloon is useful to postdilate short stents and sometimes to dilate very focal lesions that are resistant. In a resistant lesion that does not have adequate stent expansion with high pressures, it is sometimes necessary to use an oversized balloon to improve the expansion. Using short balloons can limit the oversizing to the stent segment and may decrease dissections that occur as a result of balloon oversizing.

When coiled stents are deployed, special attention must be given to stent site optimization. Most of the noncompliant balloons on the market at present have a problem with balloon winging after balloon deflation. This creates a condition in which there is a large deflated profile of the balloon, which can cause the stent coils to stretch or modify when the balloon catheter is pulled back into the balloon and thus create gaps between the stent struts. Allowing for full balloon deflation before withdrawing the balloon can prevent or limit potential stent modification, especially when the stent has not been fully expanded with a high-pressure balloon dilatation. Once the balloons are fully deflated, releasing the negative force on the indeflator may make the balloon wings softer than when there is continuous negative aspiration by the indeflator. This technique may prevent coiled-stent strut modification. Using a minimally compliant balloon for final stent optimization is another tactic to use for final dilation of the coiled stents. The minimally compliant balloon has a more favorable deflated balloon profile than noncompliant balloons.

In the Milan experience the balloon that is most suitable for coil stent optimization is the Europass (Cordis, Europe), the Olympix (Cordis, USA), the Sleek (Cordis, USA), the Speedy (Schneider), the Cruiser (Nycomed), and the Pronto (USCI). These balloons are dependable to 15 atm and although they are compliant, the deflated profile is low and they can be withdrawn into the guiding catheter after balloon deflation without causing stent coil modification.

Vasospasm with High-Pressure Balloon Dilation

Vasospasm was noted more prominently during the procedure when high pressures, above 15 atm, were used for stent optimization. This phenomenon was self-limiting, always resolved with time or after high doses of intracoronary nitroglycerin, and was not associated with any unfavorable clinical events.

Special Techniques

Bare Palmaz-Schatz stent implantation and how to crimp the stent on a delivery balloon. Bare stent implantation provides the advantage of improved flexibility and trackability. The absence of a sheath also gives a lower profile, which can improve visibility and security of precise stent placement. It may be a more cost-effective strategy to use in some countries.

One of the most important aspects of using this technique is mounting a Palmaz-Schatz stent on a balloon while avoiding trauma to the delivery balloon, which can cause low-pressure balloon rupture and subsequent potential problems with stent embolization. To avoid this problem, the following technique is described.

1. Advance the stent on a 16-gauge venous catheter (Veinflow). Keep the needle in the catheter to help guide the stent over the venous catheter (Fig. 5-3A). Carefully advance the stent over the needle and on to the venous catheter. While

advancing the stent, it is important not to pinch the stent, as this may preclude placing the stent on the catheter. Slight resistance may be encountered initially while advancing the stent on the venous catheter, but gentle forward pressure will help flare the end of the stent slightly and then the stent will slide on the venous catheter without difficulty.

2. Remove the introducer needle from the 16-gauge venous catheter (Fig. 5-3B).

3. Insert the distal tip of the previously expanded but well-wrapped balloon inside the venous catheter (Fig. 5-3C). Inflating the balloon before the stent crimping adds bulk to the balloon and will prevent the stent from sliding on the balloon. Another important tip is to wipe off any slippery coating (usually silicone based) from the balloon, again, to help prevent any balloon-stent slippage.

4. Hold the balloon between the palm and the fourth and fifth fingers and the stent between the thumb and forefinger (Fig. 5-3D).

5. Pull back only the venous catheter carefully.

6. Compress the stent manually on the balloon. Be sure the balloon is over the guidewire, so that crimping is not so tight as to prevent the guidewire from being inserted or moving. When hand crimping, it is important to press the stent and then turn the balloon and press again. Avoid rolling compression, as this may damage the balloon and precipitate a balloon burst at low pressure before effective stent expansion. The crimping device may also damage the balloon and is not effective in tightly crimping the stent on a low-profile balloon. To test how snug the stent is on the balloon, the stent can be gently tugged back and forth. There should be minimal or no stent movement. After this final evaluation, the stent is ready to be delivered. Usually, one last test to be sure the stent is on the balloon firmly is made before advancing the stent in the Touhy-Bourst connector. If it is necessary to remove the stent from the delivery system balloon, this can be done in the same fashion.

Short lesions and short stents.   In short lesions, the stent articulation site should not be at the center or tightest point of the original lesion. In some instances, two short, overlapping

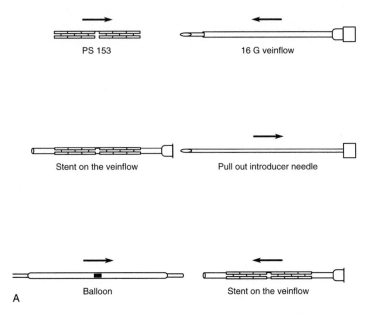

Fig. 5-3. Method of loading Palmaz-Schatz stent on a balloon catheter. **A,** 16G short plastic intravenous catheter receives the stent. The needle introducer is removed and the balloon catheter inserted into the plastic catheter.

Palmaz-Schatz stents are used to provide maximum support at the center of the lesion.

There are several indications for the short stent. These include stent insertion in very focal lesions, stent implantation to avoid placing the articulation site at the tightest point in the stent, and additional stent deployment to complete the coverage at the site of a previously deployed stent. The 8-mm Palmaz coronary stent is presently available in some international markets but is not available in the United States. A short stent can be made, however, by cutting the articulation of the Palmaz-Schatz stent with a pair of tissue scissors. It is important to place the cut articulation so that it is pointing to the proximal end of the balloon. This eliminates vessel trauma from advancing the sharp edge of the stent and may prevent the stent from becoming snagged. In very unusual circumstances, such as with extreme proximal tortuosity, the

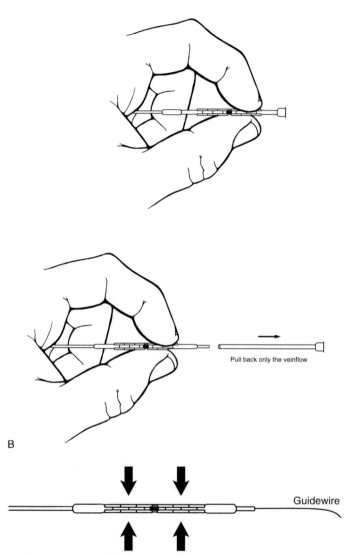

Pull back only the veinflow

B

Guidewire

Compress stent by finger on the balloon with guidewire

C

Fig. 5-3. (*Continued*). **B,** The stent is held in position on the balloon catheter and the plastic catheter withdrawn leaving the stent on the balloon. **C,** The stent is hand crimped on the balloon applying finger pressure with the angioplasty guidewire in the balloon catheter. Do not roll the stent, just compress.

short Palmaz-Schatz stents cannot be advanced to the intended stent site. In these cases, a half-stent can be cut in half to provide a single 4-mm stent. When doing this, the stent slots are cut so that a single 4-mm segment is formed. Only one 4-mm stent can be formed from this process, which will have a preserved (or closed) diamond configuration when it is expanded.

Stent implantation for acute vessel closure. When emergency stent implantation is performed for acute or threatened closure, it may be important to consider early stent implantation. A policy of early intervention with stents will decrease the percentage of patients who have stent implantation performed for acute closures and increase the number with threatened closure. The clinical effect of a prompt stent intervention policy is a decrease in the rate of myocardial infarction, and a reduction in the number of patients with hemodynamic and flow compromise, which can facilitate thrombus formation and worsen the environment for a successful stent implantation procedure. It is the presence of hemodynamic compromise or cardiogenic shock rather than the emergency bailout indication for stent implantation that is associated with higher incidence of stent failure. In the experience in Milan, early intervention may be a factor in improving the short-term results and reducing the complications of stent thrombosis after bailout stent implantation. The process of stent site optimization is perhaps more important with emergency stent implantation than with elective stent implantation. It also seems to be more dependent on intravascular ultrasound. After angiographic success has been obtained in patients with acute or threatened closure, 70% of lesions require further intervention based on information from the initial intravascular ultrasound evaluation. In contrast, after an optimal angiographic result is achieved in patients with elective stent implantation, 30% of lesions need further intervention based on the initial intravascular ultrasound evaluation. Further intervention includes additional dilation at higher pressures, with a larger balloon, or insertion of additional stents.

Technical factors that are important when stent implantation is performed for acute or threatened closure cover the full extent of the dissection. Securing the distal extent of the dissection is essential and is most easily accomplished with the first stent deployed. If the dissections are long or tortuous, short stents may be necessary to secure the distal vessel and the distal end of the dissection. If dissection is still evident distal to the stent, additional stent implantation distal to the deployed stent is necessary. When more than one stent is used, slight (2- to 3-mm) overlap is helpful to prevent dissection flaps between the stents, which may compromise flow.

Stent implantation distal to a deployed stent.   One of the most challenging problems encountered with stent implantation is dissection distal to a previously deployed stent. Securing the distal extent of a dissection or lesion with the first stent is always the best policy. When stent implantation distal to a stent is necessary, the proximal stent must first be expanded optimally with high pressure to facilitate distal delivery through a stent. A delivery system or a short stent should be strongly considered. At times the best option is the short Palmaz-Schatz stent (7 mm) or even the Micro stent. The Micro stent is ideal when the vessels are small or there is extensive proximal or lesion tortuosity and it is also necessary to deliver a stent distal to a stent. Unnecessary force should not be applied if the operator is unable to advance through the stent. Consider changing the angle of the approach, adjusting the wire position, or changing the wire to an extra-support wire. Proximal stent deployment may be necessary if the operator is unable to advance through the stent. Above all, PTCA of a distal dissection should never be considered a surrogate for distal stent deployment, especially if stent implantation is performed without subsequent anticoagulation.

Bend lesion.   Stent implantation on bend lesions presents a challenge. This is especially true for the Palmaz-Schatz stent, which tends to straighten vessels more significantly than other stents. When deploying stents on arterial bends, it is particularly important to evaluate for lesions at the stent margins. Dissection or plaque fractures at the stent margins occur more frequently when stent implantation is performed on arterial bends. Lesions on significant bends with greater than 45° angulation may need to have stents placed in the entire bend. The Wiktor and Gianturco-Roubin stents are more flexible and longer than the Palmaz-Schatz stent and may be better suited for this type of lesion. The use of flexible stents on bend lesions often provides the advantage of using only one stent and may limit dissections at the stent margins.

Severe lesion calcification by angiogram. For heavily calcified lesions, as may be seen in older patients, rotational atherectomy should be considered prior to stent implantation, though perhaps with more caution than when stent implantation is not intended. In using this approach, some caution should be given to performing rotational atherectomy on long lesions, and the number and size of the burrs should be conservative. Generally, only one burr that is slightly undersized (burr/vessel ratio of 0.5/1) is used when stent implantation is planned. The intent of this approach is not to debulk the lesion significantly but to modify the lesion compliance to avoid or decrease the phenomenon of embolization, which contributes to slow flow, while still facilitating improved stent expansion. The rotablation is followed by stent predilation with an attempt to inflate the balloon to full expansion and subsequent stent deployment. There were two early postprocedure events (one stent thrombosis and one embolic myocardial infarction) associated with prestent rotablation. As a result, we strongly consider treatment with anticoagulation for 12 to 24 hours after the procedure if rotational ablation is performed prior to stent implantation, especially if there is any evidence of slow flow at the completion of the stent procedure.

Bifurcations. There is a role for stent implantation of bifurcation lesions, because angioplasty at a lesion with a side branch is associated with a high complication rate. In addition, it is often difficult to obtain effective lumen expansion in both the main vessel and the side branch because of the problem of plaque shifting and lesion recoil, which impact on restenosis. Despite the fact that the stent is a suitable device for decreasing the procedural complications and improving long-term results by preventing lesion recoil, the implantation of a stent at a site of bifurcation had been traditionally viewed as a potential limitation to blood flow and access to the side branch. The term "stent jail" is often used to describe this concept. In this respect, the tubular slotted Palmaz-Schatz stent is felt to have a higher risk of side-branch vessel entrapment, where the stent prevents or limits access to the side branch. Most cases of failure to gain access to a side branch through a deployed stent are due to failure to cannulate the side-branch vessel and not to entrapment of the branch vessel by the stent. The risk of side-branch compromise is increased in two anatomical situations. First, when there is an eccentric lesion at the bifurcation site, asymmetric stent expansion can cause either plaque shifting or dissection at the side-branch ostium. Second, the side branch can be compromised when there is a stenosis in the ostium of the side branch. In both angiographic situations, the limit to effective side-branch access is anatomical rather than actual stent entrapment of the side branch, regardless of the type of stent that is used.

Prior to coronary stent implantation of a lesion that involves the origin of a side branch, two questions need to be addressed: (1) Is the side branch important as far as size and distribution? (2) Does the origin of the side branch have a stenosis? If the side branch is important and has a stenosis, guidewires are placed in the side branch and the major vessel and balloon dilation is performed. This prevents or minimizes vessel narrowing due to plaque shifting and facilitates side-branch access after stent implantation. The guidewire is removed from the side branch and stent implantation is performed in the major vessel. Following stent implantation, a balloon inflation of the side branch and the main vessel is performed. When the balloons are used to dilate a side branch after stent implantation, an important safety tip to limit potential balloon entrapment in the stent struts is to advance only the distal part of the balloon through the stent struts. Balloon entrapment can lead to stent dislodgement if excessive force is used in withdrawing the balloon catheter. Balloons on a wire (Probe III from USCI, and ACE from SciMed) can also be used to dilate side branches. It is especially important not to advance the balloon on a wire distal after the side-branch inflation has been performed, as is common practice with angioplasty. When attention is paid to this detail, the balloon can be more easily withdrawn in the event of a balloon rupture or a partial deflated balloon wrap. Sometimes kissing balloon dilation can be performed of the side branch and the major vessel. If there is a dissection of the side branch, stent implantation is considered when the angiographic size of the branch is at least 2.5 mm and the vessel has suitable anatomy for stent implantation. When stent implantation of the side branch is planned, the origin of the side branch is fully dilated with a high-pressure balloon and then stent implantation is performed of this branch with a Palmaz-Schatz stent delivery system.

Lesions with important side branches that do not have a baseline stenosis are generally not predilated prior to stent implantation in the major vessel. In this situation, balloon dilation is performed only if needed after stent deployment in the main branch. Stent implantation of the side branch prior to deployment of the stent in the major branch is rarely performed, because protrusion of the stent from the side branch into the major vessel may cause difficulties when trying to stent the major vessel. Nonetheless, it is a consideration if there is a dissection in an important side branch after a predilation. In this situation, guidewires are advanced into both the major vessel and the side branch, and predilation is performed in both vessels. The predilation can be performed with slightly undersized balloons. The guidewire is removed from the major branch, and stent implantation is performed in the side branch. When an optimal angiographic result is obtained after postdilation of the lesion, an intravascular ultrasound evaluation can be performed to confirm the result. The wire is then removed from the side branch and advanced to the distal major vessel, and stent deployment is performed in this lesion.

It is also possible to deliver a stent through the struts of a stent into a side branch. While it may be more easily performed when coiled stents are used, it is also possible to deliver a stent through the struts of a Palmaz-Schatz to a side-branch lesion. There are several essential points to the technique of delivering a stent through stent struts. It is important to achieve an effective area in the stent struts through which a stent can be advanced. Intravascular ultrasound at the side-branch site may help in this regard. The use of a stent delivery system can limit snagging that occurs when a bare stent is delivered through the struts of an implanted stent and can also allow safe stent retrieval when there is insufficient dilatation of the second stent to pass through the implanted stent.

The use of these techniques may broaden the safe application of stent implantation for these types of bifurcation lesions.

Troubleshooting During the Stent Procedure

Balloon rupture during initial stent deployment.   One of the most difficult problems during stent deployment is balloon rupture at low pressure. The stent is partially expanded but not large enough for the ruptured balloon to be retrieved without also withdrawing the stent. This situation occurs rarely but is an important cause of stent embolization. A partially expanded stent will almost invariably embolize if pulled into the guiding catheter. Usually, the partially expanded stent can be more readily visualized than the expanded stent, even when the stent is stainless steel. Pulling the balloon and partially expanded stent to (but not into) the guiding catheter and then withdrawing both the guiding catheter and the stent balloon as a unit back to the femoral sheath will prevent stent embolization into the cerebral circulation, but there is still a high likelihood that the stent will embolize during withdrawal through the sheath. If the balloon has a slow or moderate leak, one solution is to connect the balloon to a power injector and inject a total of 5 cc of a solution that is half-saline and half-contrast at 20 ml/sec at 300 psi maximum. This may expand the stent well enough for the balloon to be retrieved.

Stent migration.   Stent migration is more likely to occur with short stents such as the Micro stent (Advanced Vascular Engineering) or with the Wiktor stent. The stent migration is also more common when the stents are underexpanded. When stents are not visible, the findings are better appreciated by intravascular ultrasound evaluation. At times, the problem can also be identified on angiography by a persistent flap or lesion at the site of previous stent placement. Additional short stent placement may be necessary.

Lost wire position.   Lost wire position during or after stent deployment can present a significant problem. If an extra support wire has been used during the stent procedure, sometimes it may be necessary to change to a normal coronary guidewire. Recrossing the central lumen of the stent is facilitated by creating a knuckle or bend in the wire and advancing the knuckle through the stent. Other suggestions include using a Magnum wire to advance through the stent. Finding the central lumen of the stent is more difficult when the stent is not fully expanded. Lost wire position with short stents such as the Micro stent or the short Palmaz-Schatz can increase the hazard, as the short stents can twist in the center of the vessel. If the central lumen is not picked up with the guidewire, a balloon dilation at the site will compress the stent into the wall of the vessel. Usually this does not disturb blood flow, but sometimes an additional stent is necessary to cover the compressed stent.

Stent embolization. Stent embolization has occurred in less than 0.5% of stent procedures in Milan despite the frequent delivery of bare stents. There has never been a clinical problem associated with stent embolization. Stent embolization occurs, typically, after stent delivery failure, when the stent is withdrawn into the guiding catheter. The guiding catheter can strip the stent off the balloon. This can be minimized by withdrawing the stent delivery balloon until it is positioned just distal to the guiding catheter and then withdrawing both the delivery balloon and the guiding catheter as a unit to the femoral sheath. Sometimes stent embolization occurs when the stent delivery balloon and guiding catheter are pulled through the sheath. This method of removing the bare stent prevents embolization of the stent into the cerebral circulation. Generally, when the stents are not visible, they cannot be found. Visible stents such as the Biliary stent (Johnson & Johnson Interventional Systems) or the tantalum stents can be identified and removed using retrieval devices that are available commercially or by fashioning a retrieval device by double looping a coronary exchange wire.

Vessel rupture. Vessel rupture is one of the most significant complications that can occur due to balloon oversizing. Coronary vessel rupture without epicardial rupture can be identified by focal contrast staining of the subepicardium and can usually be sealed with a prolonged balloon inflation with a perfusion balloon. Coronary rupture with epicardial bleeding is more ominous and can have hemodynamic consequences by causing cardiac tamponade. The tear should be sealed immediately with a balloon or perfusion balloon catheter. Sometimes this can seal even a complete vessel tear. Another potential solution is fashioning a stent graft by overlaying the stent with a harvested vein and suturing it to the stent. This technique has been used successfully in one case of complete vessel rupture (verbal report, Dr. Gerald Dorros). Surgical repair and bypass are frequently necessary. Of importance in the case of vessel rupture that requires surgical repair, the coronary balloon or perfusion balloon should remain inflated during transport to the operating room and probably until the chest is opened to prevent cardiac tamponade.

Postprocedural Medications

If the intravascular ultrasound criteria for optimal stent expansion are met and the angiographic result is also acceptable, no further heparin is administered. When procedures are performed in the evening, heparin is infused overnight and stopped the morning following the procedure. Patients receive either one of two regimens. One regimen is Ticlopidine, 250 mg bid for 1 month, with aspirin 325 mg/day for 5 days. These patients are then treated with aspirin, 325 mg/day, after the 1-month regimen of Ticlopidine. The other regimen is aspirin, 325 mg/day, indefinitely. Patients do not receive Dextran or Persantine prior to, during, or following the stent procedure.

Patients who did not have intravascular ultrasound performed, patients who had an attempted but unsuccessful intravascular ultrasound evaluation, and patients who had a final suboptimal intravascular ultrasound performed were treated with a standard postprocedure anticoagulation and antiplatelet regimen. In these patients, at the completion of the stent procedure, the heparin was discontinued briefly to allow for sheath removal, then reinstituted within 4 to 6 hours. Warfarin was initiated on the day of the procedure, and both heparin and warfarin continued until the PT was over 16 (INR 2.0-3.5), after which the heparin was stopped. Starting on the day of the procedure, these patients received aspirin, 325 mg/day, indefinitely. These patients also did not receive Dextran or Persantine prior to, during, or following the stent procedure.

Sheath Removal

Sheath removal is generally performed 3 to 4 hours after the stent procedure, when the ACT is less than 150. If procedures are performed at night, sheaths are removed the following morning. Manual compression is used following sheath removal. More recently, collagen plug devices have been used to facilitate sheath removal immediately after the stent procedure.

Hospital Discharge

In the first 2 months of this protocol (first 60 patients), patients were observed in the hospital for 7 to 10 days and did not have any short-term clinical events (i.e., stent thrombosis). In the subsequent 300 patients, patients were discharged from the hospital within 2 days. More recently, patients have been discharged after one day or on the same day. Early discharge has been facilitated by the use of an arterial puncture device that allows sheath removal immediately after the procedure, even while the patient is fully anticoagulated.

INTRAVASCULAR ULTRASOUND (IVUS)
Equipment

The IVUS system with the monorail (0.018 guidewire compatible CVIS) 2.9F 30 MHz ultrasound catheter is the primary intravascular ultrasound system used in Columbus Hospital. The recommended zoom setting is scale 31 (the automatic setting is 37, so it is necessary to change every time). Usually, adjustment in gain control is not necessary, but when the image is too dark, the overall gain can be increased.

Environment

If there is electric interference, the IVUS catheter acts like an antenna and picks up noise artefacts. When this occurs, it may help to use an electricity source from outside the catheterization lab. Turning off the electric device that causes the artifact is sometimes necessary. Cleaning the connection between the catheter and the motor drive unit may help reduce the interference. Occasionally, a notch filter is needed to prevent an artifact from a specifically identified source.

The IVUS monitor is best positioned in front of the operator and beside the angiographic monitors. A separate monitor can be used in addition to the monitor on the IVUS unit if there is a problem with space in the catheterization laboratory. The extra monitor can be positioned on the wall or on a separate table for ease of visualization by the primary operator. The convenience of having the IVUS and the angiographic monitors near or adjacent to each other facilitates the fluoroscopic correlation between the two imaging modalities.

Preparation of the IVUS Machine

The IVUS assistant enters the patient name and the type of procedure. We describe the procedure in the patient ID space on the IVUS machine. After each IVUS imaging sequence, the procedure note is changed on the IVUS machine (ID space). The description should include a note of the additional dilation procedure.

Before recording new images, check the videotape. Make sure you are at the end of the previous patient study. If the tape is near to the end, exchange it for a new videotape. Sometimes during the procedure, the tape reaches the end and the video recorder automatically rewinds the tape. If the assistant does not recognize the automatic rewind, he or she may overrecord and erase the previous IVUS studies. After on-line measurements, the assistant has to forward the tape to the available place before recording additional images.

It is helpful for the IVUS assistant to provide a running discourse during the IVUS imaging. This facilitates evaluation if the tape is reviewed after the procedure is completed. Recording the digital angiogram images on the IVUS tape is also helpful when the tape is reviewed.

Poor Imaging Quality

Image quality can be variable, but several tips are generally helpful. A hard saline flush with a small syringe provides a good image. Flushing with a mixture of the patient's blood and saline is thought to cover the IVUS probe tip with serum protein and may limit or prevent air bubble adhesion. A distorted image (nonuniform rotational distortion) sometimes occurs in complex lesions, with calcified plaque lesions, or very distal in a tortuous vessel. These lesions interrupt the constant rotation of the ultrasound probe. Further dilation at the lesion can improve the image. Sometimes a deeply engaged guiding catheter blocks blood flow in the vessel and causes slow flow around the IVUS catheter, which can produce artefacts or poor image quality near the catheter. Image quality can be improved by improving the flow with backing out of the guiding catheter. In some instances the lumen is difficult to image clearly. Resolution improves with a saline or contrast flush and the lumen surface can be more readily identified.

IVUS Study

After successful stent implantation is confirmed by an angiographic assessment of results (less than 10% to 20% diameter stenosis and no residual dissections on the angiogram), the first IVUS study is attempted. The IVUS catheter is advanced distal to the stent. If the operator feels a resistance, the IVUS catheter should be pulled back and the angle of the guiding catheter should be adjusted or the guidewire should be repositioned if it is too distal. This will change the approach angle of the imaging catheter and may help in advancing the catheter more easily. In contrast to angioplasty, where power positioning of the guiding catheter is often essential, excessive force should not be applied when advancing the IVUS catheter. It is especially important not to use force when advancing the imaging catheter through coiled stents. The IVUS catheter can modify the coil stent shape and create gaps between the stent struts. Sometimes the resistance to advancing the catheter is because the stent is not well expanded and an additional balloon dilation is necessary prior to attempting IVUS imaging again.

After advancing the IVUS catheter distal to the stent, record the distal position on cine film to document from where the IVUS trip is started. This is helpful when reviewing the cine, because the operator can appreciate the time of IVUS study. The IVUS images are recorded from distal to the stent to proximal. The images can be recorded during slow manual pullback of the IVUS catheter or, more recently, automated pullback systems. Periodic fluoroscopic updates are helpful to correlate the IVUS imaging site and angiographic position. For the operator, it is very important to try to build up a mental picture of where the critical lesions are relative to the angiogram at the same time as the IVUS images are being mentally processed.

Measurements

Measurements are performed at the distal reference site, the tightest point in the stented site, and the proximal reference site using the computerized planimetry on the IVUS machine. After the first IVUS images are recorded, the following measurements are made at the proximal or distal reference sites, generally within 5 to 10 mm of the stented segment: vessel cross-sectional area (CSA), vessel minimal and maximal diameters, lumen CSA, and lumen minimal and maximal diameters. The reference site measurements are made at sites that do not appear severely diseased upon intravascular ultrasound image and that have a minimum of balloon trauma from prior balloon dilation. Thus, these measurements are felt to be a reasonable and practical reflection of the true lumen or vessel size by intravascular ultrasound. The border of the vessel (as distinguished from the lumen) is defined on the ultrasound image as the outer boundary of the echo-lucent media surrounding the plaque. Lumen measurements are made at the inner border of the echo-dense plaque. Intrastent lumen CSA and diameter measurements are made at the tightest position within the stent. The average of the proximal and distal vessel CSA can be used to estimate the vessel dimensions of the stented segment, because intense echo reverberations from the metallic struts frequently prevent measurements of the vessel boundary beyond the stent. Intravascular ultrasound imaging is performed in the reference sites and in the stented segment at the initial intravascular ultrasound evaluation and after each series of balloon dilations. Measurements are made at the tightest point within the stented segment after each series of balloon dilations. The tightest site within the stent is sometimes selected from several measurements performed within the stented segment. The measurements at the reference site are done on the initial intravascular ultrasound evaluation to minimize the potential balloon dilation effect that might increase the dimensions of the reference site. The benefit of intravascular ultrasound is that it can provide a cross-sectional assessment of results (Figs. 5-4A and 5-4B). Cross-sectional area measurements are preferable to diameter measurements for assessing the result at the site. Although it is easier to perform one-dimensional diameter measurements, this method is the same as the angiographic method of measuring diameter stenosis and does not take into account the eccentricity that can be seen at the stent site. The use of intravascular ultrasound diameter measurements defeats the bene-

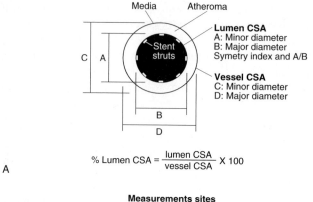

$$\% \text{ Lumen CSA} = \frac{\text{lumen CSA}}{\text{vessel CSA}} \times 100$$

A

Measurements sites

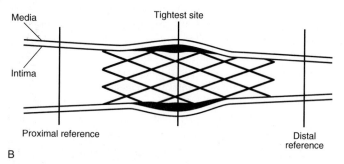

B

Fig. 5-4.   Intravascular ultrasound imaging (IVUS) measurements after stent placement. **A,** Vessel structure in cross-sectional area (CSA) A, B, C, D diameters by IVUS. **B,** Measurement sites along the course of the vessel. The most severe narrowings (tightest site) in the proximal and stent segments are compared to the distal reference site.

fit of the cross-sectional assessment of results that intravascular ultrasound provides.

General Concepts of IVUS Evaluation of Optimal Stent Expansion

The criteria for optimal stent expansion are governed by the principles of achieving full stent expansion and covering the extent of the lesion so that potential impairment to flow that could contribute to stent thrombosis is minimized and long-term results are optimized. A decision to perform further dilation based on the IVUS image measurements done at the time of angiographic success should take into account the lumen and vessel CSA. A determination of optimal stent expansion on IVUS involves an assessment of how large the stent lumen CSA is relative to the vessel CSA at the stent site and also how large the stent lumen CSA is relative to the reference lumen CSA. The concept is to expand the stent to the extent that it is safe to dilate. IVUS measurements at the stent and reference sites contribute to the scientific acceptance of using intravascular ultrasound to guide interventional procedures. From a practical standpoint, however, the assessment of IVUS results after stent implantation can be made using visual evaluation once an understanding of these two basic principles is reached. The interplay of these two methods of assessing IVUS results is illustrated in the examples in Fig. 5-5.

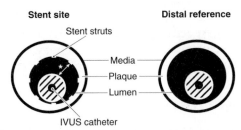

*Narrow space between IVUS catheter and the lumen surface

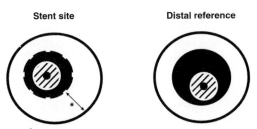

*Wide space between stent struts and the media

Fig. 5-5. Intravascular ultrasound imaging (IVUS) comparison of area of deployed stent relative to distal reference area and amount of plaque in each segment.

The IVUS evaluation reveals that the stent cross-sectional area is less than the reference lumen cross-sectional area (Fig. 5-5, top). Based on this result, the stent should have further dilation so that the stent is expanded to larger than the distal lumen CSA. This result can be confirmed by actual measurements of each site or by visual estimation. Once visual estimation as a pullback from the reference site through the stent site is performed, it can be appreciated that the stent site lumen is smaller than the reference lumen. Observing that the space between the IVUS probe and the lumen border narrows inside the stent can demonstrate that the stent is underexpanded and needs further dilation.

The IVUS evaluation also reveals that the stent lumen cross-sectional area is dilated well in comparison to the reference lumen cross-sectional area but the stent is relatively small compared to the vessel size due to plaque burden or compensatory dilation at the stent site (Fig. 5-5, bottom). In this example, further balloon dilation was performed to compress the plaque at the stent site. This can be observed visually by noting the wide space between the stent struts and the media. Frequently, the plaque will appear either not well compressed or, less commonly, there is incomplete stent-to-wall apposition.

Guidelines for IVUS Success

Assessment based on the IVUS reference lumen. Successful stent expansion on IVUS is clearly achieved when there is no significant lumen size difference between stent site and reference site lumen (particularly the distal reference) and there is good stent expansion relative to the vessel size at the stent site. In the cumulative experience in Milan since October 1993, the stent lumen area curve is larger than the distal reference lumen cross-sectional area. The percentile curve (Fig. 5-6) reveals that in small vessels, the stent lumen cross-sectional area was always larger than the distal reference lumen. In large vessels with lumen cross-sectional area in the stent segment greater than 8 mm^2, the final stent lumen cross-sectional area is slightly less than the distal reference lumen cross-sectional area. There were three stent thrombosis events (0.66%) in the Palmaz-Schatz cohort. The stent thrombosis was due to residual dissection in the unstented segments

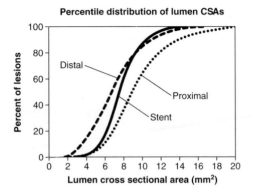

Fig. 5-6. Percentile distribution of lumen cross-sectional area (CSA) along the course of the stented vessels. Distal reference CSA is dashed line; proximal CSA is dotted line.

in two patients, and in one patient was related to stenosis within the stent site relative to the distal reference lumen. The final balloon inflation was performed with a 3.0-mm balloon in all three patients, a reflection of the decreased margin for error that exists in small vessels, especially if stent implantation is performed without subsequent anticoagulation. The practical aspects of these observations and clinical results are that when stent implantation is performed in small vessels, the IVUS criteria of achieving a final stent lumen CSA larger than the distal reference lumen CSA are strictly followed. In contrast, in larger vessels the criteria of achieving a final stent lumen CSA greater than the distal reference CSA are less vigorously enforced, but the stent site is still optimized relative to the IVUS vessel size. This is accepted because the reference sites in large vessels commonly have less disease in the reference segments than do the small vessels. This makes the safe achievement of a final stent lumen larger than the distal CSA more difficult in the large vessels than in small vessels. Typically, a final stent lumen CSA of 80% of the distal reference vessel is accepted.

Assessment based on the IVUS reference vessel. The IVUS vessel measurements can also be used to assess if optimal stent expansion has been achieved. Using criteria based only on IVUS vessel size has the inherent flaw of not incorporating an assessment of how well stents are expanded relative to the reference lumen cross-sectional area. If the criteria are too easy to achieve, the stent may be relatively underexpanded, which can cause stent thrombosis and possibly increase restenosis. Conversely, if the criteria are too rigid they cannot be achieved in a high percentage of patients. The failure to achieve rigid criteria based on vessel size is in part due to the compensatory dilation that can occur even in reference vessel sites. In the initial experience, the achievement of 50% to 60% of the average of the proximal and distal vessel measurements was the primary criterion used to determine success. The application of this criterion to the same cohort of patients performed after October 1993 is shown in Fig. 5-7. The use of a 50% average vessel criterion would have left a significant number of patients with a stent that was underexpanded compared to the distal reference lumen. The use of a 60% average vessel criterion would have positioned the final stent lumen between the proximal and distal reference lumen CSA. In our experience, this is a very difficult criterion to achieve, particularly in large vessels and in lesions with significant plaque burden or calcification. The use of reference vessel criteria has the disadvantage of requiring multiple additional measurements in contrast to using the

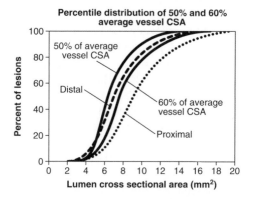

Fig. 5-7.   Percentile distribution of 50% and 60% average vessel cross-sectional area (CSA). Distal reference CSA is dashed line; proximal CSA is dotted line.

reference lumen criterion, which requires only several measurements.

Assessment based on final balloon size. There is another simplified guideline for assessing the adequacy of the final stent lumen CSA using the balloon chosen for final stent optimization. The interventionist usually selects an appropriate size balloon based on visual estimation of the reference vessel diameter. The minimum stent lumen cross-sectional area should be greater than 70% of the calculated balloon cross-sectional area that was selected based on the angiogram. The percentile curve in Fig. 5-8 shows the distal and proximal reference lumen CSA and 70% of balloon cross-sectional area. The target stent lumen cross-sectional area should be considered based on use of a quarter-size balloon for final balloon dilations (Table 5-3). The percentile curve of the balloon cross-sectional area is almost between the distal and proximal reference lumen cross-sectional areas. Importantly, the simplified criterion provides a safety buffer in the small vessels where the risks for stent thrombosis are higher, and is less strict for the larger vessels where the risks of stent thrombosis are reduced. The curve using the 70% final balloon method generally follows the stent lumen CSA curves in the cumulative Milan cohort.

IVUS assessment based on MUSIC trial criteria. Recently, the MUSIC (Multicenter Ultrasound Study in Coro-

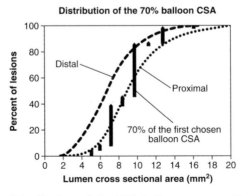

Fig. 5-8. Distribution of the 70% balloon cross-sectional areas (CSA).

TABLE 5-3.   Balloon diameter and cross-sectional area

Diameter (mm)	CSA (mm²)	70% of balloon CSA (mm²)
2.5	4.9	3.4
2.75	5.9	4.2
3.0	7.1	5.0
3.25	8.3	5.8
3.5	9.6	6.7
3.75	11.0	7.7
4.0	12.6	8.8
4.25	14.2	9.9
4.5	15.9	11.1

CSA, Cross-sectional area.
From Centro Cuore Columbus, Milan, Italy.

nary stenting) trial recommended 90% of the average reference (proximal and distal) lumen cross-sectional area as a target stent minimum lumen cross-sectional area. In this trial, patients in whom this target criterion is achieved will not receive anticoagulation after the stent procedure. Patients who do not achieve this criterion will be continued on a standard post-stent implantation anticoagulation regimen. The percentile distribution using an estimate of the 90% average reference lumen cross-sectional area based on the cumulative Milan cohort of patients undergoing IVUS guided stent implantation is shown in Fig. 5-9. The percentile distribution from an

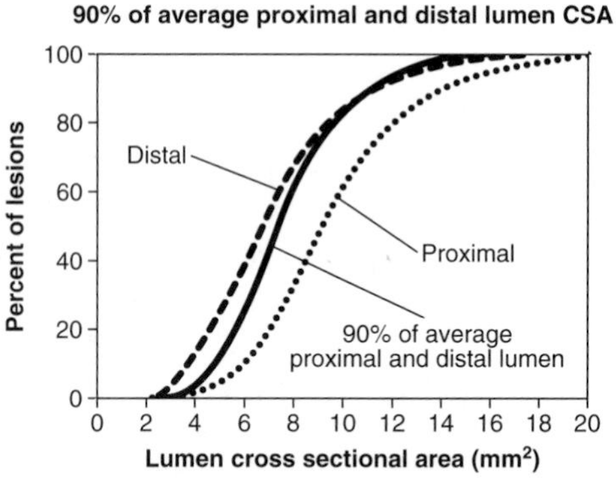

Fig. 5-9.   Distribution of the 90% average proximal and distal lumen cross-sectional areas (CSA).

estimate of this criterion is very similar to the actual percentile distribution of final stent CSA from the Milan cohort.

The reference lumen CSA shown in Figs. 5-6 and 5-8 were obtained from the same 275 stented lesions from October 1993. These results are a reflection of a strategy of using appropriate balloons for final dilations.

Stent Expansion Strategies

There are two methods for optimizing stent expansion and improving the stent lumen cross-sectional area. One method is to use high pressure, the other is to use a large-diameter balloon. In performing final optimization dilations, it is important to work within the natural limitations of the vessel. When an oversized balloon is used, there is an increased likelihood that the limitations of the vessels can be exceeded, leading to complications of coronary vessel rupture or dissection. Using high pressure with a balloon that is appropriately sized to the vessel allows stent expansion to occur within the natural confines of the vessel. To avoid stent optimization complications, the balloon/angiographic reference vessel ratio should be approximately 1.0. If an angiographic balloon-vessel ratio of greater than 1.0 is used then a short, noncompliant balloon with medium pressure (12-16 atm) is preferable. When a balloon larger than the angiographic vessel diameter is used for final stent optimization, it should never be larger than the distal IVUS minimum vessel diameter (measured media to media). When there is a large differential between the size of the proximal and distal vessels, as may occur in the left anterior descending artery before and after the second diagonal, careful balloon selection is important. Generally, using slightly lower pressure in the distal part of the stent segment and a higher pressure for the proximal portion of the stent is all that is necessary. Care should be given not to dilate beyond the distal edge of the stent with an oversized balloon. Occasionally, if there is significant vessel tapering, dilation with two different-diameter balloons should be considered. Noncompliant balloons are preferable to compliant balloons for final dilations for several reasons. Noncompliant balloons will expand and dilate uniformly, even in focal areas of resistant lesions, and are more likely to maintain a uniform diameter even at high pressures. Thus noncompliant balloons allow for optimal stent expansion without overexpansion of the balloon in adjacent unstented segments that contribute to dissection. Additionally, experience with intravascular ultrasound has shown that 25% of stents have improved stent expansion with an increase in pressure from 15 to ≥18 atm. There are no compliant balloons presently available that are consistently dependable at pressures above 16 atm when used for stent implantation procedures.

Lesion Morphology Assessed by IVUS

Asymmetric expansion. The information from IVUS evaluation has also revealed information that has helped in the understanding of the subtleties of improving stent expansion and the avoidance of complications. Typically, the stent expansion is symmetric in soft plaque, especially soft plaque with lipid pool. Very hard plaque (fibrotic or calcified) is seen in approximately 20% to 30% of lesions. In this type of lesion, the plaque is not easily compressed by balloon dilation of the stent struts, and stent expansion is asymmetric into the normal arc of the vessel. In lesions with a significant arc (≥270°) of dense or hard fibrocalcified disease, the stent expansion can be markedly asymmetric, with a minimum to maximum lumen diameter ratio (symmetry index) <0.7. In these lesions, further inflation leads to focal overstretching in the less diseased arc of the vessel. The symmetry index can worsen after further dilation, especially if an oversized balloon is used (Fig. 5-10A). Using a balloon that is 0.25 to 0.5 mm smaller than the size of the vessel and very high pressures may improve the symmetry index but will not necessarily increase the lumen cross-sectional area at the stent site.

It is important to recognize the stent that has marked asymmetric expansion because it is this type of lesion that is at a higher risk of vessel rupture. The risks are highest if a larger balloon is used for dilation, due to the concentration of asymmetric balloon expansion in a focal direction. If the stent lumen CSA is acceptable relative to the distal lumen CSA and the stent is well opposed to the intimal surface, it is better not to try to make the stent symmetry perfect. When high-pressure dilations are performed, suboptimal stent expansion is rare. Generally, patients with suboptimal stent expansion are placed on a standard anticoagulation therapy after the stent procedure.

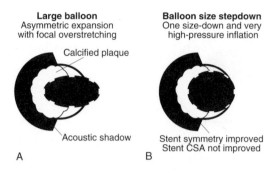

Large balloon
Asymmetric expansion
with focal overstretching

Calcified plaque

Acoustic shadow

A

Balloon size stepdown
One size-down and very
high-pressure inflation

Stent symmetry improved
Stent CSA not improved

B

Fig. 5-10.   Balloon inflation strategy based on intravascular
ultrasound image (IVUS) after stent placement. **A**, Asymmetric
stent expansion may require larger size balloon. **B**, Stent symmetry is improved but cross-sectional area (CSA) is not increased; use smaller balloon at very high inflation pressure.

Stent expansion also appears to be dependent on the plaque
burden. Optimal coronary stent expansion in lesions with
50% to 70% diameter stenosis or in lesions with a spiral dissection can be accomplished with relative ease because there is
not much atheroma. Optimal stent expansion in lesions with
greater than 90% diameter stenosis is more difficult to achieve,
is associated with a higher percentage of asymmetric stent
expansion, and commonly requires higher pressure.

Incomplete stent expansion.   Incomplete stent expansion
when the stent struts do not attach to the intimal surface is
not common but can occur particularly in ectatic vessels (at
poststenotic dilation or aneurysm sites) and in the ostial LAD,
where the operator is cautious about performing a balloon
inflation in the left main trunk (Fig. 5-11). In the latter case,
dilation of the ostial lesion with the balloon shoulder sometimes does not provide sufficient expansion force to dilate
the stent.

Plaque fracture at the stent margin.   The benefit of intravascular ultrasound also extends to providing a cross-
sectional assessment of the adjacent unstented segments after
stent implantation procedures. Final stent dilations sometimes cause a distal plaque fracture, which requires further
short stents to stabilize fractured plaque (Fig. 5-12). The addi-

Incomplete stent expansion

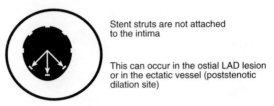

Stent struts are not attached
to the intima

This can occur in the ostial LAD lesion
or in the ectatic vessel (poststenotic
dilation site)

Fig. 5-11.   Intravascular ultrasound image (IVUS) of incomplete stent expansion.

tional stents are placed to prevent flow limitation from these lesions, which may contribute to stent thrombosis.

Plaque fracture may result from misplacement of a balloon, especially if there is clear balloon oversizing relative to the angiographic vessel size. Plaque fracture can also occur even when balloon position is within the stented segment. Based on ultrasound measurements, this most commonly is due to plaque fracture at the stent margins in noncompliant (calcified or fibrotic) vessels. In more elastic or soft lesions, this is less likely to occur, but it can be seen at the stent margins when the stents are deployed on bend lesions.

Plaque prolapse.   Plaque prolapse is found in 5% of coil stent implantation. Although the coiled stents have advantages in flexibility, the stent structure provides less complete radial support to the vessel wall. At times, fractured plaque or flaps appear within the stented lumen. When this problem is encountered, further dilation does not improve the stent

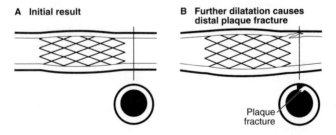

A   **Initial result**

B   **Further dilatation causes distal plaque fracture**

Plaque fracture

Fig. 5-12.   **A, B,** Overexpansion of stent may cause distal dissection.

lumen CSA and additional short stent deployment within the stent is necessary. Generally, a short Palmaz stent is the preferred method of treating this problem. A short Gianturco-Roubin stent is also an option in this situation.

OPTIMIZATION COMPLICATIONS

The importance of appropriate balloon sizing cannot be underestimated. From an experience with 535 lesions in 421 patients, the most significant predictor of stent optimization angiographic complications of vessel rupture or dissection that resulted in major clinical complications (myocardial infarctions, emergency bypass surgery, or death) was a high balloon-vessel ratio. Inflation pressure was not a significant factor (Table 5-4). By stepwise logistical regression, the balloon-vessel ratio was the only independent predictor of stent optimization (postdeployment balloon dilations) complications.

General Impressions on Stent Implantation with IVUS Guidance

The use of IVUS prolongs the stent procedure time but provides valuable information that has clinical impact on improving both short-term and long-term results. It is also instructive to correlate the angiographic and the IVUS results and can help interventionists appreciate the angiographic subtleties of an underexpanded stent. One of the factors associated with increased time of procedure is performing the IVUS

TABLE 5-4. Effect of balloon dilation strategies

	Oversized balloon	Appropriate balloon	p value
Patients	263	210	
Lesions	339	232	
Reference vessel	3.30 ± 0.57	3.30 ± 0.47	ns
Balloon-vessel ratio	1.23 ± 0.19	1.07 ± 0.16	0.0001
Maximal pressure (atm)	14.6 ± 3.0	16.0 ± 3.0	0.001
Final percent diameter stenosis	-10 ± 15	-0 ± 12	0.0001
Procedure complications	15 (6%)	2 (1%)	0.006
Optimization complications	8 (3%)	1 (0.5%)	0.05
Stent thrombosis	2 (0.8%)	2 (0.9%)	ns

From Centro Cuore Columbus, Milan, Italy.

measurements. With experience, an interventionist can begin to visually estimate the lumen cross-sectional area after coronary stent implantation when there is symmetric stent expansion. In the same IVUS imaging run, mental comparisons of the stent site lumen to the reference lumen cross-sectional areas as well as an assessment of the adequacy of plaque compression at the stent site can be made. In this sense, the intravascular ultrasound can be used in a manner similar to angiography to provide information that can be utilized to confirm good stent expansion. When the lumen is markedly asymmetric, which occurs in less than 5% of procedures, it is sometimes more difficult to estimate the stent lumen cross-sectional area and measurements may still be necessary.

After experience with IVUS guided stent implantation, it may not be necessary to perform intravascular ultrasound in all lesions. For elective stent implantation in focal lesions in vessels larger than 3.5 mm that have a perfect angiographic result with less than 10% stenosis and no evidence of residual dissection, it may be reasonable not to use intravascular ultrasound. The heparin-coated stent currently under clinical investigation in Europe may provide an additional safety margin in preventing stent thrombosis. However, in more complex lesions, such as stenosis in small vessels or diffuse disease, emergency (bailout) stent implantation, or when more than one stent is used, there is an increased benefit to using IVUS to confirm an optimal result. For all these complex stent implantation indications, additional balloon dilation with higher pressure or a larger balloon and sometimes additional stent implantation was necessary in more than 70% of the procedures after an acceptable angiographic result was obtained. The additional interventions were based on information from intravascular ultrasound. In contrast, for the straightforward case in large vessels with focal lesions, additional intervention at the stent site based on IVUS information was necessary in fewer than 30% of procedures after an acceptable angiographic result was achieved.

ANTICOAGULATION FOR STENT PLACEMENT
Pre- and Periprocedural Anticoagulant Regimens

Anticoagulation is commonly used in stent implantation. Inadequate or overzealous use of anticoagulants is responsible for most morbidity and mortality associated with stent implantation.

Steps taken in clinical trials to minimize the risk of thrombosis include:

1. Prior to stent implantation:
   a. Aspirin (nonenteric coated, nonbuffered), 325 mg PO qd for 48 hours before procedure
   b. Dipyridamole, 75 mg PO, tid for 24 to 48 hours before procedure
   c. Coumadin, 10-15 mg PO, given night before or morning of procedure*
   d. Low-molecular-weight dextran (Dextran 40), 100 cc/hr IV infusion, 2 to 3 hours before procedure*
   e. Ticlopidine, 250 mg PO, bid
2. During stent implantation:
   a. Heparin, 10,000 to 15,000 μ IV bolus depending on patient weight, then as needed to maintain ACT above 300 sec
   b. Low-molecular-weight dextran (Dextran 40), continue 100 cc/hr IV infusion during stent placement; the usual total dose of Dextran 40 is approximately 1 L.* For patients with renal insufficiency or congestive heart failure, a lower infusion dose may be appropriate and is left to physician discretion.
3. Immediately after stent implantation:
   a. Discontinue heparin
   b. Low-molecular-weight dextran (Dextran 40), continue at 50 cc/hr IV infusion for the first 6 to 12 hours after stent implantation until heparin is restarted.* The usual total dose of Dextran 40 is approximately 1 L. For patients with renal insufficiency or congestive heart failure, a lower infusion dose may be appropriate and is left to physician discretion.
4. Anticoagulation with coumadin and dipyridamole for a minimum of 1 month and aspirin indefinitely poststent implant are used.*
5. Careful monitoring of the patient's anticoagulation and antiplatelet medication (PT level of 16 to 18 sec [1.5× control] or INR values of 2 to 3) is required.

* Stenting without coumadin or dextran can be performed. See discussion on p 172.

The recommended protocol is based on empirical testing. Prospective randomized trials are presently assessing the risk/benefit ratio of using heparin, dextran, coumadin, dipyridamole, or aspirin in stent patients. Anticoagulant regimens for stenting are summarized in Table 5-5.

Postprocedural Care Sheath Removal, and Resumption of Anticoagulation

Sheaths are usually removed on the same day, after allowing the ACT to decrease to 150 sec. Prolonged manual and assisted femoral artery compression, as well as bed rest (strict bed rest for 24 hours with minimal activity allowed for the next 24 hours), is necessary. Heparin infusion is resumed after puncture-site hemostasis is obtained. The PTT is kept between 60 and 80 sec for several days until an INR of 3 to 4 is achieved by oral daily doses of coumadin. Heparin should be continued for another 24 hours after INR and PT are in the desired range for two successive measurements 24 hours apart. Despite all efforts, some patients may develop late bleeding, hematoma, retroperitoneal bleeding, and false aneurysms of the femoral artery.

In-Hospital Anticoagulation Phase

1. Aspirin (nonenteric coated, nonbuffered), continue 325 mg PO, qd.
2. Dipyridamole, continue 75 mg PO, tid.
3. Following sheath removal and access-site hemostasis, restart continuous heparin infusion for 3 days or longer to maintain PTT at 1.5 to 2.0× control (target range of 50-70 sec) until PT is between 16 and 18 sec (1.5× control) or an INR of 2 to 3. Usual heparin dose is 600-1200 U/hr based on body weight.
4. Titrate coumadin dose to achieve and maintain PT at 16 to 18 sec (1.5× control) or an INR of 2 to 3.*

Long-Term Poststent

1. Aspirin (nonenteric coated, nonbuffered), 325 mg PO, qd indefinitely.

* Stenting without coumadin or dextran can be performed. See discussion on p 172.

2. Dipyridamole, 75 mg PO, tid, continue for at least 1 month.
3. Coumadin, continue appropriate dose to maintain PT at 16 to 18 sec ($1.5\times$ control) or an INR of 2 to 3 for at least 1 month.
4. Ticlopidine, 250 mg PO, bid.

Safety of Magnetic Resonance Imaging

A magnetic resonance imaging (MRI) scan should not be performed until the implanted stent has been completely endothelialized (8 weeks), in order to minimize the risk of migration of the stent under a strong magnetic field. The stent may cause susceptibility artifacts in MRI scans due to distortion of the magnetic field.

CLINICAL RESULTS: STRESS AND BENESTENT TRIALS

Two randomized trials were conducted at 47 North American and European institutions involving 923 patients. Procedure success in the STRESS trial (Table 5-6) was defined as the reduction of stenosis severity to $<50\%$ by visual estimate and the absence of major complications (death, myocardial infarction, bypass surgery, or bailout stenting) during the hospital stay. A core laboratory using quantitative coronary angioplasty (QCA) later reviewed the angiographic films. Procedure success was defined similarly for the BENESTENT trial, except that the angiographic result was assessed by QCA (Table 5-7). Angiographic restenosis was defined as a $\geq50\%$ stenosis at 6-month follow-up using QCA in both trials. Event-free survival was defined as freedom from death, myocardial infarction, emergency bypass surgery, emergency stent bailout during the angioplasty, and repeat angioplasty. For the STRESS trial, target lesion revascularization was defined as any balloon angioplasty or bypass surgery performed for restenosis of the study lesion after documentation of recurrent angina and/or objective evidence of myocardial ischemia by stress testing at >30 days. In the BENESTENT trial, event rates began at the end of the initial procedure when the guiding catheter was removed from the arterial sheath. Bleeding/peripheral vascular complications consisted of cerebrovascular accidents, bleeding requiring transfusion, or bleeding requiring surgical repair of the vascular access site.

TABLE 5-5. Anticoagulant regimens

Drug	Aspirin nonenteric-coated nonbuffered	Dipyridamole	Low-molecular-weight dextran (Dextran 40)*	Heparin	Coumadin*
Before stent implantation	325 mg PO, qd 48 hr before	75 mg PO, tid 24-48 hr before	100 cc/hr IV infusion 2-3 hr before		10-15 mg PO, night before or morning of procedure
During stent implantation			Continue 100 cc/hr IV infusion	10,000-15,000 units IV bolus depending on patient weight, then as needed to maintain ACT above 300 sec	
Immediately after stent implantation			Continue 50 cc/hr IV infusion for the first 6-12 hr after stent implantation until heparin is restarted	Discontinue	

206

Remaining in hospital poststent	Continue 325 mg PO, qd	Continue 75 mg PO, tid	Following sheath removal and access-site hemostasis, restart continuous heparin infusion for ≥3 days to maintain PTT at 1.5-2.0× control (target range 50-70 sec) until the PT is between 16 and 18 sec (1.5× control) or an INR of 2-3. Usual heparin dose is 600-1200 U/hr based on body weight	Titrate dose to achieve and maintain PT at 16-18 sec (1.5 control) or INR of 2-3
Long-term poststent	325 mg PO, qd indefinitely	Continue 75 mg PO, tid for at least 1 month		Continue appropriate dose to maintain PT at 16-18 sec (1.5× control) or INR of 2-3 for at least 1 month

---

* Stenting without coumadin or dextran can be performed.

TABLE 5-6. STRESS trial—principal effectiveness and safety results: all patients treated ($n = 407$)

Effectiveness measures	Stent	Balloon	p value	Relative risk (95% confidence intervals)
Procedure success (QCA)	92%	85%	0.018	1.09 (1.01-1.17)
Percent DS after device	19 ± 11%	35 ± 14%	<0.001	
Percent DS 6-month follow-up	42 ± 18%	49 ± 19%	<0.001	
Restenosis rate	31%	42%	0.037	0.74 (0.55-0.98)
Target lesion revascularization	10%	15%	ns	0.67 (0.40-1.12)
Safety measures				
In-hospital clinical events	3%	10%	0.005	0.33 (0.14-0.76)
Out-of-hospital clinical events	17%	23%	ns	0.73 (0.50-1.09)
No clinical events	81%	73%	ns	1.10 (0.99-1.22)
Cerebrovascular accident	1%	0.5%	ns	1.97 (0.18-21.56)
Bleeding complications requiring transfusion	5%	2%	ns	2.46 (0.79-7.73)
Vascular complications requiring surgery	4%	2%	ns	1.97 (0.60-6.44)
No bleeding/vascular complications	93%	96%	ns	0.97 (0.92-1.01)
Total hospital stay (days)	8.3 ± 5.6	5.3 ± 4.2	<0.001	

Numbers are mean ± 1 SD or number (%) for the indicated group; *p* values (two-tailed) based on *t* test or chi-square analysis. QCA, Quantitative core lab angiography; DS, diameter stenosis; clinical event = death, nonfatal myocardial infarction, coronary bypass surgery, or stent bailout; target lesion revascularization, balloon angioplasty or bypass surgery performed at least 30 days postprocedure in STRESS trial or postinitial procedure in BENESTENT trial for restenosis of the study lesion after documentation of recurrent angina and/or myocardial ischemia by stress testing; no bleeding/ vascular complications, no cerebrovascular accident, bleeding requiring transfusion, or vascular complication requiring surgery.

TABLE 5-7. BENESTENT—principal effectiveness and safety results: all patients treated ($n = 516$)

Effectiveness measures	Stent	Balloon	p value	Relative risk (95% confidence intervals)
Procedure success (QCA)	86%	87%	0.821	1.99 (0.93-1.06)
Percent DS after device	22 ± 8%	33 ± 8%	<0.001	
Percent DS 6-month follow-up	38 ± 18%	43 ± 16%	<0.001	
Restenosis rate	22%	32%	0.013	0.68 (0.40-1.28)
Target lesion revascularization	18%	27%	0.014	0.67 (0.48-0.92)
Safety measures				
In-hospital clinical events	7%	10%	ns	0.71 (0.40-1.28)
Out-of-hospital clinical events	14%	24%	0.003	0.58 (0.40-0.84)
No clinical events	80%	67%	0.002	1.18 (1.06-1.31)
Cerebrovascular accident	1%	0.5%	ns	1.97 (0.18-21.56)
Bleeding complications requiring transfusion	4%	1%	0.045	3.31 (0.92-11.88)
Vascular complications requiring surgery	10%	2%	<0.001	4.96 (1.93-12.6)
No bleeding/vascular complications	86%	97%	<0.001	0.89 (0.85-0.94)
Total hospital stay (days)	8.5 ± 6.8	3.1 ± 3.3	<0.001	

Numbers are mean ± 1 SD or number (%) for the indicated group; p values (two-tailed) based on t test or chi-square analysis. QCA, Quantitative core lab angiography; DS, diameter stenosis; clinical event, death, nonfatal myocardial infarction, coronary bypass surgery, or stent bailout; target lesion revascularization, balloon angioplasty or bypass surgery performed at least 30 days postprocedure in STRESS trial or postinitial procedure in BENESTENT trial for restenosis of the study lesion after documentation of recurrent angina and/or myocardial ischemia by stress testing; no bleeding/ vascular complications, no cerebrovascular accident, bleeding requiring transfusion, or vascular complication requiring surgery.

Comparisons of patients who received elective stents to patients who received balloon angioplasty are summarized in the following text for both the STRESS and BENESTENT trials. Analysis of safety and effectiveness data indicated no differences between the genders, hence the data presented are representative for both genders.

Restenosis in Stents

Restenosis rates after stent implantation in selected patients are similar to those after balloon angioplasty. However, the peak restenosis rate may be delayed. Restenosis can be managed by repeat angioplasty. Restenosis and reocclusion are affected by the artery diameter and the degree of residual narrowing. Achieving a residual narrowing <20% in a 3-mm or larger artery decreases the risk of restenosis after elective implantation.

Many patients who exhibited angiographic restenosis at follow-up received redilation of the stent. However, the long-term effects of redilation of a stent in the event of restenosis are not well characterized. In the STRESS trial, of the 22 patients with repeat balloon angioplasty, one patient had a coronary artery bypass graft procedure performed 3 months after the repeat angioplasty. In the stent Registry ($n = 1141$), 33 patients had an event (death, CABG, or another balloon angioplasty) within 6 months of the repeat procedure.

Acute and Chronic Complications of Coronary Stenting

Vascular complications (Table 5-8).   Anticoagulation regimens required to prevent stent thrombosis are associated with a higher incidence of vascular complications than conventional coronary angioplasty. Reported complications include pseudoaneurysm, arteriovenous fistula, major bleeding requiring transfusion, retroperitoneal hematoma, and the development of femoral neuropathy. In the STRESS trial, hemorrhagic complications were significantly higher in patients treated with Palmaz-Schatz stents compared to balloon angioplasty (9.3% versus 4.0%). In the multicenter Gianturco-Roubin stent trial, 16.8% of patients required blood transfusions secondary to hemorrhagic complications. Same-day sheath removal decreased vascular complications.

The incidence of vascular complications requiring surgical repair after stent placement procedures in the STRESS investi-

TABLE 5-8. Principal adverse events—STRESS, BENESTENT, and Registry trials: total patients ($n = 2064$)

Complication	STRESS		BENESTENT		Registry
	($n = 205$) Stent (%)	($n = 202$) Balloon (%)	($n = 259$) Stent (%)	($n = 257$) Balloon (%)	($n = 1141$) Stent (%)
Death total	1.5	1.5	0.8	0.4	1.2
Early (in hospital)	0.0	0.0	0.0	0.0	0.26
Late (out of hospital)	1.5	1.5	0.8	0.4	0.94
CABG total	4.9	8.4	6.2	4.3	6.6
Early (in hospital)	1.5	4.0	3.9	1.9	1.8
Late (out of hospital)	3.4	4.5	2.3	2.3	4.7
Myocardial infarction total	6.3	6.9	4.2	4.3	3.4
MI (in hospital)	2.9	4.0	3.5	2.7	1.9
MI (home)	3.9	3.5	0.8	1.6	1.3
Stent thrombosis total*	3.4	N/A	3.5	N/A	5.0
Early (in hospital)	1.0	N/A	3.5	N/A	3.6
Late (out of hospital)	2.4	N/A	0.0	N/A	1.3
Cerebrovascular accident	1.0	0.5	0.0	0.8	0.4
Vascular complications					
Requiring surgery	3.9	2.0	9.7	2.7	7.2
Requiring transfusion	4.9	2.0	3.9	1.2	7.4
Stent delivery failures					
On patient basis					2.8
On delivery attempt basis					0.96

* Includes only patients who received a stent.

Note: In cases where patients experienced both an in-hospital event and an out-of-hospital event, they are counted once in each group. They are counted only once in the event total. Hence, the sum of the in-hospital event rate and the out-of-hospital event rate may not equal the total event rate.

A count of delivery failure modes was available only in the Registry group. There were 37 stent delivery failures, which included 18 successful withdrawals (49%), 13 stent embolizations (35%), and 6 proximal stent deployments (16%). There were no clinical sequelae as a result of stent embolization.

gation was 4%, compared with 2% following balloon angioplasty ($p = 0.091$). The incidence of vascular complications requiring surgical repair in the BENESTENT trial was 10% for the stented patients and 2% for balloon angioplasty ($p < 0.001$). The rates for bleeding requiring transfusion were 4% in the stent group and 1% in the angioplasty group ($p = 0.045$). The risk of vascular complications may be minimized by careful adherence to the sheath-removal procedure.

Nonsurgical management using ultrasound-guided compression may be successful for treating pseudoaneurysms, depending on their size and location, even in patients on anticoagulants.

Stent thrombosis.   The following factors are associated with an increased risk of stent thrombosis (Fig. 5-13):
1. Presence of thrombus
2. Dissection not covered by the stent
3. Poor distal runoff
4. Inadequate stent expansion
5. Subtherapeutic anticoagulation
6. Vessels <2.5 mm in diameter

Elective stent thrombosis. Subacute stent thrombosis is defined as any thrombotic event occurring >24 hours after implantation. The incidence of subacute thrombosis ranges from 0% to 30%. In the STRESS trial, the incidence of stent thrombosis was 3.4% for elective stenting and 21% after stenting for abrupt closure. In the case of stenting for abrupt closure, thrombosis may occur at an average of 5 to 6 days (range 0 to 29) after implantation. It is often temporally associated with discontinuation of heparin. Using the Gianturco-Roubin

Refolding of the deflated balloon

Fig. 5-13.   Diagram of refolding deflated balloon to prevent snagging during balloon catheter removal.

stent, the incidence of thrombosis was 25% for 2-mm stents, 8.7% for 2.5-mm stents, 7.6% for 3-mm stents, 11.4% for 3.5-mm stents, and 0% for 4-mm stents.

Emergency stent thrombosis. In bailout stent procedures (i.e., stenting performed under emergency conditions after failed balloon angioplasty), the incidence of thrombosis was as high as 21%. Major risk factors for bailout stent thrombosis include poststent dissection, persistence of thrombus at the treatment site, small vessel diameters, lesions located in the LAD, and use of the stent as a bailout device (relative risk = 6.3 with 95% confidence intervals of 1.8 to 21.7).

Patients who develop stent thrombosis are at a particularly high risk for major complications including death, myocardial infarction, and emergent coronary artery bypass surgery.

Postdischarge stent thrombosis. Subacute thrombotic occlusion may occur in a small but significant proportion of the patients, usually about the third to fifth day of the implantation, but may also happen within the week following discharge. Risk factors for subacute occlusion include small vessels (<3 mm), presence of dissection after stenting, presence of filling defects, and stent placement in infarct-related vessels. Emergency (for treatment of acute closure) rather than elective (primary) implantation itself is a risk factor for late subacute occlusion. The risk of subacute thrombosis is increased when multiple overlapping stents are used, probably due to the abnormal hemodynamics and biological environment produced. Patients with these risk factors may require prolonged simultaneous intravenous and oral anticoagulation. Subacute occlusion is treated with repeat balloon dilatations and urokinase infusion.

Stent thrombosis is usually associated with electrocardiographic changes consistent with acute myocardial infarction. If stent thrombosis is suspected, a bolus of heparin should be given to help restore flow. Systemic thrombolytic therapy, an alternative to emergency coronary angioplasty, may be given. There is increased risk of hemorrhage in patients on warfarin. Emergency coronary angioplasty is usually successful in reestablishing distal vessel patency, and continuous overnight intracoronary thrombolytic infusion may prevent reoccurrence.

The most recent studies indicate stent thrombosis is 3% without the use of oral anticoagulants when optimal stent deployment in vessels 3.0 mm is achieved. Heparin-coated stents may further reduce the incidence of acute and subacute stent thrombosis.

PERIPHERAL VASCULAR STENTS

Following the techniques of percutaneous transluminal angioplasty for peripheral vascular disease as described in Chapter 11, stent placement in peripheral arteries can easily be performed.

Iliac Stent Indications

1. A stenotic or occluded atherosclerotic lesion or lesions of the common or external iliac arteries
2. A lesion that is *de novo* or restenosed after a previous PTA
3. If the balloon dilatation produces an inadequate angiographic and/or hemodynamic result, defined as an intimal dissection and/or residual stenosis ≥30% and/or a trans-stenotic mean pressure gradient of ≥ 5 mm Hg

Iliac Stent Contraindications

1. Extravasation at the target site
2. Marked tortuosity
3. Densely calcified lesions

Equipment Needed

1. Balloon catheter (or qualified stent delivery system)
2. Inflation device
3. Stent
4. Sheath introducers
5. 10F 30-cm introducer sheath
6. Crimping tool (optional)
7. 0.035-in. or 0.038-in. guidewire

Stent Preparation

1. Placing stent on balloon: Apply negative pressure to the balloon catheter using a syringe containing 10 cc of diluted contrast and clamp. The stent is slipped on the delivery catheter and positioned between the two radioopaque markers. The stent fits exactly between the two markers.

2. Crimp the stent onto the balloon with gentle manual finger compression. The plastic crimping tube (designed to protect the stent/balloon assembly during crimping) is slipped over the stent/balloon assembly. With the plastic crimping tube covering the stent/balloon assembly, it is slipped into the hole of the crimping tool. The stent should be carefully aligned within the jaws of the crimping tool. Squeeze the handles of the crimping tool until it comes to a fixed stop. The crimping tool is specially designed to stop at the precise position necessary for a secure crimp of the stent onto the balloon. Gently remove the crimping tube and stent/balloon assembly. Discard the crimping tube.

3. Visually inspect the postcrimped stent on the balloon to ensure proper placement of the stent between the markers. A gentle tug will test the stent for a secure crimp.

4. Inserting the stent into the sheath: The metal introducer tube is slipped over the stent/balloon assembly to prepare for insertion into the hemostatic valve of the 10F sheath. The stent/balloon assembly and introducer tube are advanced over the guidewire to the hemostatic valve of the sheath. The tip of the balloon catheter is then advanced into the hemostatic valve and the pointed end of the metal introducer tube protects the stent/balloon as it is advanced across the valve. Once the stent is past the hemostatic valve, the metal introducer tube is pulled out of the valve and pushed to the back end of the catheter shaft.

Stent Placement in Single Lesions

1. Vascular access and guidewire across lesion.
2. Sheath with dilator advanced across lesion.
3. Dilator removed. Sheath protects the lesion and vessel.
4. Stent/balloon assembly is advanced through sheath over guidewire and positioned at lesion. Balloon expands stent.
5. Sheath is retracted, exposing stent to lesion. Balloon is inflated, deploying the stent. Balloon is then deflated.
6. Sheath and deflated balloon are removed, leaving expanded stent in the artery creating a widely patent artery.

Techniques for Stent Placement in Chronic Iliac Artery Occlusion

1. Lesions <6 cm long:
   a. Guidewire probing
   b. Urokinase, 240,000 U/hr × 3 hours
   c. Balloon dilatation
   d. Stent
2. Lesions >6 cm long:
   a. Contralateral urokinase infusion (240,000 U/hr × 3 hr; 120,000 U/hr × 10 to 15 hours)
   b. Balloon dilatation
   c. Stent

Multiple Iliac Stents

1. When placing multiple stents, the proximal stent is placed first with the more distal stent placed second. This method is recommended to prevent equipment (e.g., sheath) from having to recross the stent lumen.
2. After the proximal stent is placed, withdraw the initial stent delivery balloon into the sheath.
3. Exchange the balloon with the sheath dilator.
4. Advance the sheath with dilator over the guidewire through the lumen of the stent past the second stent.
5. Exchange the dilator with the second stent/balloon assembly and advance through the sheath into position for placement. Slight overlapping of the stents is typically done.
6. After confirming stent position via contrast injection, pull back the sheath, exposing the stent to the vessel wall, and inflate balloon to expand stent.

Difficult Situations and Useful Techniques for Peripheral Stent Placement

Situation	Technique
Mild tortuosity	Stiff guidewire
Impaired pain sensation	Cautious stent expansion
Diseased common femoral artery	Intraoperative place
Concomitant aortoiliac aneurysm	Diagnosis by sectional imaging
Poor femoral runoff	Enhanced anticoagulation
Hypercoagulability	Prolonged anticoagulation

Medication Regimen

1. Aspirin-persantine, 48 hours before to 3 months after procedure

2. 4000-8000 units heparin/procedure (ACT 200 to 250 sec)
3. Antibiotics: routine prophylaxis if indicated

Technical Problems and Solutions

Ruptured balloon.   Exchange ruptured balloon for a new one. Loss of inflation pressure during expansion of the stent can indicate balloon perforation. If this occurs after the ends of the stent are flared and anchored in the artery wall, the balloon is deflated, rotated two or three times inside the stent, and gently pulled back inside the sheath and removed. A new balloon catheter is introduced through the sheath and positioned inside the partially expanded stent. Inflation of the new balloon catheter then completes stent expansion and deployment.

Stent deployment and balloon withdrawal.   Refolding of the deflated balloon before its withdrawal ensures that the balloon wings are not "tethered" or caught on the stent struts (Fig. 5-14):
a. Balloon inflated within artery and stent expanded
b. Deflated balloon illustrating wings of balloon flattened
c. Rotation of balloon is counterclockwise direction within stented artery to refold wings

Tethered balloon.   Sometimes the stent tends to move out of target. If by pulling back the catheter the stent moves (meaning the ends of the stent have not been expanded and anchored securely in the arterial wall), the sheath tip should be advanced to the stent to stabilize it while the balloon catheter is withdrawn into the sheath and exchanged for a new one. The new balloon catheter is advanced through the sheath into the stent lumen. Inflation of the balloon then completes stent expansion and deployment.

Stent migration.   If the delivery balloon ruptures and the stent has migrated from the target area, the sheath tip is advanced to the stent to stabilize it. The balloon catheter is then removed through the sheath and exchanged. The new balloon is then advanced through the stent lumen and partially inflated with contrast to "catch" the stent. The inflated ends of the balloon, in a dumbbell or dog-bone configuration, will apply pressure against the ends of the stent struts and prevent snagging at the lesion site. Forward motion can be attempted over the wire if no resistance is met. After reaching the target area, stent deployment is completed. If resistance

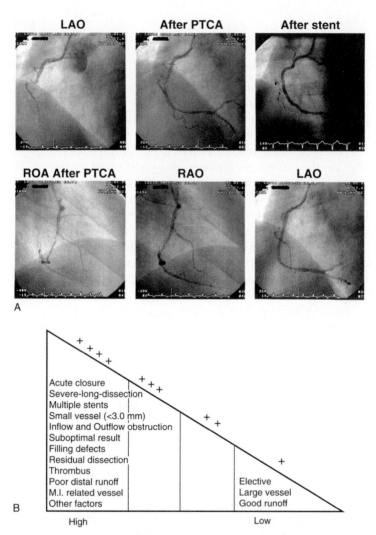

Fig. 5-14. **A,** Case example of stent thrombosis. Angiograms show proximal total right coronary artery occlusion. Recanalization by PTCA is performed with evidence of dissection (top middle). A stent is placed and a lucent filling defect is seen at the distal end of the stent (top right). Further balloon inflations reduced the presumed thrombus. LAO, Left anterior oblique view; RAO, right anterior oblique view. **B,** Diagram of factors contributing to risk of stent thrombosis. Factors associated with highest risk are shown at left. (From Gary Roubin, M.D., University of Alabama, Birmingham, Ala.)

is met when advancing the stent, do not continue. Deploy the stent. A second stent can then be introduced through the sheath and deployed at the lesion.

SUGGESTED READINGS

Argawal S, Hearn JA, Liu MW, et al.: Stent thrombosis and ischemic complications following coronary artery stenting (abstr), *Circulation* 86:I-113, 1992.

Back MG, Kopchok G, Mueller M, Cavaye D, Donayre C, White RA: Changes in arterial wall compliance after endovascular stenting, *J Vasc Surg* 19(5):905-911, 1994.

Capers Q IV, Thomas CN, Weintraub WS, King SB III, Douglas JS Jr, Scott NA: Emergent stent placement: worse outcome in patients with a recent myocardial infarction (abstr), *J Am Coll Cardiol* 71A, February 1994.

Cavaye DM, Diethrich EB, Santiago OJ, Kopchok GE, Laas TE, White RA: Intravascular ultrasound imaging: an essential component of angioplasty assessment and vascular stent deployment, *Int Angiol* 12(3):214-220, 1993.

Cavaye DM, Tabbara MR, Kopchok GE, Termin P, White RA: Intraluminal ultrasound assessment of vascular stent deployment, *Ann Vasc Surg* 5:241-246, 1991.

Cavaye DM, White RA, Kopchok GE, Mueller MP, Maselly MJ, Tabbara MR: Three-dimensional intravascular ultrasound imaging of normal and diseased canine and human arteries, *J Vasc Surg* 16:509-519, 1992.

Cavaye DM, White RA, Lerman RD, et al.: Usefulness of intravascular ultrasound imaging for detection of experimentally induced aortic dissection in dogs and for determining the effectiveness of endoluminal stenting, *Am J Cardiol* 69:705-707, 1992.

Colombo A, Hall P, Almagor Y, et al.: Results of intravascular ultrasound guided coronary stenting without subsequent anticoagulation (abstr), *J Am Coll Cardiol* 335A, February 1994.

Crowley RJ, Mann MA, Joshi SH, Lennox CD, Roberts GT: Ultrasound guided therapeutic catheters: recent developments and clinical results, *Int J Cardiol Imag* 6:145-156, 1991.

Davidson CJ, Sheikh KH, Kisslo KB, et al.: Intracoronary ultrasound evaluation of interventional technologies, *Am J Cardiol* 68:1305-1309, 1991.

Deaner ANS, Cubukcu AA, Rees MR: Assessment of coronary stent by intravascular ultrasound, *Int J Cardiol* 36:124-126, 1992.

de Feyter PJ, de Scheerder IK, van den Brand M, Laarman GJ, Suryapranata H, Serruys PW: Emergency stenting for refractory acute coronary artery occlusion during coronary angioplasty, *Am J Cardiol* 66:1147-1150, 1990.

de Jaegere PP, Serruys PW, Bertrand M, et al.: Wiktor stent implantation in patients with restenosis following balloon angioplasty of a native coronary artery, *Am J Cardiol* 69:598-602, 1992.

Diethrich EB: Endovascular treatment of abdominal aortic occlusive disease: the impact of stents and intravascular ultrasound imaging, *Eur J Vasc Surg* 7:228-236, 1993.

Fischman DL, Leon MB, Baim DS, et al., for the STRESS trial investigators: A randomized comparison of coronary stent placement and balloon angioplasty in the treatment of coronary artery disease, *N Engl J Med* 331:496–501, 1994.

Fischman DL, Savage MP, Leon MB, et al.: Angiographic predictors of subacute thrombosis following coronary stenting (abstr), *Circulation* 84:II-588, 1991.

Fischman DL, Savage MP, Leon MB, et al.: Fate of lesion related side branches after coronary stenting, *J Am Coll Cardiol* 22:1641-1646, 1993.

George BS, Voorhees WD III, Roubin GS, et al.: Multicenter investigation of coronary stenting to treat acute or threatened closure after percutaneous transluminal coronary angioplasty: clinical and angiographic outcomes, *J Am Coll Cardiol* 22:135-143, 1993.

Goy JJ, Sigwart U, Vogt P, Stauffer JC, Kappenberger L: Long-term clinical and angiographic follow-up of patients treated with the self-expanding coronary stent for acute occlusion during balloon angioplasty of the right coronary artery, *J Am Coll Cardiol* 19:1593-1596, 1992.

Haude M, Erbel R, Issa H, et al.: Analysis of risk factors for the occurrence of subacute stent thrombosis after intracoronary implantation of Palmaz-Schatz coronary stents (abstr), *J Am Coll Cardiol* 19:77A, 1992.

Haude M, Erbe R, Straub U, Dietz U, Schatz R, Meyer J: Results of intracoronary stents for management of coronary dissection after balloon angioplasty, *Am J Cardiol* 67:691-696, 1991.

Hearn JA, King SB III, Douglas JS Jr, Carlin SF, Lembo NJ, Ghazzal ZMB: Clinical and angiographic outcomes after coronary artery stenting for acute or threatened closure after percutaneous transluminal coronary angioplasty: initial results with a balloon expandable, stainless steel design, *Circulation* 88:2086-2096, 1993.

Herrmann HC, Buchbinder M, Clemen MW, et al.: Emergent use of balloon-expandable coronary artery stenting for failed PTCA, *Circulation* 86:812-819, 1992.

Holmes DR, Garratt KN, Schwartz RS, White C, for the Medtronic Wiktor Stent Investigators: Timing of stent occlusion/thrombosis after stent placement (abstr), *J Am Coll Cardiol* 70A, February 1994.

Isner JM, Rosenfield K, Losordo DW, et al.: Percutaneous intravascular US as adjunct to catheter-based interventions: preliminary experience in patients with peripheral vascular disease, *Radiology* 175:61-70, 1990.

Keren G, Douek P, Oblon C, Bonner RF, Pichard AD, Leon MB: Atherosclerotic saphenous vein grafts treated with different interventional procedures assessed by intravascular ultrasound, *Am Heart J* 124:198-206, 1992.

Keren G, Pichard AD, Kent KM, Satler LF, Leon MB: Failure or success of complex catheter-based interventional procedures assessed by intravascular ultrasound, *Am Heart J* 123:200-208, 1992.

Laskey WK, Brady ST, Kussmaul WG, et al.: Intravascular ultrasonographic assessment of the results of coronary artery stenting, *Am Heart J* 125:1576-1583, 1993.

Marsico F, Kubica J, DeServi S, et al.: The evaluation of intracoronary stents by intravascular echography, *Giornale Italiano di Cardiologia* 3(11):1091-1096, 1993.

Mintz GS, Pichard AD, Satler LF, Popma JJ, Kent KM, Leon MB: Three dimensional intravascular ultrasonography: reconstruction of endovascular stents in vitro and in vivo, *J Clin Ultrasound* 21:609-615, 1993.

Moon MR, Dake MD, Pelc LR, et al.: Intravascular stenting of acute experimental type B dissections, *J Surg Res* 54:381-388, 1993.

Mudra H, Blasini R, Regar E, Klauss V, Rieber J, Thiesen K: Intravascular ultrasound assessment of the balloon-expandable Palmaz-Schatz coronary stent, *Coro Artery Dis* 4(9):791-799, 1993.

Muller DW, Shamir KJ, Ellis SG, Topol EJ: Peripheral vascular complications after conventional and complex percutaneous coronary interventional procedures, *Am J Cardiol* 69:63-68, 1992.

Nath FC, Muller DW, Ellis SG, et al.: Thrombosis of a flexible coil coronary stent: frequency, predictors and clinical outcome, *J Am Coll Cardiol* 21:622-627, 1993.

Palmaz JC, Garcia O, Kopp DT, et al.: Balloon-expandable intraarterial stents: effect of antithrombotic medication on thrombus formation, *in* Zeitler E, Seyferth W, editors: *Pros and cons in PTA and auxiliary methods,* Berlin, Heidelberg, 1989, Springer-Verlag, pp 170-178.

Palmaz JC, Sibbitt RR, Tio FO, et al.: Expandable intraluminal vascular graft: a feasibility study, *Surgery* 99:199-205, 1986.

Palmaz JC, Windeler AS, Garcia F, et al.: Expandable intraluminal grafting in atherosclerotic rabbit aortas, *Radiology* 160:723-726, 1986.

Popma JJ, Satler LF, Pichard AD, et al.: Vascular complications after balloon and new device angioplasty, *Circulation* 88:1569-1578, 1993.

Roubin GS, Cannon AD, Agrawal SK, et al.: Intracoronary stenting for acute and threatened closure complicating percutaneous transluminal coronary angioplasty, *Circulation* 85:916-927, 1992.

Schryver TE, Popma JJ, Kent KM, Leon MB, Eldredge S, Mintz GS: Use of intracoronary ultrasound to identify the "true" coronary lumen in chronic coronary dissection treated with intracoronary stenting, *Am J Cardiol* 69:1107-1108, 1992.

Serruys PW, de Jaegere P, Kiemenij F, et al., for the BENESTENT study group: A comparison of balloon-expandable-stent implantation with balloon angioplasty in patients with coronary artery disease, *N Engl J Med* 331:489–495, 1994.

Sigwart U, Urban PH, Gold S, et al.: Emergency stenting for acute occlusion after coronary balloon angioplasty, *Circulation* 78:1121-1127, 1988.

Slepian MJ: Application of intraluminal ultrasound imaging to vascular stenting, *Int J Cardiol Imag* 6:285-311, 1991.

Spaedy TJ, Wilensky RL: Coronary stenting, *ACC Curr J Rev* 59-62, November/December 1994.

Sutton JM, Ellis GS, Roubin GS, et al., for the Gianturco-Roubin Intracoronary Stent Investigator Group: Major clinical events after coronary stenting: the multicenter registry of acute and elective Gianturco-Roubin stent placement, *Circulation* 89:1126-1137, 1994.

Tenaglia AN, Kisslo K, Kelly S, Hamm MA, Crowley R, Davidson CJ: Ultrasound guide wire-directed stent deployment. *Am Heart J* 125:1213-1216, 1993.

Trerotola SO, Lund GB, Samphilipo MA, et al.: Palmaz stent in the treatment of central venous stenosis: safety and efficacy of redilation, *Radiology* 190(2):379-385, 1994.

van der Giessen WJ, Slager CJ, Gussenhoven EJ, et al.: Mechanical features and in vivo imaging of a polymer stent, *Int J Cardiol Imag* 9(3):219-226, 1993.

6

CORONARY ATHERECTOMY, ROTATIONAL ABLATION, AND TRANSLUMINAL EXTRACTION CATHETER TECHNIQUES

Frank V. Aguirre, Ubeydullah Deligonul, and Morton J. Kern

Because atherosclerotic plaque remains in the artery after balloon dilatation, physical removal of the plaque, atherectomy (athero = plaque; ectomy = cut) from inside the coronary artery, was thought to improve the results of balloon angioplasty. Three devices developed for the purpose of plaque removal are approved for coronary intervention: the directional atherectomy catheter (DCA), the high-speed Rotablator, and the transluminal extraction catheter (TEC) (see Table 6-1). These three devices have unique mechanisms and specific indications.

223

TABLE 6-1.   Recommended DCA device selection according to vessel diameter

Atherocatheter	Maximum working diameter (mm)	Recommended artery diameter (mm)
5F	3.0	2.5 to 2.9
6F	3.5	3.0 to 3.4
7F	4.0	3.5 to 3.9
7F graft	4.5	4.0 or larger

Housing / Inflated balloon   B   −0.55 mm =   A

Circumference   Circumference

DCA, Directional coronary atherectomy.

DIRECTIONAL CORONARY ATHERECTOMY

Directional coronary atherectomy is performed using a specially designed catheter with a cylindrical metal cutting chamber that contains a rapidly rotating cylindrical cutter. The cutting chamber is 5 to 10 mm long and is pushed against the coronary lesion by a supporting balloon located on the opposite side of the cutting chamber opening. The cutter is rotated by a hand-held motor at 2000 rpm and is advanced within the cutting chamber. The operator shaves the plaque and deposits it in the nose cone of the catheter (Fig. 6-1).

Mechanisms

1. The Dotter (pushing) effect created by the bulk of the catheter (5 to 7 French) pushes the plaque aside.
2. A balloon dilatation effect caused by inflation of supporting balloons.
3. Cutting or shaving removes the plaque. This mechanism is usually the dominant one.

Indications

1. Single or multiple coronary stenoses located in vessels ≥3.0 mm in diameter in proximal segments. Patients with large vessels (>3.0 mm) and ostial or eccentric lesions that decrease the success rate with balloon cathe-

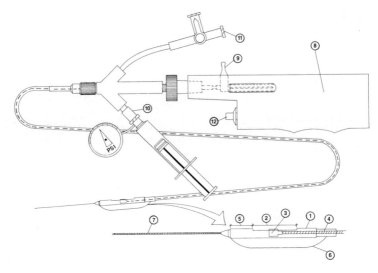

Fig. 6-1. Directional atherectomy catheter system. Components include: (1) cylindrical housing, (2) opening along housing, (3) cutter, (4) cutter drive cable, (5) specimen collection chamber, (6) balloon, (7) guidewire, (8) drive motor, (9) cutter advance lever, (10) balloon inflation port, (11) flush port, and (12) motor switch. (From Simpson JB, et al.: Directional coronary atherectomy: a symposium in interventional cardiology, *Am J Cardiol* 61:97G, 1988.)

ter dilatation are candidates for DCA. Calcified, angulated, long (>20 mm) narrowings, spiral dissections, and friable graft lesions are not suitable for DCA. Bifurcation lesions may be approached using special guidewires, but extra caution must be exercised to avoid perforation.
2. Saphenous vein graft stenoses with the following characteristics:
   a. Discrete
   b. Subtotal
   c. Accessible

Generally, lesions that are most accessible to DCA are those in the proximal or mid portion of coronary vessels. As with most angioplasty patients, patients selected for coronary atherectomy should be acceptable candidates for coronary-artery bypass graft surgery.

There is insufficient experience from multicenter studies to document the use of DCA for treatment of unstable angina or acute myocardial infarction patients. Patients who have severe peripheral vascular disease are considered at high risk for complications due to potential limb ischemia from insertion of the large (10F) sheath and guiding catheter system.

Contraindications

Contraindications for DCA are the same as for coronary balloon angioplasty. Relative contraindications include:
1. Left main coronary artery disease.
2. Lesions located in or distal to severely tortuous or densely calcified coronary vessels.
3. Calcified aorto-ostial lesions.
4. Significant ilio-femoral occlusive disease precludes insertion of large catheters and, therefore, is a relative contraindication for coronary DCA.
5. Absolute contraindications include:
   a. Patients who are not suitable for coronary artery bypass surgery
   b. Patients with totally obstructed arteries where a guidewire cannot be passed through the lesion

Equipment

1. Atherectomy catheter
2. Motor drive unit
3. Guide catheter
4. Long large sheath (10 or 11F)
5. Hemostatic valve
6. Exchange guidewire
7. Specimen preparation materials

Selection of Guide Catheters

Because of the large size of the DCA catheter and rigid cutter housing, large-lumen guide catheters with specially designed curves are needed. The right coronary catheters are 9.5 French and the left coronary catheters are 10 or 11 French. An appropriate size long sheath and a large-bore rotating hemostatic adapter are also required. The DCA guiding catheters are designed to provide more torque and more support compared to angioplasty/diagnostic catheters. Each guiding catheter is packaged with a guiding catheter introducer. It is important to use the guiding catheter introducer to ensure that there is minimal guiding catheter trauma during insertion and to maintain hemostasis. Six unique tip shapes are available, designed to accommodate the rigid housing of the DCA catheter (Fig. 6-2).

Right coronary artery DCA guides.   The three different right tip shapes are designed for various anatomical takeoffs. The most frequently seen horizontal takeoff of the right ostium requires the standard Judkins right configuration (JR) 4.0 guiding catheter. If the takeoff is oriented in an upward (superior) direction, a preferred guide is the Judkins right configuration graft (JRGRF). For the inferiorly oriented right ostia, the JR 4.0 inferior (IF) may work best.

Left coronary artery DCA guides.   The choice of a guide for engagement of the left coronary system is determined by the aortic root size. The tip shapes for the left side have a

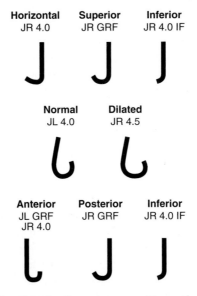

Fig. 6-2.   Directional atherectomy guide catheter shapes. JR, Judkins right configuration; GRF, graft; IF, inferior; JL, Judkins left configuration. (Modified from Freed M, Grines C, editors: *Manual of interventional cardiology*, 1992, Physician's Press, Birmingham, Michigan, p 277.)

more circular shape without acute angles in comparison to the standard Judkins curve. The circular shape accommodates the rigid housing of the DCA. The JL 3.5 is the most commonly used left DCA guide catheter. For selectively engaging the circumflex artery, a Judkins left configuration (JL) 4.0 is recommended, whereas the left anterior descending artery is readily engaged using a JL 3.5.

Vein graft DCA guide catheters.   For saphenous vein grafts placed posteriorly in the aorta, use a JRGRF. For grafts situated anteriorly, a Judkins left configuration graft (JLGRF) is recommended.

DCA guide catheter placement.   See *The Cardiac Catheterization Handbook,* pp 530-532.

The guide catheter is straightened with the long introducer catheter (7 or 8F) and advanced over a 0.038-in. J guidewire to avoid aortic vessel trauma (Fig. 6-3). This guide catheter and introducer system is advanced into the aortic root with the guidewire several centimeters in front of the introducer catheter tip. The guidewire and inner catheter introducer are then removed. The guide catheter is connected to a manifold and large-diameter Y connector flushed. The Y connector accommodates larger catheters than those used for balloon angioplasty. Because of the size and stiffness of the guide catheter, special care should be taken in manipulation, especially avoiding deep engagement of the coronary vessel. Contraindicated techniques for guiding catheter placement include:
1. Deep engagement
2. Vigorous torquing
3. Noncoaxial alignment of the guiding catheter to the ostium

The Atherectomy Catheter

Catheter sizing.   Selection of the cutting atherectomy catheter size depends on the diameter of the vessel lumen: 5F for 2.5- to 2.9-mm-diameter vessels, 6F for 3.0- to 3.4-mm, 7F for 3.5- to 3.9-mm, and 7F "graft" for 4-mm or larger vessels. In general, most vessels selected should be large enough to be treated with the 7F or 7G catheters (Table 6-1).

Atherectomy catheter preparation
1. Attach low-pressure inflation device to balloon port.
2. Aspirate 15 sec.

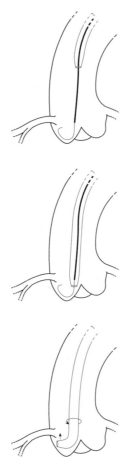

Fig. 6-3. Technique of advancing directional atherectomy catheter to the coronary ostium. Top panel shows guidewire extending to the aortic root through the guide catheter obturator within the guide catheter. Middle panel shows guide catheter advancing over the obturator with the guidewire in place. Bottom panel shows guide catheter with obturator and guidewire removed. (Modified from Freed M, Grines C, editors: *Manual of interventional cardiology*, Birmingham, Michigan, 1992, Physician's Press, p 280.)

3. Purge forward, holding end of atherocath up until the balloon is completely filled and all air bubbles are expelled (newer balloons are aspiration prep only).
4. Deflate the balloon and leave the inflation device in neutral position.
5. Inject heparinized saline into the flush port.
6. Load a 0.014-in. guidewire, either from the proximal end (cutter is kept forward) or backward from the nose cone (cutter is kept in the middle of the chamber).
7. Attach the motor drive unit over the guidewire until it snaps into the catheter adapter with the thumb toggle up.
8. A rubber band pulling the cutter thumb handle (on motor drive) forward is a helpful accessory.

Atherectomy catheter placement.   The target coronary stenosis is crossed in the usual manner with a coronary guidewire (0.014-in. diameter). The DCA catheter is advanced over the guidewire slowly by keeping constant forward tension and rotating the catheter slightly as the catheter is moved forward. Do not "jack-hammer" the catheter. The guide catheter may back up in the aorta at this time. Do not try to bring the guide catheter deep into the vessel. Slight removal of the coronary guidewire while advancing the DCA device is helpful. It may be necessary to predilate a tight lesion to allow easy passage of the cutting device. While advancing the cutting catheter over the artery curves, keep the cutting chamber opening toward the outer curvature and keep the cutter blade in a forward locked position at all times.

Atherectomy cutting sequence.   Once the cutting window is in place within the lesion (Fig. 6-4):

1. The cutter is retracted using the thumb lever on the motor drive.
2. The balloon pressure is increased to 20 to 30 psi. (**Caution:** Balloon rupture may occur at more than 60 psi or 4 atm.)
3. The motor is turned on.
4. The cutter is advanced in a slow and steady manner until it is at the end of the cutting chamber. (Failure to advance and lock the cutter fully in place risks tissue embolization and/or produces an incomplete cut, leaving an intimal flap with the potential for abrupt reclosure.)
5. The motor is turned off.
6. The balloon is deflated.

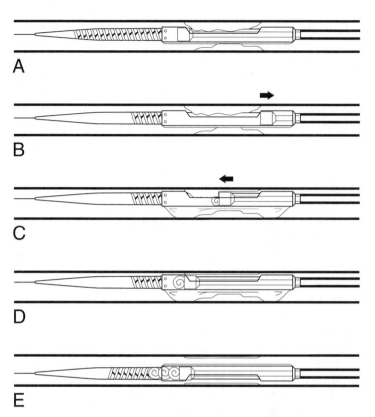

Fig. 6-4. Directional atherectomy catheter cutting sequence. **A,** Catheter housing is positioned in the coronary lesion. Cutter is forward. **B,** Cutter is retracted. **C,** Balloon is inflated and cutter motor turned on and cutter slowly advanced shaving tissue. **D,** Cutter is advanced to deposit the specimen into the nose cone chamber. **E,** Balloon is deflated. Keep the cutter forward until after the catheter is rotated to the next position. Repeat steps A to E. (From Simpson JB, Selmon MR, Robertson GC, et al.: Transluminal atherectomy for occlusive peripheral vascular disease, *Am J Cardiol* 61:96G-101G, 1988.)

7. The cutting catheter is rotated about a quarter turn and the sequence is repeated.
8. During cutting, it is important to keep the wire a few centimeters distal to the catheter tip to avoid entrapment in a small vessel.

Cautionary notes. Several cuts in at least four different directions should be made during a single passage of the device.

1. Cuts should be made principally where angiographic evidence of disease is seen. This technique will minimize the possibility of cutting into or through normal vessel wall. During catheter manipulations, the arterial pressure and electrocardiogram should be monitored for signs of ischemia. The device should be removed promptly to minimize ischemia.

2. The collection chamber is full when the cutter cannot be fully advanced within the distal housing, as seen during fluoroscopic evaluation of housing components. The position of the fully advanced cutter will be separated from the distal window edge. Cuts should not continue to be made once the collection chamber is full, since subsequent cuts may not be completed and embolization of tissue may result because the cutter cannot be fully advanced. The collection chamber may also be full when the guidewire becomes immobilized. Guidewire fracture may result when the wire becomes fixed and the motor drive unit is activated. Therefore, check guidewire freedom often, and empty the chamber when the guidewire is immobilized.

3. When there is residual narrowing (more than 20% diameter), the same device can be reintroduced to make cuts by applying higher balloon pressures. Alternatively, a larger-size device can be introduced. However, attempts to improve results by overinflating the balloon or oversizing the device increase the risk of vessel perforation. Recently, intravascular ultrasound imaging has been used to verify the amount of plaque removed. Better clinical results appear to accompany more tissue extraction.

Removal of DCA catheter. There are two ways to remove the DCA catheter. Both ways require the cutter be located in the distal section of the housing.

1. Use a 300-cm exchange guidewire.

2. Remove the guidewire and DCA together. A guidewire can be left across the lesion if it is not fixed in the distal nose cone. Experience has shown that it is best to use an exchange technique when:
   a. Wire negotiation was difficult at the initial pass
   b. Working in vein grafts

    c. Working in dissections

    d. Following predilatation

When removing the DCA catheter, put tension on the guiding catheter to prevent deep seating. If the guidewire becomes fixed, remove the guidewire with the DCA and empty the distal collection chamber. Guidewire recrossing is generally easy, because of the smooth surfaces at the atherectomy site.

Atherectomy tissue removal. Removal of tissue from the DCA catheter is best accomplished by pulling the cutter blade proximal, inserting the nose cone into a saline-filled syringe, and flushing specimens into a collection cup. Once they are dislodged from the collection chamber, specimens in the chamber may be retrieved with tweezers. Check for tissue specimens in the cutter cup. After removing tissue, the DCA catheter may be reinserted for further atherectomy. Prior to reinsertion, the guidewire lumen should be flushed with saline.

Team management for DCA

    1. One physician, one scrub technician

      a. Physician role

        (1) Guiding catheter manipulation

        (2) Wire negotiation

        (3) DCA negotiation

        (4) Cutter control

        (5) Wire control during advancement of cutter

      b. Scrub technician role

        (1) Balloon inflation/deflation device

    2. Two physicians, one scrub technician

      a. Physician$_1$ role

        (1) Guiding catheter manipulation

        (2) DCA negotiation

      b. Physician$_2$ role

        (1) Wire negotiation

        (2) Cutter control

        (3) Wire control during cutting

      c. Scrub technician role

        (1) Balloon inflation/deflation device

Saphenous Vein Graft Atherectomy

Equipment selection

    1. Guiding catheter (JR4, right bypass, left bypass); remember that coaxial alignment of guiding catheter and minimizing deep seating are important.

  2. Atherectomy catheter
     a. 7F devices with 3.5-mm and 4.0-mm working diameters
     b. 7G devices with 4.5-mm working diameters

Case selection

Operator experience is the most important factor in patient selection.
  a. Old, diffusely diseased grafts should be avoided.
  b. Restenotic vein graft lesions have a higher restenosis rate.
  c. DCA of internal mammary artery grafts has not been reported.

Restenosis rates after DCA in saphenous vein grafts are not better than those after balloon angioplasty.

Criteria for Successful Atherectomy

Three criteria are used in combination to evaluate atherectomy results:
  1. An artery with angiograpically smooth borders
  2. Residual stenoses in the range of 5% to 20%
  3. An average number of tissue samples removed ranging from 5 to 13 samples weighing >5 mg

Anticoagulation and Sheath Removal

Administration of heparin follows standard balloon angioplasty technique (10,000 U IV bolus, 1000 U/hr infusion). During the procedure, the patient should be well anticoagulated, with an activated clotting time (ACT) over 350 sec. Early sheath removal (≥4 hour after the procedure) has been advocated. However, the occurrence of some late subacute occlusions must be balanced against the risk of keeping the sheath in overnight with intravenous heparinization.

Because of the large size of the sheaths, distal leg pulses should be checked frequently. In case of limb ischemia, the atherectomy sheath should be removed promptly. Longer arterial puncture-site compression and periods of bed rest are necessary after atherectomy sheath removal. A vascular clamp or other mechanical artery compression system may be helpful.

Complications

Because of the large size of atherectomy sheaths, arterial complications are the most significant source of morbidity and mortality, especially in elderly patients. Other complications of DCA include proximal vessel dissection, thrombotic or atherosclerotic emboli to uninvolved adjacent branches, vasospasm, coronary ostial injury, myocardial infarction, or death.

Several helpful points to remember to minimize complications with DCA are:
1. Cut only where disease is present.
2. Avoid large devices in small vessels.
3. Avoid extensive angioplasty dissections.
4. Use low inflation pressures (≤30 psi).
5. Avoid bifurcation and ostial techniques prone to perforation (Fig. 6-5).

For management of DCA-induced dissection:
1. Evaluate type of dissection and vessel wall integrity.
2. If a discrete flap or a minor linear dissection is present, DCA may help.
3. Use a small device (6F), low pressure, and accept an adequate lumen without pristine borders.
4. Do not use atherectomy on spiral dissections.
5. Consider stenting.

Postatherectomy Follow-up and Restenosis (Table 6-2)

Routine follow-up is similar to that for regular balloon angioplasty. Restenosis after atherectomy occurs at a rate and time similar to that for balloon angioplasty. A recent randomized study suggested a small restenosis benefit with DCA as com-

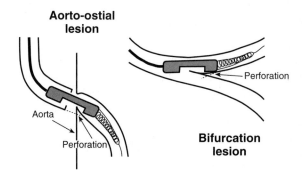

Fig. 6-5.   Diagram of directional atherectomy catheter positioning in the ostial lesion (left panel) and at bifurcation points (right panel). Extra caution is needed to avoid perforating the vessel at these high-risk locations. (From Topol EJ: *Textbook of interventional cardiology,* 2 ed, Philadelphia, 1994, W. B. Saunders, p 594.)

TABLE 6-2. Distribution of angiographic restenosis for lesions initially treated successfully using DCA device and for which follow-up angiograms are available

Lesion characteristic	Denovo lesions			Restenotic lesions		
	n	RST	%	n	RST	%
Native arteries:	112	34	30	206	94	46
RCA	26	7	27	57	26	46
LAD	75	26	35	133	65	49
LCX	8	1	13	13	2	15
LM	3	0	0	3	1	33
Ostial location	17	8	47	7	2	29
Proximal location	60	16	27	118	49	42
Mid location	29	9	31	72	39	54
Distal location	6	1	17	9	4	44
Focal lesion (<10 mm)	62	15	24	95	30	32
Tubular lesion (10 to 20 mm)	38	16	42	91	54	59
Diffuse lesion (>20 mm)	12	3	25	20	10	50
Eccentric lesion	78	23	29	110	42	38
Concentric lesion	34	11	32	96	52	54
Calcified lesion	16	2	13	26	16	62
Noncalcified lesion	96	32	33	180	78	43
Saphenous vein grafts	32	10	31	34	23	68

DCA, Directional coronary atherectomy; LCX, left circumflex coronary artery; LAD, left anterior descending coronary artery; LM, left main coronary artery, RCA, right coronary artery; RST, restenosis.

pared to balloon angioplasty in patients with proximal left anterior descending artery lesions. Restenosis after DCA is less in patients with <20% residual narrowing in those with reference-vessel lumen diameter of ≥3 mm. Since some studies indicated increased complications with DCA, the risk/benefit ratio should be carefully evaluated in each patient.

Figure 6-6 illustrates an angioplasty with adjunctive DCA guided by intravascular ultrasound imaging (IVUS).

ROTATIONAL ATHERECTOMY (ROTABLATOR)

The Rotablator is made of an olive-shaped steel burr (1.25 to 2.5 mm in diameter) (Fig. 6-6) that is embedded with microscopic diamond particles on the front half and is rotated with a torque wire at ≤200,000 rpm by an external air turbine (Fig. 6-7). The device is inserted through 8F to 10F guide catheters over a special 0.009-in. steel guidewire. A continuous pressurized heparin saline infusion is flushed through the device drive shaft to aid lubrication and heat dissipation.

Indications

Percutaneous transluminal coronary rotational atherectomy (PTCRA) with the Rotablator system as a sole therapy or with adjunctive balloon angioplasty is indicated in patients with coronary artery disease who are acceptable candidates for coronary artery bypass graft surgery and who meet one of the following selection criteria:

1. Single-vessel atherosclerotic coronary artery disease with a calcified stenosis that can be passed with a guidewire
2. Low-risk, multiple-vessel coronary artery disease
3. Restenosis of the native vessel
4. Native vessel atherosclerotic coronary artery disease that is <25 mm in length

Complementary or adjunctive balloon therapy is used ≥75% of the time. Larger vessels (>2.5 mm) may require the use of complementary or adjunctive balloon dilation more frequently than smaller vessels, since the largest Rotablator burrs are 2.50 mm in diameter.

High-Risk Rotablator

Operators should be aware of the higher risk conditions for PTCRA and the current lack of scientific evidence for these applications. High-risk conditions and patients include:

1. Patients who are not candidates for coronary artery bypass surgery
2. Patients with severe, diffuse, three-vessel disease (multiple diseased vessels should be treated in separate sessions)
3. Patients with unprotected left main coronary artery disease
4. Patients with ejection fraction <30%
5. Lesions longer than 25 mm in length
6. Angulated (≥45° lesions)

Contraindications

Contraindications to the use of the Rotablator include:

1. Occlusions through which a guidewire will not pass
2. Last remaining vessel with compromised left ventricular function
3. Saphenous vein grafts

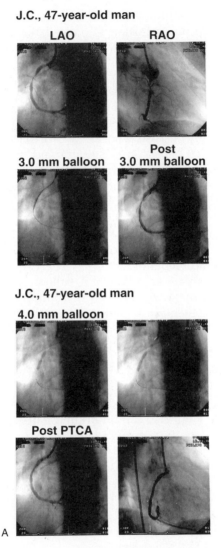

Fig. 6-6. Case example of sequential PTCA and directional atherectomy catheter guided by intravascular ultrasound imaging (IVUS). (A, top panels) Angiograms demonstrating severe proximal right coronary stenosis in a 47-year-old man with rest angina. Calcifications are not visible angiographically. A 3.0-mm balloon is inadequate at 12 atm, and a 4.0-mm balloon is used at high pressure (lower panels) with a marginal result.

J.C., 47-year-old man

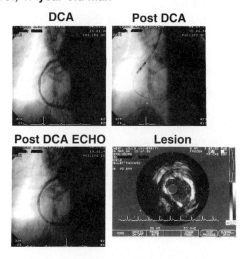

Fig. 6-6. (*Continued*). (**B,** top panels) IVUS images with corresponding angiography. IVUS in lesion shows considerable residual plaque. Lower panels show the DCA catheter in place with angiography after DCA cutting and IVUS. The IVUS image is considerably improved and now shows deep calcifications not previously identified.

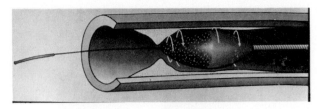

Fig. 6-7. Diagram of the rotational ablation catheter (From Rotablator manual of operations, Heart Technology, Bellevue, Washington.)

4. Angiographic evidence of thrombus
5. Angiographic evidence of significant dissection at the treatment site. (The patient may be treated conservatively for approximately 4 weeks to permit the dissection to heal before treating the lesion with the Rotablator system.)

Complications

Complications associated with the use of the Rotablator system have been compiled from the multicenter registry as of April 1993. PTCRA is associated with the following procedural complications:

Clinical events

1. Access-site bleeding of significance (1.9%)
2. Distal embolization (0.3%)
3. Intimal dissection (13.7%)
4. Acute vessel closure (4.0%)
5. Vessel perforation or tear (0.7%)
6. Emergency surgery; vascular repair or bypass (2.5%)
7. Contrast reaction (0.07%)
8. Stroke (0.0%)
9. Myocardial infarction (1.1%)
   (creatine phosphokinase [CPK] enzyme elevation without myocardial infarction [13.0%])
10. Arrhythmia requiring treatment (2.7%)
11. Cardiac tamponade (0.1%)
12. Death (1.0%)

Angiographic complications

1. No reflow (0-7%)
2. Intimal dissection with dye stain (3%)
3. Intimal dissection without dye stain (11%)

4. Acute vessel closure (5%)
5. Vessel perforation or tear (1%)
6. Arrhythmia (3%)

No or slow flow after Rotablator ablation.   No/slow flow is the occurrence of no blood flow (no flow) or blood flow reduced by one angiographic thrombolysis in myocardial infarction study (TIMI) flow grade (slow flow) in the treated artery despite the fact that the treated segment is patent. No or slow flow is believed to occur because of the transient increase in blood viscosity due to the presence of microparticles or vasospasm at the level of the distal microvasculature. No or slow flow has been observed in 6% to 7% of PTCRA patients (Figs. 6-8A and 6-8B). No or slow flow can be minimized by:

1. Advancing the burr slowly
2. Using a stepped burr approach (smaller, then larger) in long or calcified lesions
3. Using a "pecking" motion at the plaque to avoid blocking the arterial lumen
4. Maintaining maximum blood flow by repeated flushing with saline (bolus of 10 to 30 cc)
5. Using guide catheters with side holes
6. Maintaining the left ventricular filling pressures (and mean arterial pressure) by appropriately increasing the volume status of the patient

No or slow flow generally resolves within a short period of time (<15 min) with the use of nitroglycerin. Intracoronary verapamil (200 μg) has been reported to improve no or slow reflow.

Equipment Needed for Rotational Ablation

1. Rotablator burr
2. Turbine motor drive unit
3. Heparinized, pressurized, warm flush solution
4. Type A, C Rotablator wire
5. Guidewire clip
6. 8F to 10F guide catheter and arterial sheath
7. Exchange catheter/guidewire
8. Temporary pacemaker

The PTCRA system (Fig. 6-9) uses a high-speed, rotating, diamond-coated burr to ablate occlusive material and restore luminal patency. The burr tracks over a 0.009-in. (0.23-mm), specially designed guidewire that can be independently ad-

J.C., 47-year-old man

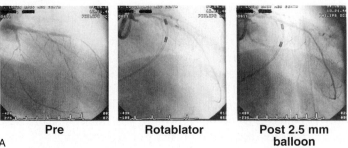

Pre	Rotablator	Post 2.5 mm
A | | | balloon |

Fig. 6-8. Case example of rotational ablation. The mid left anterior descending artery has a calcified 99% stenosis associated with reversible ischemia after myocardial infarction. Long-standing coronary artery disease in the circumflex was not symptomatic. **A,** Angiograms of left coronary artery before (left), during Rotablator 1.75-mm burr (middle), and after Rotablator (right). **B,** Although the initial Rotablator result was satisfactory, angiographic and measured flow velocity (Doppler guidewire velocity trend) showed slow then no reflow, subsequently treated with balloon inflations, intracoronary nitroglycerin, and verapamil. Flow was restored and the procedure completed without complication. Flow velocity trend scale 0 to 100 cm/sec. (From Khoury AF, Bacj RG, Kern MJ: Influence of adjunctive balloon angioplasty on coronary blood flow after rotational atherectomy, *Cath CV Diagn* 35: 272-276, 1995.)

vanced and steered. The guidewire comes with a 0.017-in. (maximum) spring tip (0.43 mm in diameter), facilitating negotiation of the wire through the vasculature.

The Rotablator burr is advanced on an independent extension, permitting accurate positioning and forward motion. A compressed-gas turbine located within the Rotablator advancer spins the flexible drive shaft and the diamond-coated burr. It is designed with minimal rotational mass so that it can be started and stopped abruptly. The controls provide good operator feedback and sensitivity.

Components of the PTCRA System

The seven main components of the PTCRA are the guidewire, the drive shaft and burr, the drive shaft sheath, the advancer,

J.C., 47-year-old man

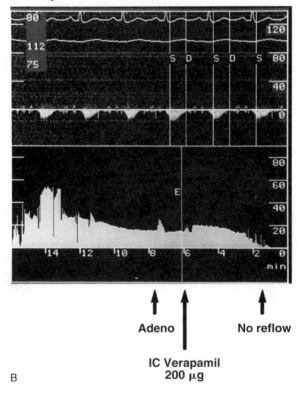

Fig. 6-8. (*Continued*).

the control console, the foot pedal, and the compressed-gas supply.

Rotablator guidewire.   Two types of guidewires are generally used. Type A has a diameter of 0.009 in. (0.23 mm) and has a spring tip (0.17 in. maximum, 0.43 mm in diameter) and a safety core that extends to the end of the spring tip. Type C is 0.0009 in. (0.23 mm) in diameter and tapers at the distal end, terminating in a flexible, formable platinum spring that is 0.017 in. maximum (0.43 mm) with a safety core that extends to within 0.5 in. (12.71 mm) of the end of the spring. The guidewire tip is atraumatic and radioopaque. The wire shaft of the guidewires is constructed of polished stainless

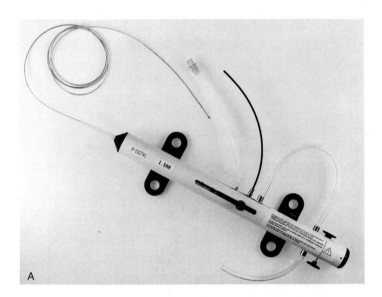

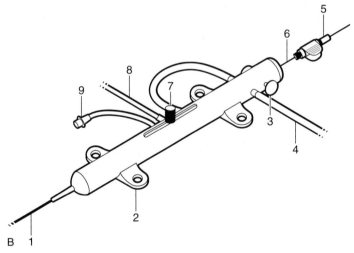

Fig. 6-9. **A,** Rotablator burr advancer unit. **B,** Diagram of components: (1) drive shaft sheath, (2) stabilizing foot, (3) break defeat knob, (4) air pressure hose for advancer, (5) wire Clip on, (6) Rotablator wire, (7) burr position control knob, (8) fiber-optic tachometer cable, (9) pressurized saline infusion port. (Modified from Rotoblator manual of operations, Heart Technology, Bellvue, Washington.)

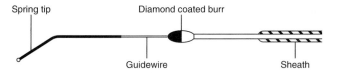

Fig. 6-10. Rotablator guidewire with burr through sheath assembly. (Modified from Rotoblator manual of operations, Heart Technology, Bellevue, Washington.)

steel. The tip can be bent or preformed to form a steerable system (Fig. 6-10). The wireClip torquer is specially designed to be used to manipulate the PTCRA wire (Fig. 6-11).

Because of the torque responsiveness, the Rotablator guidewire is more difficult to handle than commercially available guidewires used in coronary angioplasty.

Burr and shaft. The diamond-coated burr consists of a tapered body coated with fine diamond abrasive. The burr spins at high speed and ablates occlusive tissue into fine particles that are carried distally and removed by the reticuloendothelial system. If too large a quantity of particles is generated per unit time, a no- or slow-flow phenomenon may occur. The burr is driven by a flexible helical shaft that has a central

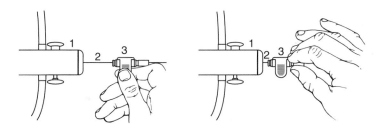

Fig. 6-11. Manipulation of the unique wire Clip on the Rotablator guidewire: (1) advancer unit, (2) Rotablator guidewire, (3) Wire Clip. (Left panel) Pinching wings of wire Clip permits attachment to guidewire. (Right panel) The end of the wire Clip can then be used as a torque tool to rotate and steer the guidewire in the distal coronary artery. (Modified from Rotoblator manual of operations, Heart Technology, Bellevue, Washington.)

lumen to permit passage of the guidewire. The shaft and burr are delivered to the coronary lesion using standard angioplasty guidewire technique. The shaft is capable of transmitting rotary motion at speeds up to 190,000 rpm. Table 6-3 provides recommended advancer turbine speeds.

Burr shaft sheath.   The sheath is 0.058 in. (1.4 mm) in diameter, constructed of Teflon, and is beveled at the tip to allow easy passage in the vessel. The proximal end of the Rotablator sheath is permanently attached to the front of the advancer body. The sheath functions are:
1. To guide the helical drive from the point of entry to the site of the lesion
2. To protect the arterial tissue from the spinning drive shaft
3. To lubricate the drive shaft.

Burr advancer.   The advancer acts as a support for the air turbine and the control for the sliding elements for burr extension. A *brake* within the advancer body is designed to hold the guidewire firmly during burr rotation to prevent the wire from spinning or moving. Manipulation of the burr control knob and the wireClip torquer allows independent

TABLE 6-3.   Recommended Rotablator advancer turbine speed

Available for:	Burr size (mm)	Burr size (French)	Design rotational speed range (rpm) [1/min]*	Optimum rotational speed range (no tissue contact) (rpm)
CV	1.25	3.75	150,000 to 190,000	180,000
CV	1.50	4.50	150,000 to 190,000	180,000
CV	1.75	5.25	150,000 to 190,000	180,000
CV	2.00	6.00	150,000 to 190,000	180,000
CV	2.15	6.45	140,000 to 180,000	160,000
CV	2.25	6.75	140,000 to 180,000	160,000
CV	2.50	7.50	140,000 to 180,000	160,000

Rotablator catheter sheath O.D.		
Size (mm)	Size (French)	Size (in.)
1.35	4.0	0.058

* Preset speed outside of the body at the higher rotational speed. (For example, for a 1.25-mm Rotablator advancer, set speed outside body at 190,000 rpm [1/min].)
From *Rotablator operations manual,* Heart Technology, Bellevue, Washington.

extension of the guidewire tip and burr. The use of compressed gas to generate the high rotational speeds necessary for ablation and low inertial mass permits the driving elements to be started and stopped quickly.

Control console. The console monitors and controls the rotational speed of the burr and provides the operator with continuous performance information during the procedure. The main features and functions on the front panel of the console are:

1. On/off switch
2. Turbine pressure (rotational speed) adjustment, to regulate the gas pressure to the turbine and, consequently, the rotational speed
3. Turbine pressure gauge: The pressure gauge displays the pressure of the compressed gas being supplied to the advancer gas turbine. The higher the gas pressure to the gas turbine, the faster is the rotational speed. The pressure should not exceed 70 psi (4.8 bar) during normal operation. A pressure-relief valve will prevent the delivery of excessive pressure to the advancer.
4. Rotational speed (tachometer): The rotational speed display indicates the speed in rpm of the burr. The display is blank when the gas turbine is not operating.
5. Stall light: Stall detection is a safety feature designed to discontinue delivery of compressed gas to the advancer in the event of excessive mechanical loading or incorrect connection of the fiber optic. Releasing the foot pedal will clear the stall condition and extinguish the stall light. The stall light, located immediately below the rotational speed display, is visible only when the rotational speed of the advancer falls below 150,000 rpm for more than 0.5 sec. When this occurs, delivery of compressed gas to the advancer is discontinued. A stall condition may also be detected if the fiber-optic connection is not engaged properly.
6. Event time: The event timer records how long the foot pedal has been continuously depressed with the air turbine and burr spinning. Depressing the foot pedal resets and restarts the timer.
7. Procedure time: The procedure time is the sum of the individual event times and indicates the total time the burr has been spinning during the procedure.

8. Fiber-optic tachometer cable connectors: The fiber-optic tachometer cable carries light pulses, which the console uses to determine the gas turbine and burr speed.

Rotational Ablation Technique
Routine technique

1. The guide catheter is placed using balloon angioplasty guide catheter technique. Table 6-4 indicates internal diameter of the guide catheter required for various burr sizes.
2. The maximum burr diameter should be no larger than 70% to 80% of the normal arterial luminal reference segment diameter.
3. The special Rotablator guidewire is positioned across the lesion. In some cases, a 0.014-in. angioplasty guidewire is needed to negotiate diffusely diseased vessels and then exchanged using a small tracking catheter for the Rotablator guidewire.
4. The infusion port on the advancer is connected to a 1-L pressurized bag of saline with macro drip tubing and used to ensure steady infusion against arterial pressure. The recommended pressure is 150 to 200 mmHg. The saline should flow through the advancer and sheath and exit from the sheath tip running bubble free.

TABLE 6-4. Recommended guide catheter sizes for use with the coronary Rotablator

Rotablator burr size (mm)	Recommended guide catheter internal diameter (in.)	Guide French size*
1.25	0.053	8
1.50	0.063	8
1.75	0.073	8
2.00	0.083	9
2.15	0.089	9
2.25	0.093	9
2.50	0.102	10

* For a given French size catheter, the inside diameter will vary from manufacturer to manufacturer. These French sizes assume thin-wall (high-volume flow) catheters with side holes, which are now being offered by a number of manufacturers. When using a guide catheter for the first time, it should be tested with the larger Rotablator advancer burr intended to be used with it.

From *Rotablator operations manual,* Heart Technology, Bellevue, Washington.

Warning: The Rotablator advancer should never be operated without saline infusion.

5. The burr is advanced through the guide catheter and tested. Be sure pressure flush is running; burr speed is ≥160,000 to 200,000 rpm.

6. After the burr is positioned immediately proximal to the lesion, advancer tension is released so the burr does not jump forward. The system is activated and the burr is advanced through the lesion in a slow and steady manner.

7. Several burr passes are performed before removal of the burr and decision for larger size burr or complementary balloon inflation is made.

8. Most (>75%) cases require additional angioplasty balloon inflations to decrease the residual stenosis.

9. Coaxial guide and burr alignment to ostium and vessel course is important.

Compressed-gas cylinder care

1. A nitrogen compressed-gas cylinder with pressure regulator capable of delivering at least 140 L/min at 90 to 100 psi is required.

2. The compressed-gas cylinder valve must be open to supply compressed gas to the console. The regulator should be adjusted so that it never supplies more than 100 psi.

Clinical Results

PTCRA is most suitable for rigid, calcified, and long lesions in which balloon angioplasty success is expected to be low. The complication and restenosis rates are similar to balloon angioplasty, although no randomized comparisons have been published. A specific complication of PTCRA is temporary no-reflow phenomenon with CK enzyme rise (non-Q-wave myocardial infarction) in some patients.

The Rotablator multicenter registry (2953 procedures and 3717 lesions) evaluated the safety and efficacy of PTCRA as a standalone procedure or with adjunctive coronary angioplasty for the treatment of coronary artery stenosis. The clinical data based on the findings from 22 clinical sites as reported to the FDA indicated primary success (defined as a <50%

luminal diameter with at least a 20% reduction in overall stenosis and no major complications, with or without complementary balloon angioplasty) was 95% with the use of adjunctive balloon angioplasty. The data showed no statistical difference in the overall primary success rate when segmented by lesion characteristics.

Restenosis

The results of most clinical studies indicate that the restenosis rate for patients treated with PTCRA is not different from the restenosis rate obtained for patients treated with balloon angioplasty or other interventional devices.

Because the procedure is relatively new, the exact long-term effectiveness of percutaneous rotational angioplasty with the Rotablator system is not fully known. A case illustration with Rotablator and IVUS luminal response is shown in Fig. 6-12.

Recommended Training

This system should be used only by physicians who are credentialed in angioplasty and who have obtained proper training in the technique of rotational angioplasty. The minimum requirements for the primary user include:

1. The physician must be accredited and qualified to perform coronary angioplasty at his or her local institution.
2. The physician must perform a minimum of 75 coronary angioplasties per year.

TRANSLUMINAL EXTRACTION CATHETER ATHERECTOMY

The TEC system operates over a guidewire and recanalizes coronary vessels by debulking and removing atherosclerotic material. The TEC is a hollow tube with a conical cutter at the tip. Cutting-tip rotation (750 rpm) with vacuum aspiration is applied to the device by means of a complex, hand-held drive unit while advancing the cutter through the lesion over the special ball-tipped, 0.014-in. guidewire (Fig. 6-13). The large size of the device (from 5.5F to 7.5F) necessitates specially designed 10F guide catheters. The microsurgical cutting component shaves intraluminal obstruction, while the vacuum feature extracts the excised debris. The device appears to be most useful in lesions complicated by thrombus.

K.L., 47-year-old man, rota, PTCA

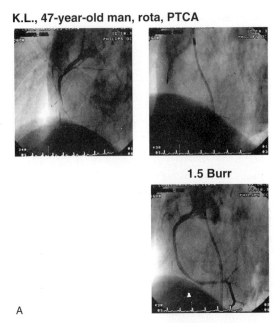

1.5 Burr

A

Fig. 6-12.   Case example of rotational ablation and PTCA with IVUS. **A,** Arteriograms of right coronary artery with 99% calcified stenosis in the mid portion of the vessel. A 1.5-mm burr is used and 3.0-mm angioplasty balloon produces an acceptable angiographic result. **B,** IVUS after PTCA shows residual plaque and heavily calcified vessel at the lesion (site *b*). Site *a* and site *c* are proximal and distal to lesion, respectively. Based on these data, no further intervention was performed.

Indications

Although lesion selection is not precisely defined for TEC, long, saphenous vein bypass graft lesions and lesions with thrombus appear to be most suitable for treatment with this device. The TEC system is also indicated for percutaneous transluminal atherectomy of native coronary arteries.

Patients should be candidates for percutaneous transluminal coronary angioplasty. In a majority of TEC cases, balloon angioplasty is used as an adjunctive procedure.

Because the TEC system operates ''over the wire,'' the TEC guidewire must be able to cross a lesion for the system to be

K.L., Post rota, post PTCA

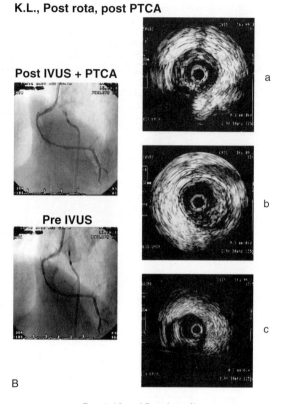

B

Fig. 6-12. (*Continued*).

utilized. In general, lesions in native coronary arteries that are located only in the proximal or mild vessels are accessible to the TEC. However, the entire length of bypass grafts usually is accessible because of the large size of the graft diameter and the absence of tortuosity and taper.

Lesion criteria include:

1. Significant atherosclerotic disease and/or thrombus in native coronary arteries and bypass grafts, whether previously untreated or restenosed from previous intervention
2. Aorto-ostial, proximal, mid, or sometimes distal target lesions that are short and discrete or long and diffuse
3. Single- or multiple-vessel disease, if treating the latter does not pose unacceptable risk to the patient, such as unpro-

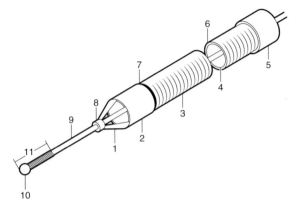

Fig. 6-13. Transluminal extraction catheter: (1) cutting blade, (2) cutting housing, (3) wire-wound catheter shaft, (4) inner liner, (5) end cap of catheter, (6) outer coating, (7) tapering connection to cutter, (8) guidewire lumen, (9) guidewire, (10) 0.020-in. ball tip, and (11) 2-cm spring coil. (From TEC operations manual, Interventional Technologies, Inc., San Diego, California.)

tected left main disease, highly calcified lesions, or total occlusions of native coronary arteries

Contraindications

Contraindications include:
1. Occlusions of any length through which a guidewire will not pass
2. Internal mammary arteries
3. Calcified lesions that have not responded to balloon angioplasty
4. Coronary ectasia
5. Relative contraindications include:
   a. Untreated, severe peripheral vascular disease
   b. Severe eccentricity or angulation of the target lesion
   c. Evidence of dissection
   d. Bleeding diathesis, including ongoing thrombolytic drug therapy
   e. Native coronary arteries with diffuse disease >20 mm in length
   f. Total occlusions in native coronary arteries
   g. Arterial segments with evidence of spasm

Complications

Percutaneous TEC may give rise to the following complications:

1. Access-site bleeding or infection
2. Hematoma
3. Angina
4. Arterial dissection
5. Arterial spasm
6. Distal embolization
7. Thrombosis
8. Acute vessel closure
9. Acute myocardial infarction
10. Ventricular fibrillation
11. Vessel perforation
12. Emergency coronary artery bypass surgery
13. Stroke
14. Death

Lesion Selection by Location, Morphology, and Type

The following lesion types may exceed TEC or experienced physician capabilities and are not recommended. Physicians performing TEC should take care to avoid the anatomical configurations listed below.

Vessel location.   As in coronary angioplasty, unprotected left main coronary arteries should always be avoided. Because of the size difference between the vein graft and the native artery, as well as the angle at which the graft is frequently sewn, distal saphenous vein graft anastomoses should be avoided.

Vessel angulation.   Both arterial and saphenous vein graft takeoffs that are sharply angled in a superior orientation should be avoided. The anatomical situation is extremely difficult to engage with a guiding catheter and causes substantial resistance to the rotation of the TEC system.

The proximal vessel anatomy should be as straight as possible to avoid sharp angles, tortuosities, sharp bends, and bifurcations within 3.0 cm of the target lesion. Special care should be taken to avoid lesions involving bifurcations associated with an acute angle. The integrity of the artery, as well as that of the cutting catheter shaft, may be compromised.

Lesion length and vessel size.   In native artery disease, it is recommended that one avoid total occlusions and lesions >20 mm in length and those containing severe ectasia. Also, avoid lesions in arteries that are smaller than 2.3 mm in diameter.

Lesion calcification.   Do not perform TEC in lesions which demonstrate severe calcium on fluoroscopy or cineangiography, especially in those lesions that appear to be cylindrical in morphology. Frequently, calcified or highly fibrous lesions are not recognized prior to choosing the treatment method.

When encountering lesions that, for any reason, do not yield to the advancement of the cutter catheter, stop. If the slide control will not move forward after significant forward pressure has been applied, and if you do not observe the cutter head to be moving forward on fluoroscopy, retract the slide control and consider choosing an alternative method of treating this lesion.

Equipment

1. TEC (catheter)
2. Motor drive with rear extension vacuum tube
3. Coronary power pack
4. TEC guidewire
5. Rotating dual hemovalve kit
6. Guiding catheter
7. Vacuum bottle

Device Components

The TEC device contains the following components (see also Fig. 6-14):

Component	Function
1. Motor	Provides cutter rotation.
2. Gears	Transfers motor rotation to the drive shaft.
3. Gear lock	Locks the motor while opening and closing the collet.
4. Collet	Locks the drive shaft onto the torque tube.
5. Drive shaft	Transmits rotational energy to the cutting catheter from the motor/gear assembly.
6. Actuator	Activates rotation of the torque tube and vacuum of excised material.
7. Slider	Advances and retracts the cutting catheter within the vessel (3.6-cm excursion).
8. Rotator	Allows the TEC drive to be connected to the dual hemovalve via a luer lock.

9. Inserter guide	A prepositioned arrowlide guide that directs the cutting catheter through the central lumen of the TEC drive during system preparation. The inserter guide protects the cutting catheter's microtome-sharp blades and prevents damage to the internal vacuum seal of the TEC drive.
10. Rear extension	The rear extension is a hollow plastic tube, 16 in. in length, which attaches to the back of the TEC drive. It is constructed with a luer-type connection at the distal end and an adjustable guidewire seal at the proximal end. The rear extension allows the guidewire to extend through the proximal end and be locked in place, while maintaining system vacuum. Another function is to contain the cutting catheter during advancement and retraction.

TEC Atherectomy Technique

Careful patient selection and device handling will reduce the possibility of dissection and vascular perforation. The TEC cutting catheter selected should not exceed the luminal diame-

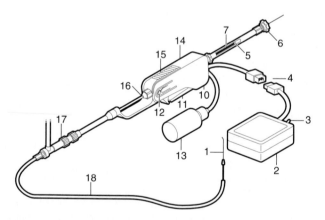

Fig. 6-14.   Transluminal extraction catheter system: (1) guide-wire, (2) power, (3) on–off switch, (4) power connection to motor drive unit, (5) wire guide in (6) connecting tube, (7) lumen, (8) and (9) not included in figure, (10) motor drive, (11) advancer release, (12) lock, (13) aspiration vacuum bottle, (14) motor drive case, (15) advancer, (16) catheter lock, (17) Y connector to guide catheter, and (18) guide catheter. (From TEC operations manual, Interventional Technologies, Inc., San Diego, California.)

ter of the artery proximal or distal to the lesion. The maximum cutter size should be 0.5 mm less than the arterial lumen diameter.

1. Heparinize the patient according to laboratory protocols for complex angioplasty.
2. Prepare a pressure bag of 1000 cc of normal saline with heparin added to use as flush solution.
3. Use a standard, percutaneous, retrograde, femoral approach to place the introducer sheath and guiding catheter.
4. Assemble the TEC catheter and aspirating system.
5. Position the tip of the guiding catheter into the ostium of the target artery or graft.
6. Introduce the TEC guidewire into the guide catheter and position the guidewire across the target lesion. Position the guidewire several centimeters beyond the target lesion to avoid cutter contact with the coiled portion of the guidewire during the procedure. Once in place, secure the guidewire by tightening the hemovalve.
7. Open the guidewire seal on the rear extension of the TEC drive to allow passage of the guidewire.
8. Back-feed the proximal end of the guidewire through the previously assembled TEC system.
9. Advance the TEC catheter to the target stenosis.
10. Activate the motor drive and slowly advance the TEC cutter while aspirating material. Repeat angiogram and TEC cutter advancement as needed.

Clinical Results

Clinical results for TEC data from a multicenter procedure registry involving 19 American institutions concluding data analysis entered by December 1991 on 1147 patients with 1318 lesions demonstrated satisfactory outcomes in normal coronary arteries (51%) and saphenous vein grafts (49%) of the population. A successful procedure was defined as the ability of the TEC device alone to cross the entire lesion with reduction of the stenosis by at least 20% and improvement in TIMI grade flow by one level. A ≤50% stenosis at the end of the procedure, with or without adjunctive balloon angioplasty, was considered angiographic success. For native coronary arteries, success rates range from 81% to 91%. TEC

TABLE 6-5.   Atherectomy device comparison

	Atherocatheter	Rotablator	TEC
Speed	Low rpm (2000)	High rpm (180,000)	Low rpm (750)
Mechanism	Side cutting	Ablation	Forward cutting
Material handling	Manual debris removal	No debris removal	Simultaneous debris removal

plus balloon angioplasty achieved a 91% success rate in both native and saphenous vein grafts. Lesion length did not affect the success rate. Six-month follow-up, available in 74% of registry patients, demonstrated an overall clinical restenosis rate of 38%. In subgroup analysis for TEC standalone cases, restenosis occurred in 40% of patients. TEC plus balloon angioplasty had a restenosis rate of 37%. The saphenous vein graft clinical restenosis rate was 42%, and for TEC standalone restenosis the rate was 47%. Angiographic follow-up available in 50% of the native arteries and 41% of the saphenous vein grafts demonstrated angiographic restenosis for TEC standalone of 54% and TEC plus adjunctive balloon angioplasty of 49%. For saphenous vein grafts, angiographic restenosis for TEC stand alone was 66% and for TEC plus adjunctive angioplasty was 59%.

A summary of the three atherectomy devices is provided in Table 6-5.

SUGGESTED READINGS

Demer L, Gould KL, Kirkeeide RL: Assessing stenosis severity: coronary flow reserve, collateral function, quantitative coronary arteriography, positron imaging, and digital subtraction angiography: a review and analysis, *Prog Cardiovasc Dis* 30:307-322, 1988.

Deychak YA, Thompson MA, Rohrbeck SC, et al.: A Doppler guidewire used to assess coronary flow during directional coronary atherectomy (abstr), *Circulation* 86:I-122, 1992.

Doucette JW, Corl PD, Payne HM, et al.: Validation of a Doppler guidewire for intravascular measurement of coronary flow velocity, *Circulation* 85:1879-1911, 1992.

Eichhorn EJ, Grayburn PA, Willard JE, et al.: Spontaneous alterations in coronary blood flow velocity before and after coronary angioplasty in patients with severe angina, *J Am Coll Cardiol* 17:43-52, 1991.

George BS, Voorhees WD III, Roubin GS, et al.: Multicenter investigation of coronary stenting to treat acute or threatened closure after percutaneous transluminal coronary angioplasty: clinical and angiographic outcome, *J Am Coll Cardiol* 22:135-143, 1993.

Kern MJ, Aguirre F, Bach R, Donohue T, Siegel R, Segal J: Augmentation of coronary blood flow by intra-aortic balloon pumping in patients after coronary angioplasty, *Circulation* 87:500-511, 1993.

Kern MJ, Bach RG, Donohue TJ, et al.: Clinical utility of continuous coronary flow velocity monitoring during interventional studies, *Cathet Cardiovasc Diagn* 29:81, 1993.

Kern MJ, Donohue T, Bach R, Aguirre F, Bell C: Monitoring cyclical coronary blood flow alterations following coronary angioplasty for stent restenosis using a Doppler guidewire, *Am Heart J* 125:1159-1160, 1993.

Kern MJ, Donohue TJ, Bach RG, Aguirre FV, Caracciolo EA, Ofili EO: Quantitating coronary collateral flow velocity in patients during coronary angioplasty using a Doppler guidewire, *Am J Cardiol* 71(14):34D-40D, 1993.

Kumar K, Dorros G, Jain A, Dufek CA, Mathiak LM: Coronary flow measurements following rotational ablation (atherectomy) (abstr), *Cathet Cardiovasc Diagn* 32(1):97, 1994.

Leon M, Richard A, Kramer B, Knopf W, O'Neill W, Stack R: Efficacious and safe transluminal extraction atherectomy in patients with unfavorable coronary lesions (abstr), *J Am Coll Cardiol* 17:219A, 1991.

Mehta S, Kramer B, Margolis JR, Trautwein R: Transluminal extraction, *Coro Artery Dis* 3:887-896, 1992.

Ofili EO, Kern MJ, Labovitz AJ, et al.: Analysis of coronary blood flow velocity dynamics in angiographically normal and stenosed arteries before and after endolumen enlargement by angioplasty, *J Am Coll Cardiol* 21:308-316, 1993.

Ofili EO, Labovitz AJ, Kern MJ: Coronary flow velocity dynamics in normal and diseased arteries, *Am J Cardiol* 71(14):3D-9D, 1993.

Phillips HR, Sketch MH Jr, Meany TB, et al.: Coronary transluminal extraction-endarterectomy: a multicenter experience (abstr). *Circulation* 82:II-827, 1991.

Sketch MH, Quigley PJ, Tcheng JE, Bauman RP, Phillips HR, Stack RS: Restenosis following coronary transluminal extraction-endarterectomy (abstr), *Circulation* 80:II-583, 1989.

Stack RS, Phillips HR, Quigley PJ, et al.: Multicenter registry of coronary atherectomy using the transluminal extraction-endarterectomy catheter (abstr), *J Am Coll Cardiol* 15:196A, 1990.

Stertzer SH, Rosenblum J, Shaw RE, et al.: Coronary rotational ablation: initial experience in 302 procedures, *J Am Coll Cardiol* 21:287-295, 1993.

Straur B: The significance of coronary reserve in clinical heart disease, *J Am Coll Cardiol* 15:775-783, 1990.

Topol E, Leya F, Pinkerton C, et al., for the CAVEAT Study Group: A comparison of directional coronary atherectomy with coronary angioplasty in patients with coronary artery disease, *N Engl J Med* 329:221-227, 1993.

Younis L, Kern MJ, Bach R, et al.: Postprocedural normalization of coronary flow dynamics following successful atherectomy, PTCA and stenting: analysis of intracoronary spectral Doppler (abstr), *J Am Coll Cardiol* 21:79A, 1993.

Warth DC, Leon MB, O'Neill W, Zacca N, Polissar NL, Buchbinder M: Rotational atherectomy multicenter registry: acute results, complications and 6-month angiographic follow-up in 709 patients, *J Am Coll Cardiol* 24:641-648, 1994.

7

RESTENOSIS

Ubeydullah Deligonul, Stanley G. Rockson, and Morton J. Kern

RESTENOSIS
Background

Restenosis is defined as the reaccumulation of material within a vessel at the site of previous coronary angioplasty. The process of restenosis appears to be initiated by injury of the vessel, with release of thrombogenic, vasoactive, and mitogenic factors. Endothelial and deep vessel injury leads to platelet aggregation, thrombus formation, inflammation, and activation of smooth muscle cells and macrophages. The production and release of growth factors and cytokines promote further synthesis of such factors and release from the cells involved. The migration of smooth muscle cells is initiated from their location within the arterial media to the endovascular lumen. These cells become a synthetic type of cell that produces extra cellular matrix; leading to cellular proliferation and mechanical obstruction of the vessel lumen.

Recoil and remodeling of the arterial wall are also important components of the restenosis process. The vessel is further affected by scar contraction, which may reduce the appearance of the lumen. This process occurs a greater or lesser degree in all patients who undergo coronary angioplasty. Restenosis is probably not device specific, but rather a function of the anatomic substrate and the type of injury produced. Figure 7-1 illustrates the various interventions and expected injury responses leading to restenosis. The variables associated with restenosis are listed in Table 7-1.

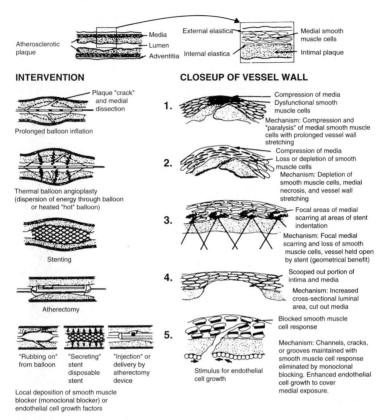

Fig. 7-1.   Interventional devices and presumed mechanisms of action on the arterial plaque and wall. The indication, immediate outcome, and restenosis rate depend on both the device and the arterial substrate encountered. (From Waller, et al.: Mechanisms of restenosis after successful balloon angioplasty, *J Am Coll Cardiol* 17:58B-70B, 1991.)

Definition of Restenosis

The two types of restenosis, angiographic and clinical, are not mutually exclusive.

Angiographic restenosis. Angiographically measured luminal renarrowing after coronary angioplasty has long been the "gold standard" for restenosis. The percent renarrowing after angioplasty shows a normal distribution. Angiographic restenosis is a continuous phenomenon, with no obvious

TABLE 7-1.   Variables associated with increased risk of restenosis after PTCA

Clinical variables

Male sex
Cigarette smoking
Diabetes mellitus
Systemic arterial hypertension
Hypercholesterolemia
End-stage renal disease
Vasospastic angina
Unstable angina
Short interval from PTCA to recurrence of symptoms

Anatomical variables

Proximal stenosis
Saphenous vein graft
Involvement of the left anterior descending artery
Chronically occluded artery
Stenosis >5 to 10 mm in length
Severe pre-PTCA stenosis

Procedural variables

Residual stenosis >30%
Small residual lumen
Use of undersized balloon

From Landau C, Lange RA, Hillis LD: Percutaneous transluminal coronary angioplasty, *N Engl J Med* 330:981-993, 1994.

threshold separating "restenosers" from "nonrestenosers." Studies have shown that percent stenosis or minimal lumen diameter has a near Gaussian distribution on follow-up angiograms after balloon angioplasty. Therefore, restenosis can best be measured as a continuous variable. Nevertheless, definitions of restenosis as a dichotomous variable are utilized, mostly because of practicality. Several different angiographic definitions of restenosis have been published. An important point is that different definitions may overlap in some patients. Some definitions use percent diameter narrowing upon follow-up angiogram (>50% or 70% restenosis), and others use percent luminal gain loss (20% to 30% loss) or some combination thereof. Quantitative angiography studies have used 0.72 mm or 0.50 mm absolute minimum lumen diameter loss. A diameter stenosis of ≥50% of the follow-up angiogram is the most widely used definition.

Restenosis is both a lumen- and a wall-related phenomenon. It appears that 40% to 60% of the acute luminal gain is lost during follow-up in all patients treated with different devices. A similar degree of intimal thickening (restenosis by wall measurement) may or may not cause a significant luminal narrowing (restenosis by lumen measurement). Therefore, some authors argue that the increased acute luminal gain (larger lumen, less stenosis immediately after angioplasty) should decrease the late "luminal restenosis," although the late loss ("wall restenosis") may even be worse.

As expected, the vessel size itself exerts a significant positive influence on minimal lumen diameter at follow-up and an equally negative effect on late loss. A larger artery will have a larger lumen at follow-up, and vice versa for a smaller artery. Using percent stenosis rather than absolute lumen diameter will neutralize this effect by correcting automatically for artery size.

Intravascular ultrasound imaging is superior to angiography for anatomic and morphologic definitions. Recent intravascular ultrasound studies have shown that an important component of restenosis is vessel recoil and that a large amount of residual plaque after angioplasty may be a predictor of restenosis.

Clinical restenosis

Symptoms. Restenosis is the most frequent cause of recurrent angina after coronary angioplasty. Disease progression in nondilated arterial segments may be important in 10% to 15% of cases late after angioplasty. Incomplete revascularization is the cause for symptoms in about 10% of patients. Recurrence of typical angina after an asymptomatic period following angioplasty is a very specific clinical indicator for restenosis. On the other hand, atypical chest pain is a poor predictor. Restenosis may be documented in 15% of asymptomatic cases.

Functional tests. Early (<1 month) exercise tests after percutaneous transluminal coronary angioplasty (PTCA) are often persistently positive and fail to predict future restenosis and recurrent events. An exercise test at 6 months in patients who have not yet presented with clinical recurrence show a modest positive predictive value. Bengtson et al. showed that, in order of importance, exercise-induced angina, clinical recurrence of symptoms, and a positive treadmill test were independent predictors of restenosis.* Despite a multivariate approach, one-fifth of restenosis cases were not recognized. Myocardial perfusion imaging stress studies, in addition to exercise testing, may improve diagnostic accuracy.

Despite known risk factors, it is not possible to predict reliably whether restenosis will occur in a given patient. Angiographic and clinical risk factors for restenosis were determined in 2500 patients by multivariate analysis, and regression was applied to a subsequent set of 1506 patients for validation.† Severe angina, left anterior descending artery lesions, diabetes, a higher degree of residual stenosis, hypertension, absence of intimal tear, eccentric lesion morphology, and older age were predictors for restenosis. Although the regression values showed very good agreement in the validation group ($r = .98$, $p < .001$), the predictive ability analyzed by receiver operating characteristic curve was very poor for individual patients. Nevertheless, the model allowed calculation of a probability range for restenosis.

Time course. In a small proportion of patients, restenosis may occur very early (>24 hour), due to acute elastic recoil. After this point, the incidence of restenosis increases rapidly up to the third month. New restenosis occurs uncommonly after this time. Restenosis after angioplasty using new devices probably follows a similar time course. The reported incidence of restenosis varies between 15% and 55%, with most studies averaging around 30%.

Restenosis versus clinical recurrence. It is difficult to obtain follow-up angiograms in all patients undergoing coronary angioplasty. Less than complete angiographic follow-up with preferential recatheterization of symptomatic patients creates a bias in that symptomatic patients artificially increase the restenosis rate in that population. At the same time, asymptomatic restenosis cases will go unrecognized. Clinical recurrence of symptoms or other events, such as fatal or nonfatal myocardial infarction, is a useful indicator of the efficacy of

---

* Bengtson JR, Mark DB, Honan MB, et al.: Detection of restenosis after elective percutaneous transluminal coronary angioplasty using the exercise treadmill test, *Am J Cardiol* 65:28-34, 1990.

† Weintraub WS, Kosinski AS, Brown CL, King SM: Can restenosis after coronary angioplasty be predicted from clinical variables? *J Am Coll Cardiol* 21:6–14, 1993.

coronary angioplasty as a therapeutic procedure. This approach may underestimate the actual angiographic restenosis rate. Target vessel revascularization rate is another surrogate for angiographic restenosis rate. Strict guidelines should be followed in proceeding with repeat revascularization once the follow-up angiogram has been completed. Incomplete revascularization as a cause of recurrent symptoms further complicates the issue.

Saphenous vein graft lesions. Saphenous vein graft lesions are associated with higher restenosis rates, particularly in the proximal anastomotic (58%) and body (52%) portions of the graft. Distal anastomotic narrowings respond to angioplasty well, especially in patients with recent coronary artery bypass graft surgery. The time course of restenosis in vein grafts is different than in native coronary vessels, with continued significant attrition beyond 6 months. The internal mammary graft anastomotic site responds very favorably to angioplasty, with 15% or less restenosis rate.

Totally occluded saphenous vein bypass grafts constitute a group with suboptimal long-term results. In a study of 83 patients with totally occluded grafts, Kahn et al. reported only 34% revascularization-free survival at 3 years.[*] De Feyter et al. reported only one long-term success in 15 patients.[†]

NEW INTERVENTIONAL DEVICES
Background

During almost two decades since the introduction of coronary angioplasty, experimental data and clinical experience convincingly support the notion that this is a highly effective, safe, and durable approach to nonsurgical coronary revascularization. Worldwide utilization of PTCA has increased confidence in the procedure to enhance coronary blood in the majority of patients, and has instilled a growing awareness of the inherent limitations to the long-term efficacy of angioplasty.

[*] Kahn JK, Rutherford BD, McConahay DR, et al.: Initial and long-term outcome of 83 patients after balloon angioplasty of totally occluded saphenous vein bypass grafts, *J Am Coll Cardiol* 23:1038-1042, 1994.
[†] De Feyter PJ, Serruys P, vanden Brand M, et al.: Percutaneous transluminal angioplasty of a totally occluded saphenous vein bypass graft: a challenge that should be resisted, *Am J Cardiol* 64:88-90, 1989.

However, the high incidence of clinical and angiographic restenosis remains a major concern. Conquering restenosis has spawned a new generation of intravascular devices and approaches. Directional, rotational, and extraction atherectomy, laser-assisted angioplasty, and catheter-mounted endovascular stents have been developed, wholly or in part, to avert restenosis, with the resultant late loss of luminal diameter after vascular intervention.

One of the difficulties of attempting to categorize the vascular restenotic effect of newer interventional devices is the inescapable comparison with the "gold standard" of balloon angioplasty. However, with the application of virtually every one of the new procedures available to the interventionist, there is a uniformly high requirement for adjunctive balloon angioplasty in concert with the new device(s) to achieve an acceptable postprocedural vessel lumen. The high frequency of these hybrid procedures makes the analysis of device-specific patterns of vascular injury and repair, in the absence of balloon-induced changes, practically impossible. In fact, data derived from the New Approaches to Coronary Intervention (NACI) Registry indicate that utilization of adjunctive balloon angioplasty to complement the effect of stents, lasers, and atherectomy catheters exceeds 75%.

It is instructive to examine the manner in which each of these newer devices is associated with restenosis.

Directional Coronary Atherectomy

Directional coronary atherectomy (DCA) was the first widely employed alternative to standard balloon angioplasty. This device was conceived to circumvent the theoretical limitations of the conventional balloon technique through lesion debulking and removal of atheromatous material from the vessel lumen.

DCA provides a de-facto biopsy of the diseased intima and practical access for histologic and cytochemical analyses of patient-derived atheromatous specimens. DCA has added important insights into the mechanisms of primary atherosclerosis, as well as the restenotic process.

It was initially assumed that excision of the intima to the level of the internal elastic lamina would remove the anatomic nidus for future neointimal reproliferation and restenosis.

Extensive clinical experience has proven DCA to be an effective treatment modality supporting the original mechanical concept. Unfortunately, restenosis following DCA has not been reduced below that of PTCA.

The overall restenosis rate after directional atherectomy is approximately 50%. The restenosis rate is reported to be 42% in those patients in whom atherectomy specimens disclosed only intimal tissue, and 63% when adventitia was obtained.

Restenosis in saphenous vein grafts. In procedures performed on vein grafts, subintimal resection virtually assured restenosis (>60%), compared to the 43% restenosis incidence in patients with only intimal resection. A similar trend was observed in patients who were subjected to DCA to correct post-PTCA restenosis. Atherectomy specimens derived from restenotic lesions after DCA disclosed typical neointimal responses in the tissue specimens, which were indistinguishable from the histologic pattern observed in the coronary restenosis which follows standard balloon angioplasty. These findings suggest that the pathologic response of restenosis after PTCA and DCA is analogous. Subintimal resection in DCA predisposes to restenosis. The restenosis response with fibrous hyperplasia is heightened in vein grafts and restenotic lesions after DCA.

The use of DCA in bypass vein grafts was associated with increased complications and no 6-month restenosis benefit as compared to balloon angioplasty (45.6% versus 50.5%, respectively, Holmes et al., 1995).

Device size and restenosis. The relationship between the size of the DCA device and long-term clinical outcome is controversial. In a study of 263 patients who underwent DCA as a sole intervention, the investigators used 7F devices with peak inflation pressures of approximately 5 atm. When the outcomes were stratified according to the size of the target vessel, there was no difference in restenosis rates (20.6% in vessels exceeding 3 mm diameter, versus 28% in vessels at or less than 3 mm). However, other studies have observed a relationship both with vessel size and with the immediate gain in lumen size after the procedure.

Randomized trials of restenosis. The coronary atheterectomy versus angioplasty trial (CAVEAT) and Canadian coronary atherectomy trial (CCAT) have provided influential data for a procedure-to-procedure comparison between DCA and balloon angioplasty. These two large-scale, randomized studies compared the initial and intermediate-term outcomes when each device was utilized as de-novo therapy. The primary procedural success rate and vessel geometry were enhanced by DCA. Despite the observed improvement in the initial outcomes, DCA did not confer any benefit in terms of angiographic restenosis. In the CCAT trial, the restenosis rates at 6 months were 46% and 41% for DCA and PTCA, respectively. In the CAVEAT trial, DCA yielded a better outcome in the subset of left anterior descending artery lesions (51% versus 63%). Despite this apparent advantage, there exists no clear mandate for the use of atherectomy over balloon angioplasty even in this subset of patients. The CAVEAT trial, in contradistinction to CCAT, also demonstrated a significantly higher complication rate for DCA than for PTCA.

Whereas the improvement in clinical outcome can be related to larger vessel size and postinterventional lumen diameter, a greater immediate gain at the time of intervention may prove to be predictive of a greater tendency to restenosis. The development of a treatment stratagem that will achieve an appropriate balance among these factors is the challenge to justify utilizing this (or any other) nonballoon interventional procedure.

Stents

Balloon-expandable endovascular stents were developed to prevent abrupt closure and restenosis after angioplasty. Primary stenting appears to improve the long-term angiographic and clinical outcome, when compared with results from standard balloon angioplasty. Several risk factors have been identified that predispose stent patients to restenosis. These variables include multiple stent implantation, deployment in a vessel with a reference diameter ≤3 mm, and a postdeployment residual stenosis diameter exceeding 8%.

It should be noted that most of the published data on the incidence of restenosis have been driven by the angiographic definition of late loss of vascular lumen diameter following coronary intervention. Restenosis within the Palmaz-Schatz stent can be treated successfully with balloon angioplasty, but the re-restenosis rate may be as high as 50%.

Randomized trials.   The BENESTENT trial (Europe) assessed clinical and angiographic outcomes in patients undergoing primary stent placement when compared to similar patients after primary balloon angioplasty. Minimal luminal diameter at follow-up was assessed by quantitative coronary angiography. The initial angiographic outcomes were superior in the stented patients, as manifested both by a reduced incidence of clinical events and by greater postprocedural arterial diameter. After 6 months of follow-up, the stented patients demonstrated a significantly lower rate of restenosis (22% versus 32% for PTCA). Coronary stenting was associated with higher primary success rates, lower rates of clinical event during postprocedural follow-up, and a reduced need for subsequent surgical intervention. In other studies, the stent restenosis rate in previously untreated lesions of the native coronary circulation has been reported to be as low as 13%. Because warfarin therapy was required in the trials, these clinical and quantitative angiographic improvements were attained at a greater risk of vascular complications, as well as a requisite prolongation of hospital stay, in the stented patients.

Saphenous vein grafts. Stent placement offers distinct advantages over angioplasty in proximal- and mid-vessel segments of degenerated saphenous vein grafts. Stenting reduces both restenosis and the incidence of distal embolization. Despite the low incidence of restenosis after stent placement for focal vein graft stenosis (17%), the long-term requirement for additional revascularization is high, presumably because of the advanced, multifocal nature of the coronary artery disease in this subset of stent recipients.

Implantation of Palmaz-Schatz stents in bypass vein grafts in a nonrandomized study was associated with a 6-month restenosis rate of only 34% in 209 bypass vein graft lesions. The restenosis rate was even lower in de novo as compared to restenotic lesions (22% versus 51%, respectively). Event-free survival at 1 year was 82% in the de novo lesion group.

Bailout stenting. There are few data on restenosis after bailout stenting. Schomig et al.* reported a 30% angiographic

---

* Schömig A, Kastrati A, Mudra H, et al.: Four-year experience with Palmaz-Schatz stenting in coronary angioplasty complicated by dissection with threatened or present vessel closure, *Circulation* 90:2716-2724, 1994.

restenosis rate at 6 months after bailout Palmaz-Schatz stent implantation in 339 patients. The restenosis rate after bailout Flexstent implantation in a multicenter study was 39%, with a subacute thrombosis rate of 8.7%.* These restenosis rates compare favorably to the high restenosis rates after conventional balloon dilatation of acute closure.

It has been observed that the 20% of patients who experience moderate forms (i.e., 40% to 70%) of restenosis after coronary stenting have, in general, a benign clinical outcome, which favors conservative management, rather than surgical or repeat catheter intervention. Existing data support the stent as the only modality associated with a lower restenosis rate than PTCA in selected patients when using a strategy of primary placement.

Percutaneous Transluminal Coronary Rotational Atherectomy

Percutaneous transluminal coronary rotational atherectomy (PTCRA) pulverizes the atheroma to create a satisfactory coronary lumen. The ablating mechanism creates smooth lumens and is postulated to cause less flow turbulence in the healing vessel and therefore less restenosis. Rotational atherectomy has distinct mechanical advantages for calcified lesions in the native coronary circulation.

PTCRA has been performed with a uniformly high primary success rate (approximately 95%), independent of lesion location or severity. Previous intervention predisposes to a slight improvement in clinical outcome.

Six-month restenosis rates after rotational coronary atherectomy approximate those observed after standard PTCA. In some circumstances, PTCRA restenosis rates exceed expected PTCA rates. According to reports from the Multicenter Registry for Rotational Atherectomy, the overall restenosis rate is about 38%, corresponding to 64% of treated lesions. A predisposition to restenosis after PTCRA occurs in patients with diabetes and those with a poorer initial increase in lumen diameter after the procedure.

* George BS, Voorhees WD, Roubin GS, et al.: Multicenter investigation of coronary stenting to treat acute or threatened closure after percutaneous transluminal coronary angioplasty: clinical and angiographic outcomes, *J Am Coll Cardiol* 22:135-143, 1993.

Ostial stenosis.   Ostial stenosis of a native coronary artery represents a selected anatomic circumstance in which rotational atherectomy seems to confer a procedural advantage over ballon angioplasty restenosis rates (approximately 39% to 43%).

Comparative trials.   The only comparative study of balloon versus Rotablator failed to show any improvement in restenosis rates despite better initial success.* The greatest applicability of this technique is in small vessels, and in lesions that are either nondistensible, calcified, eccentric, or located in distal segments of the vessel.

Transluminal Extraction Atherectomy

Transluminal extraction atherectomy is another device iteration that addresses the theoretical advantage of removing diseased material from the vascular lumen. The transluminal extraction catheter (TEC) consists of a torquing tube with a conical rotating blade designed to cut and remove excised atherosclerotic plaque through vacuum suction. Direct visualization of the vascular lumen through an angioscope confirms the removal of thrombus and atheromatous material from the coronary artery or bypass conduit. The characteristic, multiple residual disruptions created by the TEC device are also easily appreciated. These luminal alterations provide a potential explanation for the typically angiographically hazy appearance of the post-TEC vessel and the predisposition to restenosis in these vessels. TEC atherectomy is used as an adjunct in the treatment of stenoses in saphenous vein bypass grafts because of its ability to aspirate both atheromatous material and thrombus.

The relatively short history of active clinical use has yet to define the utility of extraction atherectomy in large-scale, long-term prospective studies. To date, the TEC procedure does not show any reduction in restenosis rates. It is notable in this procedure that loss of lumen diameter early after the atherectomy appears to contribute to early, but not to late, restenosis.

---

* Vandormael M, Reifart N, Preusler W, et al.: Comparison of excimer laser angioplasty and rotational atherectomy with balloon angioplasty for complex lesions: ERBAC study final results, *J Am Coll Cardiol (Abstr)* 57A, 1994.

The procedure does appear to avert many of the embolic sequelae of other techniques employed for saphenous vein graft intervention, with a suitably high success rate, but restenosis estimates are also high, approximating 52%. In old, diseased vein grafts, the restenosis rate is observed to be even higher (60%).

Laser-Assisted Balloon Angioplasty

Laser-assisted balloon angioplasty has been promoted as a specific technique for anatomically difficult lesions where the risk of adverse outcomes is high, such as thrombotic, angulated, or eccentric lesions, or complete vessel occlusion. In these settings, it is postulated that an ideal device for revascularization would do so while minimizing vascular trauma, thereby reducing the likelihood of a significant injury response that predisposes to restenosis.

The restenosis rate after excimer laser angioplasty at 4 ± 2 months was 58% in 3000 patients treated with excimer laser angioplasty.[*] In 168 patients who were treated with a different brand of excimer laser, the angiographic restenosis rate was similarly 50%. The restenosis risk was higher in smaller vessels, and it was not related to the laser fluence levels.[†] Restenosis after excimer laser angioplasty appears to be related directly to the final diameter achieved after intervention, with the lowest restenosis rates observed in vessels with the largest postprocedural minimal lumen diameters. However, the restenosis rates after excimer laser-facilitated angioplasty do not differ from those observed after angioplasty alone. In all likelihood, this absence of an observed difference is explained by the fact that the laser does not ablate a great deal of atheromatous tissue but simply forges a channel to facilitate the passage of the PTCA catheter, which then creates the ultimate enlarged lumen diameter. Whether laser energy alone influences the restenosis process is unknown.

[*] Litvack F, Eigler N, Margolis J, et al.: Percutaneous excimer laser coronary angioplasty: results in the first consecutive 3,000 patients, *J Am Coll Cardiol* 23:323-329, 1994.
[†] Bittl JA, Kuntz RE, Estella P, Sanborn TA, Baim DS: Analysis of late lumen narrowing after excimer laser-facilitated coronary angioplasty, *J Am Coll Cardiol* 23:1314-1320, 1994.

Patient Subsets at Higher Risk for Restenosis

Diabetes mellitus.   Several studies have shown that diabetes mellitus is a risk factor for restenosis. Restenosis is more prominent in insulin-dependent diabetics, as shown in a recent study comparing acute and 5-year outcomes in 1133 diabetic and 9300 nondiabetic patients.* Although acute success and complication rates were only slightly worse than for nondiabetics, 5-year survival was significantly shorter in diabetics, with only 36% surviving 5 years without reinfarction or a repeat revascularization. There was significant attrition within the first year, indicating a high restenosis rate. Outcome was worse in insulin-dependent diabetics for each end point as compared to non-insulin-dependent diabetics.

Chronic renal failure.   Patients with chronic renal failure who undergo PTCA have an almost prohibitively high restenosis rate (80%).

Transplantation.   Restenosis is frequent after balloon angioplasty in heart transplant recipients. In a recent multicenter study, the restenosis rate 8 ± 5 months after balloon angioplasty of 76 lesions was 55%.† Importantly, early or late failure of angioplasty had serious consequences. In this series of 162 patients, 3-year survival was less than 50%. The results with new devices such as DCA in this population are not well known.

Acute myocardial infarction.   Although the immediate and intermediate-term clinical outcome is very favorable, the angiographic restenosis rate after angioplasty in an acute myocardial infarction setting is not well known. Compared to elective angioplasty, late restenosis after emergent angioplasty for acute myocardial infarction was found to be lower (35% versus 19%). Since the rate of in-hospital reocclusion (13% versus 2%) was higher in the myocardial infarction group, the lower late restenosis rate may reflect a difference in the time course of restenosis. In a more recent study, 6-month restenosis rate after primary angioplasty for acute

* Stein B, Weintraub WS, Gebhart SSP, et al.: Influence of diabetes mellitus on early and late outcome after percutaneous transluminal coronary angioplasty, *Circulation* 91:979-989, 1995.
† Halle AA, Disciascio G, Massin EK, et al.: Coronary angioplasty, atherectomy and bypass surgery in cardiac transplant patients, *J Am Coll Cardiol* 26:120-128, 1995.

myocardial infarction was 52%, similar to elective PTCA results.*

Total occlusion. Total occlusion angioplasty is known to be associated with a high restenosis rate. Moreover, the restenosis rate after total occlusion angioplasty may not plateau at 6 months. In an (incomplete) angiographic follow-up study after total occlusion angioplasty, 41% of patients had restenosis within 65 months and 66% had restenosis within 12 months.[†] In two studies, the angiographic restenosis rate was 54% to 59%, including total occlusion in 25% to 30% of the patients 6 months after total occlusion dilatation.[‡] A more recent and more complete angiographic follow-up study showed similar results in that the restenosis rate was 45% for total occlusions compared with 34% in stenoses. In this series, 19% reocclusion was noted.[§] The recurrence of total occlusion seldom results in myocardial infarction.

Management of Restenosis

Restenosis can be treated successfully with repeat coronary angioplasty. The success and complication rates are lower than for the initial procedure because the restenosis lesion is primarily fibro-proliferative rather than an atherosclerotic plaque. Restenosis after a second angioplasty ranges from 30% to 35%, although sustained revascularization may be present in >80% of patients after two procedures. Early (<3 months) restenosis, proximal left anterior descending location, and multivessel disease increase the restenosis risk after a second angioplasty procedure. Asymptomatic restenosis

* O'Neill W, Brodie BR, Ivanhoe R, et al.: Primary coronary angioplasty for acute myocardial infarction (the Primary Angioplasty Registry), *Am J Cardiol* 73:627-634, 1994.

† Ellis SG, Shaw RE, Gershony G, et al.: Risk factors, time course and treatment effect for restenosis after successful percutaneous transluminal coronary angioplasty of chronic total occlusion, *Am J Cardiol* 63:897-901, 1989.

‡ Ivanhoe RJ, Weintraub WS, Douglas JS, et al.: Percutaneous transluminal coronary angioplasty of chronic total occlusions. Primary success, restenosis and long-term clinical follow-up, *Circulation* 85:106-115, 1992.

Bell MR, Berger PB, Bresnahan JF, Reeder GS, Bailey KR, Holmes DR: Initial and long-term outcome of 354 patients after coronary balloon angioplasty of total coronary artery occlusions, *Circulation* 85:1003-1011, 1992.

§ Violaris AG, Melkert R, Serruys PW: Long-term luminal renarrowing after successful elective coronary angioplasty of total occlusions: a quantitative angiographic analysis, *Circulation* 91:2140-2150, 1995.

TABLE 7-2. Pharmacologic agents evaluated in randomized trials to reduce the incidence of restenosis after PTCA

Antiplatelet agents
Aspirin and dipyridamole
Ticlopidine
Prostacyclin
Ciprostene
Thromboxane synthetase inhibitor
Serotonin-receptor antagonist

Antithrombotic agents
Heparin
Warfarin

Calcium-channel blockers
Nifedipine
Diltiazem

Antiproliferative agents
Corticosteroids
Colchicine

Lipid-lowering agents
n-3 Fatty acids
Lovastatin

Angiotensin-converting-enzyme inhibitor
Cilazapril

Growth inhibitor
Trapidil

From Landau C, Lange RA, Hillis LD: Percutaneous transluminal coronary angioplasty, *N Engl J Med* 330:981-993, 1994.

may require only careful monitoring. The incidence of recurrent angina and the need for repeat revascularization are lower in this group. There are no successful pharmacologic or device approaches to reduce restenosis with the exception of data from the primary stent trials.

A summary of pharmacologic agents evaluated for restenosis is listed in Table 7-2.

SUGGESTED READINGS

Adelman AG, Cohen EA, Kimball BP, et al.: A comparison of directional atherectomy with balloon angioplasty for lesions of the left anterior descending coronary artery, *N Engl J Med* 329:228-233, 1993.

Baim DS, Kent KM, King SB III, et al.: Evaluating new devices. Acute (in-hospital) results from the New Approaches to Coronary Intervention Registry, *Circulation* 89(1):471-481, 1994.

Baim DS, Levine MJ, Leon MB, Levine S, Ellis SG, Schatz RA: Management of restenosis within the Palmaz-Schatz coronary stent (the U.S. Multicenter Experience), *Am J Cardiol* 71:364-366, 1993.

Bell MR, Berger PB, Bresnahan JF, Reeder GS, Bailey KR, Holmes DR: Initial and long-term outcome of 354 patients after coronary balloon angioplasty of total coronary artery occlusions, *Circulation* 85:1003-1011, 1992.

Bengtson JR, Mark DB, Honan MB, et al.: Detection of restenosis after elective percutaneous transluminal coronary angioplasty using the exercise treadmill test, *Am J Cardiol* 65:28-34, 1990.

Bensing BJ, Hermans WR, Deckers JW, de Feyter PJ, Tijsen JGP, Serruys PW: Lumen narrowing after percutaneous transluminal coronary balloon angioplasty follows a near Gaussian distribution: a quantitative study in 1,445 successfully dilated lesions, *J Am Coll Cardiol* 19:939-945, 1992.

Bittl JA, Kuntz RE, Estella P, Sanborn TA, Baim DS: Analysis of late lumen narrowing after excimer laser-facilitated coronary angioplasty, *J Am Coll Cardiol* 23:1314-1320, 1994.

de Feyter PJ, Serruys P, vanden Brand M, et al.: Percutaneous transluminal angioplasty of a totally occluded saphenous vein bypass graft: a challenge that should be resisted, *Am J Cardiol* 64:88-90, 1989.

de Feyter PJ, van Suylen RJ, de Jaegere PPT, Topol EJ, Serruys PW: Balloon angioplasty for the treatment of lesions in saphenous vein grafts, *J Am Coll Cardiol* 21:1539-1549, 1993.

Deligonul U, Vandormael M, Shah Y, et al.: Prognostic value of early exercise stress testing after successful coronary angioplasty: importance of the degree of revascularization, *Am Heart J* 117:509-514, 1989.

Ellis SG, Shaw RE, Gershony G, et al.: Risk factors, time course and treatment effect for restenosis after successful percutaneous transluminal coronary angioplasty of chronic total occlusion, *Am J Cardiol* 63:897-901, 1989.

Fenton SH, Fischman DL, Savage MP, et al.: Long-term angiographic and clinical outcome after implantation of balloon expandable stents in aortocoronary saphenous vein grafts, *Am J Cardiol* 74:1187-1191, 1994.

Fischman DL, Leon MB, Baim D, et al., for the STRESS trial investigators: a randomized comparison of coronary stent placement and balloon angioplasty in the treatment of coronary artery disease, *N Engl J Med* 331:496-501, 1994.

Foley DP, Melkert R, Serruys PW: Influence of coronary vessel size on renarrowing process and late angiographic outcome after successful balloon angioplasty, *Circulation* 90:1239-1251, 1994.

Garratt KN, Holmes DR Jr, Bell MR, et al.: Restenosis after directional coronary atherectomy: differences between primary atheromatous and restenosis lesions and influence of subintimal tissue resection, *J Am Coll Cardiol* 16(7):1665-1671, 1990.

George BS, Voorhees WD, Roubin GS, et al.: Multicenter investigation of coronary stenting to treat acute or threatened closure after percutaneous transluminal coronary angioplasty: clinical and angiographic outcomes, *J Am Coll Cardiol* 22:135-143, 1993.

Ghazzal ZM, Burton E, Weintraub WS, et al.: Predictors of restenosis after excimer laser coronary angioplasty, *Am J Cardiol* 75(15):1012-1014, 1995.

Gordon PC, Friedrich SP, Piana RN, et al.: Is 40% to 70% diameter narrowing at the site of previous stenting or directional coronary atherectomy clinically significant? *Am J Cardiol* 74(1):26-32, 1994.

Halle AA, Disciascio G, Massin EK, et al.: Coronary angioplasty, atherectomy and bypass surgery in cardiac transplant patients, *J Am Coll Cardiol* 26:120-128, 1995.

Holmes DR Jr, Topol EJ, Adelman AG, Cohen EA, Califf RM: Randomized trials of directional coronary atherectomy: implications for clinical practice and future investigation, *J Am Coll Cardiol* 24(2):431-439, 1994.

Holmes DR, Topol EJ, Califf RM, et al.: A multicenter, randomized trial of coronary angioplasty versus directional atherectomy for patients with saphenous vein bypass graft lesions, *Circulation* 91:1966-1974, 1995.

Ishizaka N, Ikari Y, Hara K, et al.: Angiographic follow-up of patients after transluminal coronary extraction atherectomy, *Am Heart J* 128(4):691-699, 1994.

Ivanhoe RJ, Weintraub WS, Douglas JS, et al.: Percutaneous transluminal coronary angioplasty of chronic total occlusions. Primary success, restenosis and long-term clinical follow-up, *Circulation* 85:106-115, 1992.

Kahn JK, Rutherford BD, McConahay DR, et al.: Initial and long-term outcome of 83 patients after balloon angioplasty of totally occluded saphenous vein bypass grafts, *J Am Coll Cardiol* 23:1038-1042, 1994.

Kearney M, Califf RM, Topol EJ: One year follow-up in the Coronary Angioplasty Versus Excisional Atherectomy Trial (CAVEAT I), *Circulation* 91:2158-2166, 1995.

Kimura T, Nosaka H, Yokoi H, Iwabuchi M, Nobuyoshi M: Serial angiographic follow-up after Palmaz-Schatz stent implantation: comparison with conventional balloon angioplasty, *J Am Coll Cardiol* 21:1557-1563, 1993.

Kuntz RE, Gibson CM, Nobuyoshi M, et al.: Generalized model of restenosis after conventional balloon angioplasty, stenting and directional atherectomy, *J Am Coll Cardiol* 21:15-25, 1993.

Kuntz RE, Keaney KM, Senerchia C, Baim DS: A predictive method for estimating the late angiographic results of coronary intervention despite incomplete ascertainment, *Circulation* 87:815-830, 1993.

Litvack F, Eigler N, Margolis J, et al.: Percutaneous excimer laser coronary angioplasty: results in the first consecutive 3,000 patients, *J Am Coll Cardiol* 23:323-329, 1994.

Moscucci M, Piana RN, Kuntz RE, et al.: Effect of prior coronary restenosis on the risk of subsequent restenosis after stent placement or directional atherectomy, *Am J Cardiol* 73(16):1147-1153, 1994.

Nobuyoshi M, Takeshi K, Nosaka H: Restenosis after successful percutaneous transluminal coronary angioplasty: serial angiographic follow-up of 229 patients, *J Am Coll Cardiol* 12:616, 1988.

O'Brien ER, Alpers CE, Stewart DK, et al.: Proliferation in primary and restenotic coronary atherectomy tissue. Implications for anti-proliferative therapy, *Circ Res* 73(2):223-231, 1993.

O'Neill W, Brodie BR, Ivanhoe R, et al.: Primary coronary angioplasty for acute myocardial infarction (the Primary Angioplasty Registry), *Am J Cardiol* 73:627-634, 1994.

Piana RN, Moscucci M, Cohen DJ, et al.: Palmaz-Schatz stenting for treatment of focal vein graft stenosis: immediate results and long-term outcome, *J Am Coll Cardiol* 23(6):1296-1304, 1994.

Safian RD, Grines CL, May MA, et al.: Clinical and angiographic results of transluminal extraction coronary atherectomy in saphenous vein bypass grafts, *Circulation* 89:302-312, 1994.

Savage MP, Fischman DL, Schatz RA, et al.: Long-term angiographic and clinical outcome after implantation of a balloon-expandable stent in the native coronary circulation, *J Am Coll Cardiol* 24(5):1207-1212, 1994.

Serruys PW, Jaegere PD, Kiemenij F, et al.: A comparison of balloon-expandable-stent implantation with balloon angioplasty with coronary artery disease, *N Engl J Med* 331:489-495, 1994.

Serruys PW, Lujiten H, Beatt KJ, et al.: Incidence of restenosis after successful coronary angioplasty: a time related phenomenon, *Circulation* 77:361, 1988.

Simonton CA, Mark DB, Hinohara T, et al.: Late restenosis after emergent coronary angioplasty for acute myocardial infarction:

comparison with elective coronary angioplasty, *J Am Coll Cardiol* 11:698-705, 1988.

Stein B, Weintraub WS, Gebhart SSP, et al.: Influence of diabetes mellitus on early and late outcome after percutaneous transluminal coronary angioplasty, *Circulation* 91:979-989, 1995.

Stertzer S, Rosenblaum J, Shaw R, et al.: Coronary rotational ablation. Initial experience in 302 procedures, *J Am Coll Cardiol* 21:287-295, 1993.

Topol EJ, Leya F, Pinkerton CA, et al.: A comparison of directional coronary atherectomy with coronary angioplasty in patients with coronary artery disease, *N Engl J Med* 329:221-227, 1993.

Umans VA, Robert A, Foley D, et al.: Clinical, histologic and quantitative angiographic predictors of restenosis after directional coronary atherectomy: a multivariate analysis of the renarrowing process and late outcome, *J Am Coll Cardiol* 23(1):49-58, 1994.

Vandormael M, Reifart N, Preusler W, et al.: Comparison of excimer laser angioplasty and rotational atherectomy with balloon angioplasty for complex lesions: ERBAC study final results (abstr), *J Am Coll Cardiol* 57A, 1994.

Violaris AG, Melkert R, Serruys PW: Long-term luminal renarrowing after successful elective coronary angioplasty of total occlusions: a quantitative angiographic analysis, *Circulation* 91:2140-2150, 1995.

Warth DC, Leon MB, O'Neill W, Zacca N, Polissar NL, Buchbinder M: Rotational Atherectomy Multicenter Registry: acute results, complications and 6-month angiographic follow-up in 709 patients, *J Am Coll Cardiol* 24(3):641-648, 1994.

8

DIFFICULT ANGIOPLASTY SITUATIONS

Morton J. Kern, Richard G. Bach, Thomas J. Donohue, and Ubeydullah Deligonul

BIFURCATION STENOSIS ANGIOPLASTY

Angioplasty of coronary lesions often involves consideration of the effect on nearby side branches. These lesions commonly require decisions to either dilate separately or, at the minimum, protect the side branch with a guidewire to gain rapid access if branch closure occurs during angioplasty of the parent branch lesion. The approach to bifurcation angioplasty is thus based on the angiographic configuration of the stenosis, the proximity of the side branch to the target lesion, the presence of significant disease in the ostium of the side branch, and the clinical consequences of side-branch loss if unprotected closure should occur. Among these considerations, the likelihood of side-branch closure is related directly to the presence of disease in the ostium of the side branch.

Common combinations of side-branch involvement during parent-branch angioplasty are shown in Fig. 8-1. Side branches with a benign relationship to the angioplasty of the parent vessel include prestenosis branches, poststenosis branches, and those branches that straddle stenoses. Angioplasty across an uninvolved side-branch carries <1% risk of occlusion. The re-

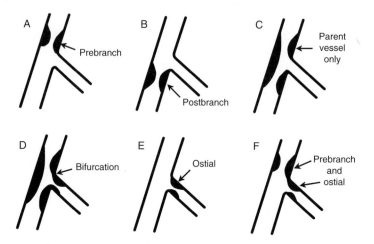

Fig. 8-1.   Schematic representation of lesion and side-branch involvement. **A, B,** and **C** represent parent vessel involvement with no disease located in the side-branch vessel. **D, E,** and **F** represent parent and side-branch involvement with >50% ostial stenosis in the side-branch. (From Freed M, Grines C: *Manual of interventional cardiology*, Birmingham, Michigan, 1992, Physician's Press.)

quirement for side-branch protection for the three benign side-branch locations is minimal, and the technical difficulty of approaching such side branches is also low. Bifurcation lesions that are at risk for side branches involve a side branch straddling the diseased target vessel, and ostial stenoses of pre- and poststenotic branches. The technical difficulty of treating these stenoses increases with the degree of side-branch involvement (narrowing). The risk of closure of a side branch with ostial narrowing exceeds 15% to 25%.

The incidence of side-branch closure is less than 15% when the side branch is not involved in atherosclerotic disease. When there is an equal distribution of coronary plaque across a bifurcation stenosis, dilatation of both branches and, in some cases, simultaneous balloon inflation in both branches to maintain vessel patency should be anticipated.

General Approach

Guide catheter selection.   Two choices of guide catheter systems are available:

1. Two guide and balloon catheter systems
2. Single guide catheter with two guidewires for two balloon catheters (Fig. 8-2)

The major advantage to using two separate guide and balloon catheter systems is the ability to select among a wide variety of dilatation/atherectomy and bailout angioplasty equipment. The major disadvantage is a second arterial access site with a commensurate increase in vascular access risks (bleeding, pseudoaneurysm, etc.). A single guide catheter system minimizes vascular access-site complications and reduces the potential for coronary ostial trauma during guide catheter manipulations. A single guide approach also minimizes x-ray exposure to the operator team and patient. A single guide catheter must accommodate all the anticipated equipment suitable to the internal dimensions of the guide catheter. Multiple balloon catheter manipulations and coronary visualization may be more difficult with this approach.

Guide catheter internal dimensions should be large enough to accommodate balloon catheters and bailout devices (including a stent). Guide catheters with internal diameters of 0.086 in. may accommodate two monorail balloon catheters or some stent systems. Smaller-diameter guide catheters often require a fixed-wire balloon for simultaneous dilation or, in some cases, the procedure must be restricted to sequential balloon inflations of the parent and side branches. Larger-lumen 8F guides (0.086 in. or 9F) may be more suitable for two simultaneous over-the-wire/monorail balloon catheter systems and can easily accommodate the use of a perfusion balloon catheter or stent, if needed.

Balloon catheter selection.   A single guide catheter system can employ:
1. Two monorail/fixed-wire balloon catheters
2. An over-the-wire and a monorail balloon catheter
3. An over-the-wire and a fixed-wire balloon catheter
4. A reperfusion balloon catheter and a second guidewire or fixed-wire balloon catheter

Guidewire Technique

To protect side branches, two guidewires can be placed in both the branch and the main vessel before beginning balloon inflations (Figs. 8-2 and 8-3). Placement of the guidewire in the side branch may lead to balloon inflation in the smaller

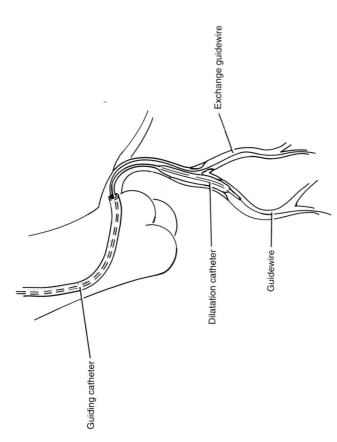

Fig. 8-2. Angioplasty procedure with single guide catheter, two wires, one balloon catheter. Exchange guidewire is positioned across bifurcation in vessel to be protected. Dilatation catheter is used for the principal lesion and the side-branch lesion in a sequential fashion. (Modified from Oesterle SN, McAuley BJ, Buchbinder M, Simpson JB: Angioplasty at coronary bifurcations: singleguide, two-wire technique, *Cathet Cardiovasc Diagn* 12:57-63, 1986.)

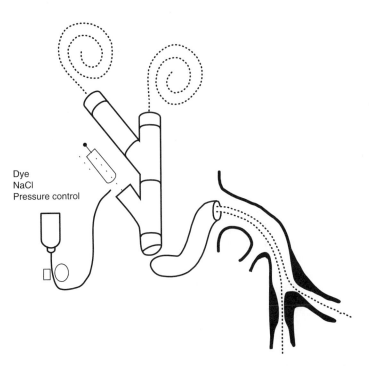

Dye
NaCl
Pressure control

Fig. 8-3. Diagram of two exchange guidewires placed through single guide catheter into the side-branch and main-branch vessel. The long exchange wires will permit either monorail or over-the-wire systems to be used sequentially. If the guide catheter is of sufficient diameter, simultaneous balloon inflation can be performed. (From Kaltenbach M, Vallbracht C, Kober G: The long wire technique for coronary angioplasty, *Cath and CV Diagn* 12:337-340, 1986.)

side branch, putting the major branch at risk (Fig. 8-4). Should a dissection occur, an unprotected major vessel will require reinstrumentation or manipulation of the guidewire, which may result in failure of reperfusion via bailout equipment. To avoid guidewire wrapping, the side branch is entered first. This may require more manipulation. Serial inflations, as opposed to simultaneous balloon inflations in both branches, may limit the need for extra balloon catheters. Coronary opacification is better with a one-balloon catheter, two-wire technique. Some operators select a long (300-cm) guidewire and

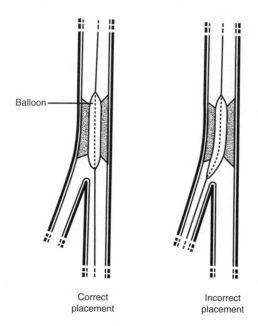

Balloon

Correct
placement

Incorrect
placement

Fig. 8-4. Correct and incorrect placement of balloon catheter in guidewire for pre-branch dilatation in a lesion with a proximate side branch. (From Kulick DL, Rahimtoola SH: *Techniques and applications of interventional cardiology,* St. Louis, 1991, Mosby, p 67.)

a fixed-wire balloon to dilate bifurcations. The fixed-wire balloon provides immediate access for dilatation of the side branch.

When using a two-guidewire system, guidewire entrapment after multiple wire manipulations may occur because of wrapping of the wires. Efforts should be made to avoid guidewire entrapment, which will prevent balloon advancement and may result in recrossing of the stenosis.

Balloon Inflation Strategies (Table 8-1)

Sequential branch inflations. Dilate the main vessel first, the side-branch second, and finish dilation in the main branch. A sequential main-branch, side-branch, main-branch balloon inflation strategy provides a safe and straightforward approach. However, shifting of atherosclerotic plaque during

TABLE 8-1. Approach to bifurcation stenosis

Approach	Advantages	Disadvantages
1. Guide catheter selection		
a. Two-guide catheter	• Large variety of catheters available	• Two artery punctures • Two guide catheter manipulation • Long procedure time
b. One-guide catheter	• One arterial puncture • Fewer catheter manipulations, low risk of ostial trauma • Reduced procedure time	
2. Balloons and guidewires		
a. Two wires, one balloon catheter	• Maintain access for balloon upsizing, perfusion catheters, or stents • Less obstruction to protected side branch coronary flow than deflated balloon-on-a-wire catheter • Less expensive • Good vessel opacification	
b. Two balloon-on-a-wire catheter	• Immediate dilatation capability during acute closure	• Expensive • Must use guide wires for exchanges
c. One over-the-wire balloon, one on-a-wire catheter	• Allows immediate dilatation of side branch • Reduces procedure time	• Expensive • Limited fixed-wire exchanges
3. Balloon inflation strategy		
a. Sequential balloon inflation	• Uses same balloon for both vessels	• More catheter manipulations • More balloons and inflation devices
b. Simultaneous balloon inflations	• Minimizes atheroma shifting to opposite branch • Allows dilatation without oversizing the balloon relative to small postbifurcation vessel diameter	

sequential inflations may result in a suboptimal main vessel dilation, requiring repeated dilatations. Simultaneous balloon inflations may be used when sequential balloon inflations are unsatisfactory.

Simultaneous balloon inflations. When a shifting plaque causes opposite branch narrowing after sequential inflations, simultaneous balloon inflations are needed. The combined diameter of two balloons in the parent branch should be considered carefully in order to avoid dissection. The loss of the side branch must be weighed against the potential damage to the main vessel by two simultaneous balloon inflations (Fig. 8-5).

Bifurcation lesions have been addressed with atherectomy or rotational ablation devices. The routine application of directional atherectomy (Simpson device) is difficult due to the cutting nature of the directional atherectomy catheter. A Nitinol wire has been recommended to protect the side branch so that metallic wire fragments will not be shaved and embolized. Clinical experience of bifurcation angioplasty with the Rotablator technique is limited.

ANGIOPLASTY OF SEVERELY ECCENTRIC CORONARY STENOSES

An eccentric lesion is a narrowing whose lumen to centerline position ratio is >0.7 (see Fig. 8-6). Moderate to severely eccentric stenoses are considered B2- or C-type lesions, depending on the involvement of side branches, calcification, vessel complexity, and morphology. A satisfactory angioplasty outcome for eccentric lesions is related to the degree of calcification, length (>20 mm), tortuosity, presence of thrombus, and vessel diameter. For most routine procedures, standard balloon angioplasty has been performed with high short- and long-term success rates. Directional atherectomy has been preferred in many of these patients, because it is thought that selective removal of the eccentric plaque can be achieved more efficiently using a directed approach. Confirmation of plaque removal after directional atherectomy with two-dimensional ultrasound imaging has been proposed to yield optimal results. For extreme eccentricity, directional atherectomy has been preferred to balloon angioplasty. Stenting may produce results with <10% residual lumen diameter.

Bifurcation PTCA

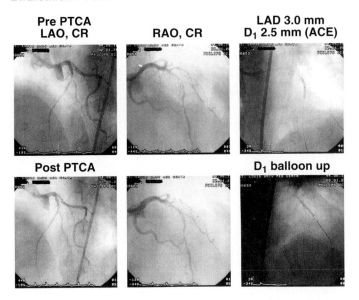

Fig. 8-5. Angiographic demonstration of bifurcation coronary angioplasty involving the left anterior descending (LAD) and first diagonal branch (D1). The LAD and diagonal are both severely involved, with long, diffuse stenoses of >90%. The procedure was performed using a single guide, one guidewire, and one fixed-wire, 2.5-mm balloon in the diagonal. Angioplasty of the LAD is shown on the top right panel. The fixed-wire balloon in the deflated configuration is positioned in the diagonal branch. Following angioplasty of the LAD and diagonal, the vessels are satisfactorily dilated (lower left and middle panels). The diagonal balloon inflation is shown in the bottom right panel. This technique is successful for complex lesions where manipulation of over-the-wire balloons may be difficult and may also require simultaneous balloon inflation.

Some interventionalists prefer laser ablation catheters, although comparative clinical outcome data are not available. Long eccentric lesions may benefit from Rotablator ablation followed with long (>30-mm) balloon dilatations. Clinical outcomes for Rotablator ablation and stent placement for eccentric lesions are still under examination.

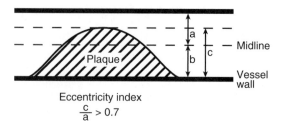

Eccentricity index
$$\frac{c}{a} > 0.7$$

Fig. 8-6.   Schematic description of lesion eccentricity.

ANGIOPLASTY OF SEVERELY CALCIFIED STENOTIC ARTERIES

Balloon angioplasty of a heavily calcified atherosclerotic artery stretches the noncalcified vessel wall, promoting dissection (or rarely rupture) originating at the border region of the calcified and elastic regions. Angiographic evidence of severe calcification is associated with reduced primary success rates and increased complications during and after balloon angioplasty. Balloon angioplasty of calcified lesions may require high-pressure balloons able to exceed 15 atm without bursting. Angioplasty balloons of noncompliant or PET balloon material are preferred. Heavily calcified lesions may puncture polyethelene terephthalate (PET) balloon catheters. Entrapment of ruptured balloon material, although rare, has been reported, making removal of the balloon catheter difficult. Some operators position the distal third of the balloon in the calcified lesion so that withdrawal of a ruptured balloon will be facilitated.

Because of the known increased complications and dissection rates, Rotablator ablation has become the technique of choice for heavily calcified lesions. Cutting of a calcified artery segment may be difficult with directional coronary atherectomy.

Device preferences:
1. Rotablator
2. High-pressure balloon/stent
3. Directional coronary atherectomy

Angioplasty of long, diffuse lesions with or without calcification was considered unsuitable for balloon angioplasty in the early years, but these lesion subtypes are increasingly being managed by long balloon catheters and new interventional techniques. Balloon lengths of 30 mm and 40 mm can cover long diseased segments with a single inflation, reducing the risk of dissection. Long balloons have a slightly larger profile than standard balloons. If necessary, a graduated balloon approach can be used by introducing smaller-diameter balloons and progressing to larger ones. Generally, systems with exchange-wire capability should be chosen because of the increased rate of dissection and the need for prolonged inflations during these procedures. If the lesion is heavily calcified, consider rotoblation first.

ANGIOPLASTY OF OSTIAL LESIONS

Narrowing of the ostium of a vessel presents a particularly difficult management problem for angioplasty because lack of guiding catheter support. The proximal location often necessitates distal perfusion. Also, inflations in the coronary ostial locations have the potential for aortic dissection during RCA angioplasty or dissection of the left main artery from dilations in the ostium of the circumflex or left anterior descending arteries. Ostial lesions are better managed by newer technologies, including atherectomy, rotablation, stent and laser excision. Balloon angioplasty works, but it should be considered a suboptimal technique.

Types of Ostial Lesions

Aorto-ostial stenoses.   The most common ostial stenosis is the aortocoronary ostial lesion, which involves the anastomotic origin of the vessel from the aortic cusp. The origin of the left main, right coronary artery, or a saphenous vein graft are specific examples.

Branch ostial stenoses.   A coronary branch ostial stenosis involves narrowing at the origin of the branch takeoff from a main coronary vessel. Left anterior descending coronary ostial, diagonal, or circumflex marginal ostial lesions are common. The most difficult lesions involve the ostial left anterior descending artery. Angioplasty (or atherectomy) may cause trauma to the left main artery during device manipulation. A left anterior descending stenosis within 2 or 3 mm of the origin should be considered as an ostial lesion with similar technical risks, because most angioplasty devices are designed to cover vessel segments >10 mm in length.

Techniques

Because elastic recoil is very common in ostial-aorto angioplasty, the effectiveness of any balloon catheter technique is limited. Rotational atherectomy, directional atherectomy, and stents minimize or eliminate elastic recoil, with correspondingly improved results.

Guide catheter selection. Angioplasty of right coronary artery ostial lesions is the most difficult, because standard right Judkins catheters often cannot provide satisfactory device support. Configurations such as modified Amplatz (left or right), multipurpose, Arani, or El-Gamal catheters have been used successfully. Ostial occlusion by the guide catheter, as seen by damping of arterial pressure, requires guide catheters with side holes. While these are adequate for coronary perfusion after reestablishment of a patent lumen, side holes permit contrast to escape and may limit coronary visualization, especially when using large devices (directional coronary atherectomy or rotablation atherectomy).

Careful engagement of the guide catheter should minimize ostial trauma to avoid complicating a difficult procedure. The use of Rotablator ablation or directional atherectomy catheters requires nearly coaxial alignment of the guide catheter (and guidewire) upon device entry in the ostium. Significant angulation between the guide catheter and the ostial takeoff will reduce the successful placement of these devices (Fig. 8-7).

Balloon catheter placement. Ostial angioplasty using balloon catheters requires appropriate seating of the balloon segment so that during balloon inflation the catheter will not be ejected from nor compressed forward past the coronary ostia (Fig. 8-8). Removal of the guide catheter into the aorta immediately before balloon inflation will permit the balloon to be inflated outside the guide catheter. The lesion will be appropriately spanned by the two ends of the balloon inflating at equal pressure. Inflation in the guide may result in failure of the distal end of the balloon to inflate properly, or rupture of the balloon.

Alternative strategies. A schematic approach to angioplasty of ostial coronary stenoses (Fig. 8-9) demonstrates an

SVG (1984) ostial lesion
90% → 10% (3.5 mm balloon + 0.018 in. flowire)

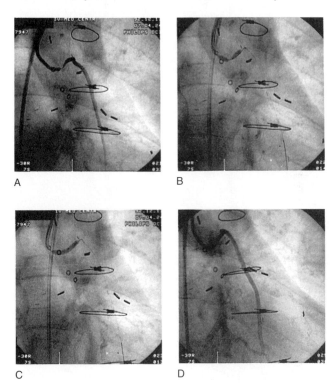

Fig. 8-7.   Example of ostial coronary artery stenosis in a saphenous vein graft. **A,** The cineangiogram shows ostial stenosis
in the right anterior oblique projection. An 8 French guide is
positioned coaxially with the origin of the graft. **B,** A 3.5-mm
high-pressure balloon was used to dilate the stenosis. **C,** The
balloon is fully inflated. **D,** The ostial lesion after balloon
angioplasty. This lesion is better treated with a stent placed
primarily. (From Kern MJ, Donohue TJ, Flynn MS, Aguirre
FV, Bach RG, Caracciolo EA: Interventional physiology: limitations of translesional pressure and flow velocity for long ostial
left anterior descending stenoses, *Cathet Cardiovasc Diagn*
33:50-54, 1994.)

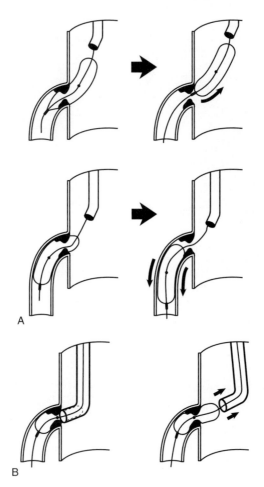

Fig. 8-8. **A,** Effect of squeezing the balloon out of an ostial lesion. The top panels show the balloon being ejected from the ostium, and the lower panels show the balloon advancing inside the artery during inflation. **B,** Proper guide catheter positioning helps to seat the balloon in an ostial lesion. (From Freed M, Grines C, Safian R, editors: *The new manual of interventional cardiology,* Birmingham, Michigan, 1996, Physician's Press.)

algorithm using rotational atherectomy (Roto), directional excimer laser coronary angioplasty (DELCA), concentric excimer laser angioplasty (ELCA), or directional coronary atherectomy (DCA). For lesions that have minimal or only mild

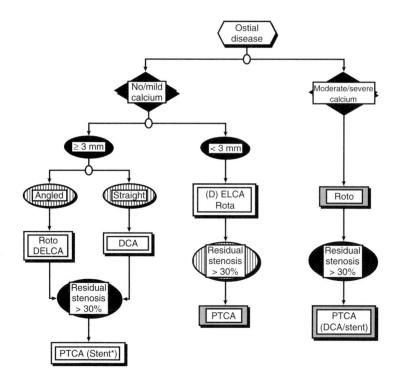

Fig. 8-9. Algorithm for approach to ostial lesions using new devices. DCA, Directional coronary atherectomy; DELCA, directional excimer laser coronary angioplasty; ELCA, concentric excimer laser coronary angioplasty; Roto, rotational atherectomy. (From Popma JJ, Leon MB: *A lesion specific approach to New-Device angioplasty* in Topol EJ, editor. Textbook of Interventional Cardiology, ed 2, Philadelphia, 1994, W. B. Saunders, pp 973-985.)

calcium >3 mm in length, rotablation and DCA are preferred. If there is a residual stenosis of >30%, coronary angioplasty with or without stent may be employed. For short (<5-mm) lesions, rotational atherectomy or laser angioplasty is recommended. For moderate to severe calcified lesions, rotational atherectomy is the technique of choice.

Clinical Results

Angioplasty results for ostial lesions are less satisfactory than angioplasty results for other arterial sites. Studies of ostial lesion angioplasty success rates are reported ranging from 74% to 90%, with complications ranging from 3% to 10%. Restenosis rates average 50% in most series.

CORONARY ANGIOPLASTY FOR VERY PROXIMAL LEFT ANTERIOR DESCENDING STENOSIS

Angioplasty of a very proximal or ostial left anterior descending artery stenosis can be very difficult. Although most studies have not identified this location as a major risk factor, a complication at this location can be life-threatening. Balloon dilatation of part of the left main coronary artery segment is unavoidable because of the proximity of the lesion. If the circumflex branch is compromised, the potential for hemodynamic instability is high. Left main coronary dissection is a forerunner to catastrophic vessel closure. Angiographic success in ostial lesions was 86%, compared to 90% for nonostial left anterior descending artery lesions.* The angiographic dissection rate for ostial stenoses was 32% versus 38% (p = NS) for other left anterior descending lesions. The incidence of coronary dissection during left anterior descending ostial angioplasty was 10%, compared to <5% for other locations in the left anterior descending artery. Of 213 patients who had very proximal LAD lesions dilated, 5 patients had left main coronary dissections. The clinical outcome was benign in 4 of the 5 patients, with one patient occluding the left anterior descending at 48 hour. No special technique for balloon angioplasty was recommended. However, sharp angulation at the left main-left anterior descending junction appeared to be a risk factor for left main dissection when the inflated balloon partially covered the left main. Based on the incidence of left main dissection and the potential for abrupt vessel closure, coronary atherectomy, rotational ablation, or stent placement has superseded the use of routine balloon angioplasty for ostial left anterior descending lesions.

ANGIOPLASTY FOR TOTAL CORONARY OCCLUSIONS

Angioplasty of coronary artery occlusions has a widely variable success rate. Success rates range from 50% to 80%, with

* Deligonul U, Vandormael M, Kern M, et al: Coronary angioplasty: a therapeutic option for symptomatic patients with two and three vessel coronary disease. *JACC* 11:1173–1179, 1988.

mortality rates of 0% to 2% and emergency coronary artery bypass surgery requirements of 1% to 3%. Abrupt vessel closure following total occlusions may occur in ≤10% of patients, but may be clinically silent depending on the collateral supply. Chronic total occlusions are perhaps the largest group of complex lesions for which angioplasty is attempted. The angiographic success rate in these lesions is 50% to 70%, which is much lower than for routine angioplasty. The restenosis rate is also higher. Procedural success rates for total occlusions depend on how long the occlusion has been in place. For occlusions <3 months old, the success rate is higher (60% to 70%), compared to 50% to 60% for those older than 3 months. Other problems in dealing with total occlusions include the potential for distal embolization, perforation, and guidewire entrapment. Chronic total occlusions represent the most technically challenging cases taken on by interventional cardiologists.

Chronic total occlusions may require specialized guidewires, including Terumo, Magnum, and stiff or standard 0.018-in. wires. The 0.018-in. wires require a 0.018-in. compatible balloon system. When crossing total occlusions, it is sometimes difficult to know whether the wire is in the true or the false lumen after crossing a distal occlusion. Catheters through which distal contrast injections can be made may be helpful. After the guidewire has been positioned across the stenosis, occasionally even a low-profile balloon catheter cannot cross the lesion. In this case, a fixed-wire system may be successful.

Anatomic and Clinical Factors

The duration of the total occlusion is the most significant factor in determining the success of angioplasty. Total occlusion >3 months' duration reduces angioplasty success rates to <50%.

The length of the total occlusion also carries significant prognostic importance with total occlusions >15 mm having success rates <45% in some studies.

Selection of arteries for total occlusion angioplasty should be based on favorable or unfavorable angiographic morphology (Fig. 8-10).

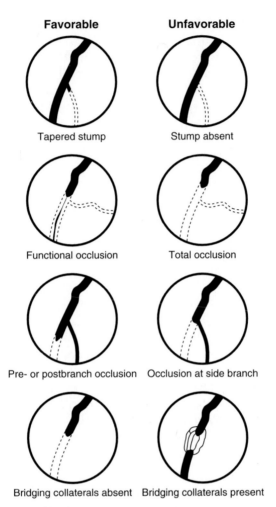

Favorable   **Unfavorable**

Tapered stump   Stump absent

Functional occlusion   Total occlusion

Pre- or postbranch occlusion   Occlusion at side branch

Bridging collaterals absent   Bridging collaterals present

Fig. 8-10. Morphology of total coronary occlusion: favorable and unfavorable morphology for procedural success. (Modified from Freed M, Grines C: *Manual of interventional cardiology,* Birmingham, Michigan, 1992, Physician's Press, p 148.)

Favorable features include:
1. Tapered stumps
2. Functional antegrade occlusions with evidence of antegrade angiographic flow

3. A post-branch location with tapered (bird beak) occlusion
4. Absence of bridging collaterals
   Unfavorable morphologic features include:
1. Flush occlusions
2. Abrupt occlusions
3. Occlusions at side-branches with no beaklike morphology
4. The presence of bridging collaterals
   Unfavorable features have been associated with poor angioplasty results. Collateral filling of the vessel in question is helpful to identify its course and potential for tolerating ischemia should reclosure occur. Contralateral collateral supply artery opacification may define the vessel course, proximal site, and length of the occluded target segment.

Techniques

Angioplasty success requires appropriate guide catheter support, selection of a suitably stiff guidewire, and identification and confirmation of the intraluminal guidewire path. An intraluminal guidewire position can be confirmed with contrast injection through the balloon catheter or a small tracking catheter (Target Therapeutics) after advancement over the guidewire through the occlusion. The balloon catheter can then be advanced safely to dilate the total occlusion (Fig. 8-11). Prolonged balloon inflations with long (>30-mm) balloons may give better results for long occlusion. In some cases, stents may be required.

Alternative Strategies

Strategies for angioplasty of total occlusions include extra stiff or coated guidewires, specialized guidewire systems (Magnum), rotablation or laser guidewires, or directional atherectomy (Fig. 8-12). These newer devices have not yet produced results exceeding those for balloon angioplasty.

Angioplasty of Total Occlusion of Saphenous Vein Grafts

Balloon angioplasty of occluded saphenous vein grafts represents a highly complex, high-risk procedure that has a low anticipated probability for success. Bypass surgery should be considered before selecting interventional percutaneous revascularization for these conditions. The recanalization of old (>3 months), totally occluded saphenous vein grafts has a low likelihood of success unless there is an antegrade channel.

A.F., 80-year-old man

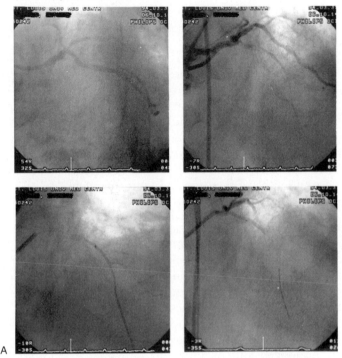

A

Fig. 8-11.   **A,** *Top left,* Left anterior caudal view showing total occlusion of the left anterior descending artery, stenosis of intermediate ramus, and patent circumflex vessel in an 80-year-old man with class IV angina. *Top right,* Right anterior oblique cranial projection with total occlusion of the left anterior descending with faint antegrade left-to-left collateral filling. *Bottom left,* Guidewire and tracking catheter successfully advanced across the total occlusion. Contrast opacification of the distal vessel confirmed intraluminal location of the guidewire. *Bottom right,* Long angioplasty balloon (2.0-mm × 30-mm) advanced and lesion dilated. **B,** *Top left,* A filling defect is prominent at the proximal left anterior descending site. *Top right,* A 3.0-mm × 20-mm Gianturco-Roubin stent placed across the proximal left anterior descending. *Bottom right,* Final result showing widely patent, previously totally occluded left anterior descending artery, now with excellent coronary blood flow. **C,** Angioplasty of second vessel (circumflex) in this multi-vessel procedure was performed after recanalization of LAD artery.

A.F., 80-year-old man

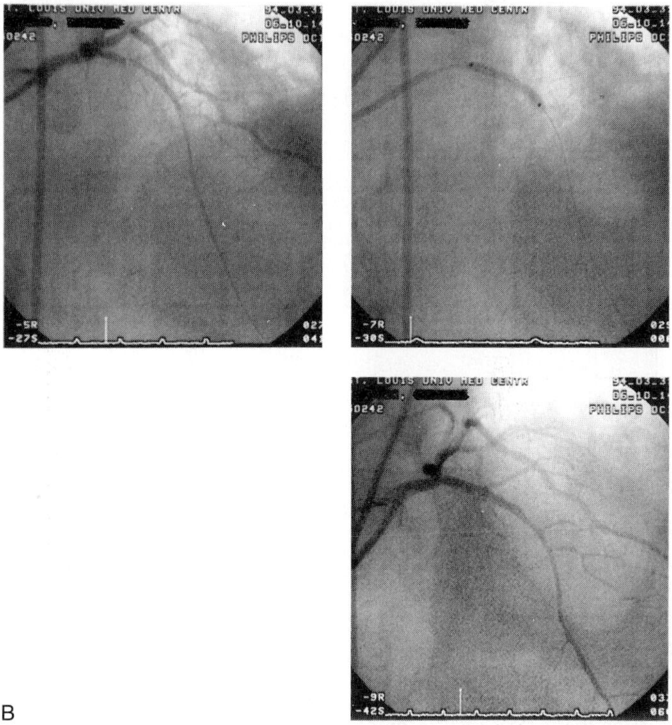

B

Fig. 8-11.   (*Continued*).

Successful angioplasty in conjunction with thrombolysis has been reported. TEC atherectomy (see Chapter 6) has been performed successfully on thrombosed saphenous vein grafts.

MULTIVESSEL CORONARY ANGIOPLASTY

Multiple-vessel coronary angioplasty approaches a series of stenoses one at a time, using any and all methods applicable to simple and complex single-vessel angioplasty. Multivessel coronary angioplasty means that coronary angioplasty is performed in at least two of the three arterial territories (left anterior descending, left circumflex, and right coronary arteries). For example, the dilatation of a mid-left anterior descending and an obtuse marginal is multivessel angio-

A.F., 80-year-old man

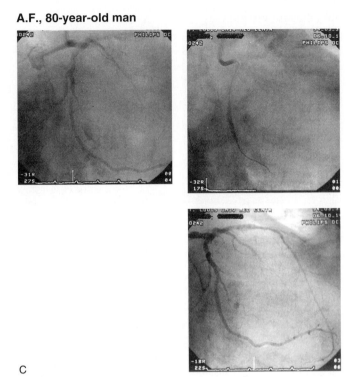

C

Fig. 8-11. (*Continued*).

plasty, but dilatation of a mid-left anterior descending and a diagonal branch should be considered single-vessel, multilesion angioplasty. Multivessel coronary angioplasty has been used instead of surgical revascularization if the coronary stenoses morphology and location are likely to yield a high level of success. Multivessel angioplasty is also selected if the operator and patient accept incomplete coronary revascularization when all stenoses cannot be dilated. The results of multicenter randomized trials between coronary artery bypass surgery and coronary angioplasty suggest that equal revascularization subgroups can be identified that have similar clinical outcomes, but angioplasty has a higher rate of repeat procedures and future surgical revascularizations. The risk of restenosis of at least one

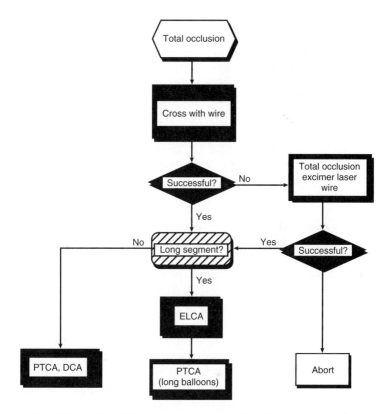

Fig. 8-12. Algorithm for angioplasty of total coronary occlusions. DCA, Directional coronary atherectomy; ELCA, concentric excimer laser coronary angioplasty. If crossing with the wire, laser angioplasty can be considered, but most interventionalists do not have this tool readily available and thus the procedure is terminated at this point. In addition, long-segment angioplasty can be used with a long balloon as noted. (From Popma JJ, Leon MB: *A lesion specific approach to New-Device angioplasty* in Topol EJ, editor. Textbook of Interventional Cardiology, ed 2, Philadelphia, 1994, W. B. Saunders, pp 973-985.)

lesion in an individual patient is related to the number of lesions dilated. This is important in making complete-versus-incomplete revascularization decisions. However, many patients will have a satisfactory long-term outcome when two or three vessels are dilated successfully.

Strategies for Multivessel Angioplasty

Complete single-setting angioplasty. The primary lesion is responsible for myocardial ischemia or is the most critical lesion supplying a moderate to large area of functioning myocardium. Multivessel angioplasty at a single setting addresses the primary target lesion first. If this is angiographically (without significant angiographic evidence of dissection or thrombus) or hemodynamically satisfactory, the secondary lesions are carefully approached and dilated consecutively (Fig. 8-11).

Staged multivessel angioplasty procedures. In some patients, only the target lesion identified by objective ischemic indicators (exercise testing or direct translesional hemodynamic assessment) is dilated. The remaining, secondary stenoses are dilated at a later date if symptoms of myocardial ischemia persist. In patients with intermediately severe multiple stenoses without objective ischemia, the culprit vessel may be identified by direct lesion assessment (see Chapter 10).

Indications. Indications for multivessel angioplasty include:
1. Patients who have clinical symptoms with evidence of ischemia during noninvasive testing
2. Patients who are resuscitated from sudden death in the absence of acute myocardial infarction
3. Patients who plan to undergo high-risk noncardiac surgery and patients with class II-IV angina with symptoms poorly controlled on medical therapy or who are intolerant of medical therapy

Target lesion angiographic morphology should preferably have low-risk features, with secondary stenoses supplying small areas of viable myocardium. In general, multivessel PTCA is best selected for low-risk lesions.

Contraindications. Relative contraindications to multivessel angioplasty are similar to those for single-vessel angioplasty for individual stenoses:
1. Left main stenosis or left main equivalent lesions
2. Type B2 or C lesions supplying large areas of viable myocardium
3. Severe lesions in two major vessels in which one is technically unsuitable for revascularization

High-risk multivessel angioplasty. Patients at high risk for death following or during coronary angioplasty include those with recent myocardial infarction, recent emergency bypass surgery, or poor left ventricular function. Patients with unprotected left main or left main equivalent disease or single-vessel disease supplying all remaining viable myocardium, high-risk angiographic morphology subsets (degenerated vein graft, intraluminal filling defect, severe angulation, severe calcification), and patients who are very elderly all present higher risk for severe complications and death.

Before considering high-risk angioplasty, discussions should be held with the referring physicians, supporting surgeons, and family members. Should disaster occur, the management approach should be already identified. High-risk angioplasty should weigh the risks versus benefits for nonoperative revascularization. Objective evidence of ischemia or myocardial viability should be present before accepting the risk of death versus the benefit of restoring patency to potentially nonfunctional myocardium.

Technical aspects of high-risk multivessel angioplasty include the following:

Identification. The target lesion should be clearly identified and characterized as ischemia producing.

Vascular access. Access to the contralateral artery and vein is maintained with 5F sheaths, in case hemodynamic support is needed.

Venous access for temporary pacing and/or monitoring of pulmonary artery pressures is required.

Lower abdominal angiography should identify patients who may not tolerate prophylactic intraaortic balloon placement.

Angioplasty equipment. Primary reperfusion balloons or stent placement should be considered early, and appropriately large guiding catheters and sheaths should be selected. Angioplasty should start with extra-support guidewires in case stenting is needed.

Hemodynamic support. An intraaortic balloon pump may be inserted prophylactically or be available on standby for immediate insertion for hypotension or ischemic complications.

Active blood perfusion pumps or perfluorocarbon perfusions have not proven more successful than autoperfusion catheters and intraaortic balloon pumping.

Portable cardiopulmonary bypass may be considered under the specific limitations described below.

Multivessel angioplasty in patients with total occlusion of one vessel. A relatively common clinical presentation is a totally occluded right coronary artery or left anterior descending artery with critical narrowing in the opposite vessel. This creates a potentially high-risk situation, especially when the totally occluded vessel is not suitable for angioplasty or when it supplies a large area. However, in selected cases the totally occluded vessel may be omitted with dilatation of the contralateral artery. A typical case may be dilatation of a left anterior descending artery in the presence of a totally occluded, small- to medium-size right coronary artery supplying an infarcted area and receiving collaterals from both the left anterior descending and circumflex arteries. For angioplasty of multivessel stenoses with one vessel totally occluded, the first approach should be to recanalize the total occlusion using standard techniques. These patients should be considered at higher than normal risk.

Revascularization should proceed with total occlusion angioplasty to restore antegrade flow to the region supplied by collaterals and potentially reverse collateral flow to the remaining target areas. If total occlusion dilatation is successful, the operator can proceed to the remaining secondary lesions. If angioplasty of the total occlusion is unsuccessful, the patient can be referred to surgery for complete revascularization.

Clinical Results

Reports of procedural success vary widely (80% to 95%) among trials based on various criteria employed for assessing the technical difficulty of the lesions. The Multivessel Angioplasty Prognosis Group recommended bypass surgery in patients with two-vessel disease who had type B2 or C lesions in large-caliber vessel or when two adverse prognostic factors were present, especially when the risk territory score was >15 or left ventricular dysfunction was present.

Restenosis for multivessel disease averages approximately 40%. Rates as high as 60% have been reported at some centers. Complex lesions are at particular risk for developing restenosis in multivessel angioplasty patients.

Complete revascularization is defined as successful dilatation of all significant coronary narrowings on bypassable vessels or branches. Incomplete revascularization is obtained either by dilating only the culprit lesion, or by attempting dilatation of all lesions that are deemed to be functionally significant, without trying to achieve anatomically complete revascularization. Identification and successful treatment of the culprit lesion are essential, otherwise the revascularization will be inadequate.

During follow-up after angioplasty, patients with incomplete revascularization experience more frequent recurrent angina and require coronary artery bypass graft surgery more often than those with complete revascularization. Some of the differences between these groups may also be related to the higher incidence of unfavorable baseline clinical characteristics of the incomplete revascularization group.

Patients who achieve incomplete revascularization may have a highly satisfactory reduction of symptoms and clinical improvement despite evidence of myocardial ischemia on future clinical evaluations. Bypass surgery for patients with complex, low-success lesion morphology, who are likely to have incomplete revascularization, may be a preferred alternative.

In patients with acute myocardial infarction and multivessel disease, the angioplasty procedure should be staged, with dilatation of only the infarct-related vessel at the first session.

ANGIOPLASTY FOR UNSTABLE ANGINA

Although unstable angina can be successfully managed medically in the majority of patients, associated morbidity and mortality are high, with in-hospital death ranging from 1% to 2%, acute myocardial infarction ranging from 5% to 9%, and 1-year mortality and recurrent infarction rates as high as 20% in some patient series. Coronary angioplasty for unstable angina is a highly effective technique despite a wide range (3% to 30%) of emergency coronary bypass surgery rates. Angioplasty mortality in this patient subset is low (0.5% to 1%).

A common strategy for patients with unstable angina begins with aggressive medical therapy (aspirin, intravenous heparin, beta blockers, calcium blockers, and intravenous nitrates). If the patient stabilizes, urgent angioplasty can be deferred. Cardiac catheterization with subsequent risk stratification can be performed. In patients with recurrent symptoms during the first 12 to 14 hour of medical management, urgent coronary angiography to identify the extent and characteristics of coronary artery disease will facilitate appropriate decisions for revascularization using either coronary bypass surgery or coronary angioplasty.

Because unstable angina is associated with thrombus and acute plaque transformation, angioplasty should be preceded by intravenous heparin infusion for ≥24 hour as tolerated. Intraprocedural thrombolytic therapy has been recommended by some operators. Angioplasty techniques for lesions with thrombus and/or type B2 or C lesions should be used. As in high-risk angioplasty, venous access is required for a temporary transvenous pacemaker, especially in patients who demonstrate intraventricular conduction delay or heart block. As indicated for high-risk angioplasty patients, hemodynamic support with intravenous fluids, pulmonary artery pressure monitoring, and intraaortic balloon pumping are also used as needed.

A recently approved antiplatelet antibody (ReoPro™, E. Lilly Co.) given as a bolus before the procedure and followed by a 12-hour infusion may decrease recurrent ischemic events after angioplasty in unstable angina patients.

ANGIOPLASTY FOR ACUTE MYOCARDIAL INFARCTION
Strategies for Angioplasty for Acute Myocardial Infarction

Direct or primary angioplasty [angioplasty undertaken without prior thrombolytic therapy]. Direct angioplasty is indicated for patients in whom thrombolytics are contraindicated, patients in cardiogenic shock, and any patient having an acute myocardial infarction who has immediate access to an interventional cardiac catheterization facility. The advantages of direct angioplasty include early and complete reperfusion, definition of associated coronary artery disease, and reduced bleeding complications of thrombolytic therapy. The disadvantages of direct angioplasty are the delay of reperfusion with 24-hour on-call services, reduced access to skilled interventionalists, and emergency surgical backup.

Rescue or salvage angioplasty [angioplasty performed in a setting of failed thrombolysis]. Rescue or salvage angioplasty is used in patients with acute myocardial infarction after failed thrombolysis. Rescue coronary angioplasty for anterior myocardial infarction reduces the risk of death and congestive heart failure and improves exercise ejection fraction. Reestablishment of coronary perfusion is directed at myocardial salvage, which is especially important in such patients who are at high risk of early mortality. The rescue angioplasty approach is supported by nonrandomized observational trials in which increased survival rates are observed in patients in cardiogenic shock or after failed thrombolysis with continued evidence of myocardial infarction. Intracoronary thrombolytic agents and intraaortic balloon counterpulsation are commonly applied adjunctive modalities for this high-risk subset.

Immediate angioplasty [angioplasty performed less than 24 hour after thrombolysis].   Immediate angioplasty following successful thrombolysis is indicated if continued myocardial ischemia is evident. Results of randomized trials of routine angioplasty after successful thrombolysis do not demonstrate benefit over elective angioplasty, based on objective ischemic indications in the postinfarction period.

Elective (or deferred) angioplasty [angioplasty performed several days after thrombolysis when indicated by evidence of myocardial ischemia].   Elective or deferred angioplasty is an acceptable approach after acute myocardial infarction in patients without complications or evidence of myocardial ischemia after they have received thrombolytic therapy. Ischemic risk stratification is performed before coronary revascularization. Catheterization and angioplasty are undertaken only if evidence of increased ischemic risk is present.

Coronary bypass surgery for patients with acute myocardial infarction.   In patients who have left main stenosis, left main equivalent stenoses, severe multivessel disease not suitable for angioplasty, or severe multivessel disease with cardiogenic shock, coronary artery bypass grafting is preferred.

Technical Considerations

Anticoagulation.   Because acute myocardial infarction always involves thromboses, medical pretreatment with oral aspirin and intravenous heparin (activated clotting time [ACT] >300 sec) is required.

Angioplasty equipment.   The operators should anticipate coronary intervention and initiate diagnostic catheterization with a large-diameter arterial sheath for both the arterial and venous accesses. Angioplasty techniques for lesions of high risk should be used. An approach to total coronary occlusion often includes intracoronary thrombolytics or a reperfusion balloon catheter. Prolonged balloon inflations may be required.

Hemodynamic support and intraaortic balloon pumping. In patients with decreased left ventricular function, an intraaortic balloon pump should be inserted before the procedure is begun. After successful angioplasty for acute infarction, intraaortic balloon counterpulsation is associated with higher rates of sustained vessel patency and reduced recurrent ischemia. Figure 8-13 illustrates angioplasty for acute myocardial infarction.

ANGIOPLASTY FOR CARDIOGENIC SHOCK

The cardiogenic shock syndrome is associated with mortality rates >90%. Prognosis and management of patients in cardiogenic shock due to myocardial infarction are determined by duration of myocardial ischemia, cardiac index, left ventricular end-diastolic pressure, and the presence of pulmonary edema. Emergency coronary revascularization with hemodynamic support, including early use of intraaortic balloon pumping, is required. Lee et al. (1991) reviewed outcomes of 69 patients in cardiogenic shock treated with emergency coronary angioplasty. Balloon angioplasty was unsuccessful in 20 and successful in 49 patients. Clinical characteristics between the two groups were similar. In patients who had unsuccessful balloon angioplasty, short-term survival rate was 20%, compared to 69% in patients who had successful coronary angioplasty. Despite successful revascularization, one-third of patients with severe left ventricular dysfunction require repeat interventions during long-term follow-up. The continued deterioration of the patient's clinical status is related to residual left ventricular function independent of angioplasty result. Emergency coronary angioplasty improves initial long-term survival for patients in cardiogenic shock complicating myocardial infarction.

ANGIOPLASTY IN THE ELDERLY

Coronary angioplasty techniques are being utilized increasingly in patients older than 75 or 80 years. Coronary angioplasty risk is increased in elderly patients. However, this risk has been improving in recent years. Careful case selection is important. Lesions with a high expected success rate should be chosen. A bailout strategy should be carefully laid out, because some emergency procedures may not be feasible or may carry a very high risk. Myocardial perfusion and hemodynamics should be optimized before the procedure. Adequate hydration and limiting the amount of contrast medium are important. Anticoagulation should be individualized, and excessive anticoagulation should be avoided. Extra precautions need to be taken in sheath removal and hemostasis.

ANGIOPLASTY IN CARDIAC TRANSPLANT RECIPIENTS

Coronary disease is a significant cause of morbidity and mortality in cardiac transplant recipients. Coronary angioplasty is used in this group of patients to treat epicardial artery obstructions. Although the acute results are similar to those in nontransplant cases, long-term effects of angioplasty on morbidity and mortality are not well known.

ANGIOPLASTY OF CORONARY ARTERY CONDUITS

Fifteen to twenty percent of all patients entering the catheterization laboratory have undergone previous coronary artery bypass graft surgery and may require revascularization. For these patients, the objective of angioplasty in general is to provide symptom rehabilitation through perfusion to ischemic zones in lieu of second or third operations. Several categories of patients who have had previous bypass surgery may be more suitable for percutaneous revascularization than undergoing a second (or third) operation. From review of surgical series, second coronary artery bypass graft operations have increased operative mortality rates (2% to 8%), postoperative myocardial infarction rates (2% to 8%), and postoperative bleeding rates (1.3% to 11%). Coronary angioplasty for saphenous vein graft stenoses has a success rate >85%, complications <10%, urgent bypass surgery 4%, myocardial infarction 3%, and mortality 1-3%. The risk/benefit ratio for angioplasty of saphenous vein grafts must be weighed against the risk/benefit ratio for repeat coronary artery bypass graft surgery.

Saphenous Vein Graft Angioplasty

A large number of patients present with recurrent angina following coronary artery bypass grafting. Balloon angio-

J.A., Acute MI with TPA

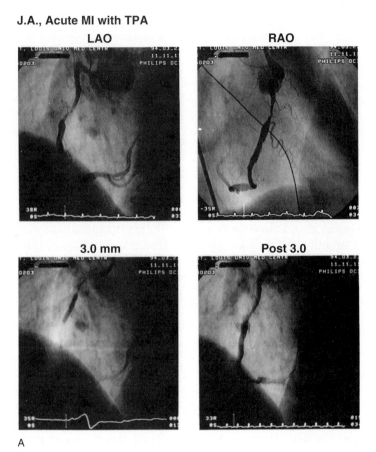

A

Fig. 8-13.   Direct coronary angioplasty for a patient with acute myocardial and angina following treatment with intravenous tissue plasminogen activator (t-PA). **A,** *Top panels,* Right coronary artery stenosis (90%) with irregular configuration and minimal evidence of intraluminal filling defect in the left anterior oblique (LAO) view. Right anterior oblique (RAO) view of the proximal right coronary artery lesion. *Bottom panels,* Direct angioplasty performed with a 3.0-mm balloon catheter. Post 3.0-mm balloon angioplasty with suboptimal result and continued accumulation of thrombotic material. **B,** *Top left,* RAO view of the postangioplasty balloon, showing a residual narrowing. *Top right,* A 3.5-mm Flow Track 40 reperfusion balloon used to dilate the long segment. The postangioplasty result is excellent (*bottom panels*) in the LAO projection and in the RAO projection. Successful patency was enhanced using intraaortic balloon pumping for 24 hours.

J.A., Acute MI with TPA

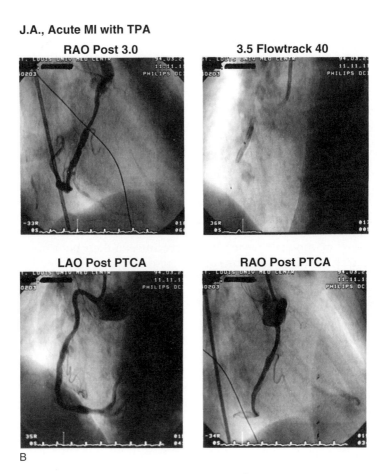

Fig. 8-13.   (*Continued*).

plasty can be performed in carefully selected patient groups. However, saphenous vein graft angioplasty has an increased risk of complications and lower long-term success rates, particularly if the vein graft has degenerated (usually associated with an irregular appearance on angiography), or if vein grafts are older than 3 years. Adequate guide catheter support for saphenous vein graft angioplasty can be difficult. Also, the saphenous veins may be too large for conventional balloon catheters with a maximum of 4 mm in diameter. The potential for distal embolization during saphenous vein graft angioplasty is high. Due to the length of saphenous vein grafts, an extremely trackable system may be required. A lesion distal to the insertion of the graft on the native vessel or through a "jump" (spanning several branches) graft may require a special balloon with a long catheter shaft length.

Likewise, internal mammary artery stenosis, particularly at the distal anastomotic site, represents a particular problem, in terms of both intubation and achieving effective placement of the balloon. A fixed-wire balloon has been advocated as a first choice. Many over-the-wire systems can now be positioned successfully in a majority of internal mammary artery stenoses, allowing for distal guidewire control in the left anterior descending artery, an extremely important vessel in all patients. Monorail systems are not particularly useful for internal mammary arteries, mainly because of their poor trackability. Similarly, because of a small-diameter internal mammary artery ostium, a small-diameter guide catheter may be needed, making visualization more of a problem.

The major factor associated with successful saphenous vein graft angioplasty is graft age. Saphenous vein grafts >3 years old have lower success rates than grafts <1 year old. Young saphenous vein grafts are often narrowed more by thrombus. Old saphenous vein grafts degenerate because of atherosclerotic material and are more prone to emboli.

Because of the predisposition to thrombosis, embolization of material within the aged vein graft to distal regions is the most common complication, resulting in a satisfactory angiographic conduit appearance with poor myocardial reflow and potential myocardial ischemia/infarction. Abrupt closure of the vein graft after angioplasty due to dissection or thrombus with poor angiographic flow has been reported in 5% to 7% of patients. Restenosis rates using conventional balloon angioplasty are ≥50% in most series. For this reason, the technique for angioplasty of saphenous vein grafts has evolved to include primary stenting to achieve maximal luminal enlargement. Stenting for saphenous vein grafts has an excellent early success rate, and lower rates of restenosis, subacute closure, embolization, myocardial infarction, and death. Restenosis rates after saphenous vein stenting are reported to be around 25% for most of the early patient series.

Saphenous vein graft angiographic morphology.   Lesion location within a saphenous vein graft is associated with different angioplasty success rates.

1. Aorto-ostial lesions have lower success rates with higher restenosis rates than saphenous vein graft mid-body stenoses.
2. Mid-body locations have lower complications and lower restenosis rates relative to aorto-ostial locations.
3. Distal saphenous vein graft-native vessel anastomosis sites can be dilated effectively with results similar to those in native vessels. For these lesions, the morphology of the stenosis carries the same implications as for those in native vessels with an increased propensity for thrombogenic complications. A strategy for saphenous vein graft angioplasty is described in Fig. 8-14.

Technique.   Guide catheters should be the large-lumen type to accommodate stents (either sheathed or hand crimped). Guide catheter support is important. Amplatz (left/right), multipurpose, or JR4 tip shapes provide excellent backup for various saphenous vein graft orientations (see Chapter 3).

Stent, directional coronary atherectomy, and prolonged balloon inflation or reperfusion balloon angioplasty are the techniques of choice.

Internal Mammary Artery Angioplasty

Internal mammary artery angioplasty presents one of the most difficult technical challenges. Lesions usually involve the anastomotic site to the native vessel. A sufficient length of the balloon angioplasty catheter and successful negotiation of the tortuosity throughout the body of the internal mammary artery are the two most common problems. Vasospasm of the arterial conduit may occur, and should be managed with appropriate dosages of intracoronary nitroglycerin.

Guide catheter selection is limited, and good seating may be difficult. Careful manipulation should prevent internal mammary artery ostial dissection.

TREATMENT OF THROMBOSIS DURING CORONARY ANGIOPLASTY

Intracoronary thrombus may occur in up to 15% of all patients undergoing coronary angioplasty (Figs. 8-15 and 8-16). Medically refractory unstable anginal syndromes have a substantially higher association with intracoronary thrombus, being observed in up to 40% of such procedures. A mechanical approach using balloon catheter dilatation of lesions associ-

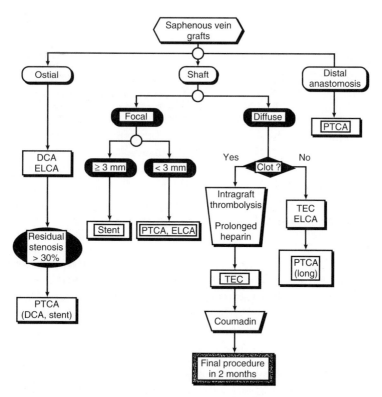

Fig. 8-14.   Approach to angioplasty in saphenous vein grafts. DCA, Directional coronary atherectomy; ELCA, concentric excimer laser coronary angioplasty; TEC, transluminal extraction catheter. Saphenous vein grafts are approached according to the location of the ostial mid-shaft or distal anastomotic lesions. For ostial lesions, DCA is performed. If the residual stenosis is >30%, angioplasty or a stent can be placed. For focal mid-shaft lesions, stent or angioplasty can be performed, depending on the length of the focal lesion. If the mid-shaft is diffusely diseased, consideration of intragraft thrombolysis with prolonged heparin followed by TEC extraction catheter treatment has been recommended. If there is no thrombus, then TEC or ELCA can be performed followed by long balloon angioplasty. For distal anastomotic lesions, angioplasty is recommended. (From Popma JJ, Leon MB: *A lesion specific approach to New-Device angioplasty* in Topol EJ, editor. Textbook of Interventional Cardiology, ed 2, Philadelphia, 1994, W. B. Saunders, pp 973-985.)

Thrombus in SVG to RCA

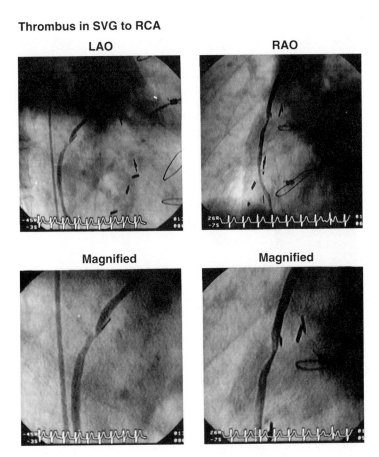

Fig. 8-15. Thrombus in a saphenous vein graft (SVG) to the right coronary artery (RCA). *Left panels,* Left anterior oblique (LAO) view of the vein graft with mid-vessel thrombus. Angiographic characterization shows irregular lucency with three sides of contrast and a longitudinal lucency in its mid-portion on the magnified view. *Right panels,* Right anterior oblique (RAO) view. On the magnified panel the filling defect can be seen extending both above and beyond the region of the stenosis. Intracoronary thrombus was treated as described.

ated with thrombus carries an increased risk of abrupt occlusion, embolization, acute myocardial infarction, emergency bypass surgery, and death compared to angioplasty for non-

B.L., 41-year-old woman, SVG

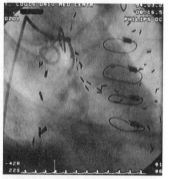
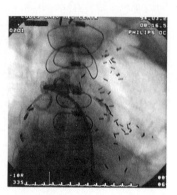
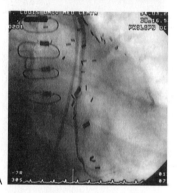

A

Fig. 8-16.   A 41-year-old woman undergoing thrombolysis and angioplasty for occluded saphenous vein graft (SVG). **A,** *Top panels,* Left and right anterior oblique projections show thrombus in the proximal segment of the vein graft to the obtuse marginal. Distal vein graft in the right anterior oblique projection (lower left) shows faint filling of the distal vessel after guidewire passage through the occluded proximal portion. **B,** Right anterior oblique (top left) and left anterior oblique (top right) view 24 hours following infusion of thrombolytic therapy into the vein graft through a tracking catheter shows a patent proximal portion of the saphenous vein graft with distal residual evidence of thrombus, which underwent successful angioplasty. *Bottom panel,* Flow velocity obtained in the distal vein graft after thrombolytic therapy, which improved from no flow prior to the procedure.

B.L., 41-year-old woman, SVG

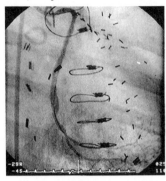
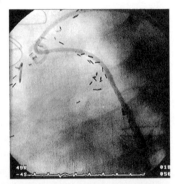

24 hours after UK

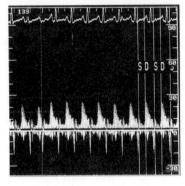

B

Fig. 8-16. (*Continued*).

thrombotic lesions. An optimal mode of therapy of angioplasty of thrombotic lesions has not been defined. Many interventionalists attempt to decrease thrombus bulk by administration of intracoronary thrombolytic agents before coronary angioplasty.

Pharmacologic Therapy

Three thrombolytic agents are available for selective intraarterial thrombolysis.

1. *Streptokinase* is a nonenzymatic protein derived from beta-hemolytic streptococci that convert plasminogen directly to the active plasmin form. Streptokinase is a nonspecific agent in that it degrades not only fibrin but also fibrinogen and other systemic coagulation factors. This results in

a systemic fibrinolytic state. In addition, because of the fact that streptokinase is a bacterial protein, patients may develop neutralizing antibodies and allergic reactions after the initial administration.

2. *Urokinase* is also a direct activator of plasminogen (i.e., it does not require binding to fibrin for activation). Thus, it also may cause significant systemic fibrinogenolysis. Unlike streptokinase, however, urokinase is not antigenic.

3. *Tissue plasminogen activator* (t-PA) is produced by recombinant DNA technology. Because t-PA requires binding to fibrin to activate plasminogen, it was initially hoped that it would lead to less bleeding. However, clinical studies have not demonstrated an advantage in terms of bleeding side effects with t-PA use relative to streptokinase. t-PA is not antigenic. Intravenous t-PA does appear to be more efficacious in opening occluded coronary arteries than intravenous streptokinase for acute myocardial infarction. However, this translates into only a small decrease in mortality in one study.

For selective intraarterial thrombolysis, there is a general consensus that urokinase is more effective than streptokinase. Less data are available for selective intraarterial thrombolysis with t-PA, but preliminary data indicate that it is approximately equal in efficacy to urokinase. In our laboratory we currently use urokinase for selective intraarterial thrombolysis.

Procedure

1. Perform arteriogram to document thrombus and branch vessel anatomy and patency.
2. Position catheter selectively in vessel to receive thrombolytic agent (Fig. 8-17).
3. A 3 French infusion catheter can be positioned adjacent to the thrombus through which the thrombolytic therapy is infused.
4. Thrombolytic therapy should be administered via catheter:

    Urokinase: 10,000- to 25,000-unit bolus, infuse at 1000 to 4000 units/min; total dose 500,000 to 750,000 units.

    Streptokinase: 25,000- to 50,000-unit bolus, infuse at 500 to 3000 units/min; total dose 750,000 to 1,000,000 units.

    t-PA: 5- to 10-mg bolus, infuse at 0.05 to 0.10 mg/kg/hr; total dose 30 to 50 mg.

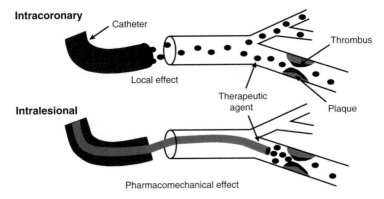

Intracoronary

Catheter

Thrombus

Local effect

Therapeutic agent

Intralesional

Plaque

Pharmacomechanical effect

Fig. 8-17. Thrombolysis for unstable angina: local delivery concepts. Method of prolonged subselective intracoronary/intragraft thrombolysis via an infusion wire.

5. The duration of thrombolytic infusion is variable and depends on a particular patient's presentation. Generally, acute thrombi, such as those that occur as a complication of angioplasty, will require a shorter infusion duration (>1 hour) than subacute thrombi, which often require prolonged infusion (8 to 12 hour). In peripheral arteries and bypass grafts, an infusion catheter may be left in a stable arterial position and the patient transferred to the ICU while the infusion is continued. Assessment of results requires repeat angiography.
6. After thrombolytic infusion is complete, continue heparin anticoagulation and consider angioplasty or surgery if significant ischemia or a stenosis persists.

Complications

Emboli. Distal vessel occlusion may result from a dislodged thrombus. This complication usually can be managed by continued thrombolysis or thrombus maceration by guidewire or balloon inflation.

Bleeding. Serious or life-threatening hemorrhage mandates termination of thrombolytic and heparin infusions. Protamine can be given to reverse heparin. Blood products, including fresh frozen plasma, may also be necessary. An example of thrombolysis in a saphenous vein graft angioplasty is provided in Fig. 8-16, in which a 41-year-old female has a thrombolytically occluded saphenous vein graft to the distal circumflex and obtuse marginal branches. The use of combined thrombolytic therapy followed by angioplasty was successfully performed using the techniques described above.

Adjunctive Agents

Heparin.   All patients with thrombus should be treated with intravenous heparin for >24 hour (if possible) before angioplasty to reduce propagation of the clot. Heparin itself will not reduce the thrombus, but it permits the intrinsic thrombolytic mechanisms to stabilize and reduce thrombus mass.

Aspirin.   To reduce platelet aggregation, aspirin should be given. Aspirin is associated with a reduced incidence of complications.

Indications

1. Patients with acute arterial thrombosis (<6 hour optimally, but in some patients as late as 24 hour) [Intravenous thrombolytic therapy is more timely but may be less effective.]
2. Selected patients with subacute thrombosis (<30 days) [Intraarterial or intragraft thrombolytic therapy may be indicated.]
3. Patients with intraarterial thrombosis complicating a coronary or peripheral angioplasty procedure

Contraindications

1. Active internal bleeding
2. Recent surgery or major trauma (within 2 months)
3. Recent stroke (<6 months)
4. Central nervous system (CNS) malignancy
5. Bleeding diathesis (check prothrombin time [PT], partial thromboplastin time [PTT], platelets, Hematocrit [Hct])
6. Severe uncontrolled hypertension (diastolic blood pressure >120 mmHg, systolic blood pressure >200 mmHg)
7. Pregnancy

SUGGESTED READINGS

Ambrose JA, Winters SL, Stern A, et al.: Angiographic morphology and the pathogenesis of unstable angina pectoris, *J Am Coll Cardiol* 5:609-616, 1985.

Cowley MJ, Vandermael M, Topol EJ, et al: Is traditionally-defined complete revascularization needed for patients with multivessel disease treated by elective coronary angioplasty? Multivessel Angioplasty Prognosis Study (MAPS) Group. *J Am Coll Cardiol* 22:1289-1297, 1993.

Deligonul U, Vandormael M, Kern M, et al: Coronary angioplasty: a therapeutic option for symptomatic patients with two and three vessel coronary disease. *JACC* 11:1173-1179, 1988.

Deligonul U, Vandormael M, Shah Y, Kern MJ: Coronary angioplasty for very proximal left anterior descending artery lesions: risk of left main dissection, *J Invas Cardiol* 1:30-38, 1988.

Ellis SG, Roubin GS, King SB III, et al.: Angiographic and clinical predictors of acute closure after native vessel coronary angioplasty, *Circulation* 77:372-379, 1988.

Ellis SG, Vandormael M, Cowley MJ, et al: Coronary morphologic and clinical determinants of procedural outcome with angioplasty for multivessel coronary disease: implications for patient selection. *Circulation* 82:1193-1202, 1990.

Ellis SG, Cowley MJ, Disciascio G, et al: Determinants of 2-year outcome after coronary angioplasty in patients with multivessel disease on the basis of comprehensive preprocedural evaluation: implications for patient selection. *Circulation* 83:1905, 1991.

Gacioch GM, Ellis SG, Lee L, et al.: Cardiogenic shock complicating acute myocardial infarction: the use of coronary angioplasty and the integration of the new support devices into patient management, *J Am Coll Cardiol* 19:647-653, 1992.

Goldberg RJ, Gore JM, Alpert JS, et al.: Cardiogenic shock after acute myocardial infarction: incidence and mortality from a community-wide perspective, 1975 to 1988, *N Engl J Med* 325:1117-1122, 1991.

Hibbard MD, Holmes DR, Bailey KR, Reeder GS, Bresnahan JF, Gersh BJ: Percutaneous transluminal coronary angioplasty in patients with cardiogenic shock, *J Am Coll Cardiol* 19:639-646, 1992.

Lee L, Erbel R, Brown TM, Laufer N, Meyer J, O'Neill WW: Multicenter registry of angioplasty therapy of cardiogenic shock: initial and long-term survival, *J Am Coll Cardiol* 17:599-603, 1991.

Mathias DW, Mooney JF, Lange HW, Goldenberg IF, Gobel FL, Mooney MR: Frequency of success and complications of coronary angioplasty of a stenosis at the ostium of a branch vessel, *Am J Cardiol* 67:491-495, 1991.

Nakhjavan FK, Goldman AP, Hutt GH, et al.: Percutaneous transluminal coronary angioplasty of the "very proximal" coronary artery stenosis, *Cathet Cardiovasc Diagn* 13:87-92, 1987.

Seydoux C, Goy JJ, Beuret P, et al.: Effectiveness of percutaneous transluminal coronary angioplasty in cardiogenic shock during acute myocardial infarction, *Am J Cardiol* 69:968-969, 1992.

Vandormael MG, Chaitman BR, Ischinger T, et al.: Immediate and short-term benefit of multilesion coronary angioplasty: influence of degree of revascularization, *J Am Coll Cardiol* 6:983-991, 1985.

9

HIGH-RISK ANGIOPLASTY

Richard G. Bach, Bruce A. Bergelson, Carl L. Tommaso, Eugene Caraciollo, and Morton J. Kern

CLINICAL AND ANATOMIC FACTORS IN HIGH-RISK ANGIOPLASTY

Retrospective reviews have identified parameters that define high-risk angioplasty procedures. Factors determining high-risk coronary angioplasty can be divided into two groups: lesion-related or anatomic factors, and patient-related clinical factors.

Lesion-Related Technical or Anatomic Factors

The American Heart Association (AHA)/American College of Cardiology (ACC) scoring system uses lesion location and morphology to assess risk and the potential for complications. The highest risk is associated with B1-, B2-, and C-type lesion classes. In addition to the location and morphology of the target stenosis, lesion severity, length, calcification, vessel tortuosity, and branching also influence the likelihood of procedural success.

Patient-Related Clinical Factors

Procedural mortality is most significantly affected by clinical parameters defining low- and high-risk patients as initially described by Hartzler et al. (Table 9-1). The two most important factors determining mortality are the amount of left ven-

TABLE 9-1. Factors increasing coronary angioplasty procedural mortality

	Mortality rate
All patients	0.7%
Low risk*	0.25%
PTCA, 3 vessels	1.3%
Age >70 years	1.4%
Left main equivalent	2.6%
Ejection fraction <40%	2.9%
Left main stenosis	3.4%

* Low risk indicates absence of characteristics cited below.
Modified from Hartzler GO, Rutherford BD, McConahay DR, Johnson WL, Giorgi LV: "High-risk" percutaneous transluminal coronary angioplasty, *Am J Cardiol* 61:33G-37G, 1988.

tricular myocardium supplied by any single target vessel and absolute left ventricular function.

Dilatation of vessels perfusing large amounts of myocardium exposes patients to higher subsequent morbidity or mortality due to vessel restenosis or occlusion. For example, the 3-year survival rate in patients with protected left main stenosis is 87%, but is only 40% in patients with unprotected left main stenosis.

Although technical success may be related to anatomic factors, procedural mortality is most significantly affected by clinical features. Patients at lowest risk have a procedure-related mortality of 0.25%. Factors such as the performance of multivessel angioplasty and patient age greater than 70 years increase risk. Data from the National Registry of Supported Angioplasty suggest a mortality rate for patients undergoing supported angioplasty of 6%. These patients all had either severe left ventricular dysfunction (left ventricular ejection fraction [LVEF] ≤25%) or had greater than two-thirds of the viable myocardium perfused by the target lesion. The highest-risk group of patients were those who had left main stenosis in addition to severe LV dysfunction or significant amounts of myocardium at jeopardy. These patients had an 18% in-hospital mortality.

The subset of patients undergoing interventional procedures who have the highest procedural risk are those in cardiogenic shock from an acute myocardial infarction. The use of angioplasty in this setting improves survival over the poor outcome statistics that were noted before the use of PTCA.

Additional clinical risk factors that increase procedural mortality include congestive heart failure, age >65 years, female gender, new-onset angina, and extent of coronary disease (0.2% in single-vessel disease compared to 2.2% in triple-vessel disease).

Data from the National Heart, Lung, Blood Institute (NHLBI) PTCA Registry and from studies of new devices suggest that these factors are becoming of decreasing importance for operators with high skill levels.

SUPPORTING THE HIGH-RISK ANGIOPLASTY PATIENT
Pharmacologic Agents

Limiting coronary ischemia during balloon inflation with pharmacotherapy addresses mechanisms to reduce regional oxygen consumption and augment collateral myocardial blood flow.

Nitroglycerin. Nitroglycerin, intravenous or intracoronary, commonly used before and after balloon dilatations, has not been demonstrated to provide prolonged ischemic benefit. Intravenous and intracoronary nitroglycerin will reduce coronary vasospasm and preload with control of blood pressure. When using nitroglycerine, an adequate margin of blood pressure (mean arterial pressure >70 mm Hg) should be maintained so that transiently induced severe ischemia does not reduce blood pressure below a critical (mean arterial pressure <60 mm Hg) level, thereby producing ischemia in other myocardial regions as a result of excessively low perfusion pressure.

Beta-adrenergic and calcium channel blockers. Beta-adrenergic blockers have also been used both systemically and regionally to prevent or reduce ischemia during coronary balloon occlusion. In this setting, beta-adrenergic and calcium channel blocking agents reduce myocardial ischemia through a local decrement in myocardial oxygen consumption. Although they are effective, these agents will not prolong the time to ischemia enough to make a substantial clinical impact.

Sublingual nifedipine does not prolong the time to ischemic ST segment changes or improve regional blood flow during balloon inflation. The beneficial effects of these agents most likely occur through a reduction in vessel spasm or indirectly by reducing myocardial oxygen demand, rather than directly by augmenting coronary blood flow through the collateral circulation. Serruys et al.* found that regional nifedipine administration was associated with a negative inotropic effect and evidence of decreased anaerobic metabolism. As with nifedipine, intravenously administered diltiazem delayed the onset of ischemic pain and ST segment elevation.

Vasopressors. In patients who develop hypotension without coexisting hypovolemia, vasopressor infusions may be necessary to restore adequate blood pressure. An intraarterial (not coronary) aramine bolus (1 mg) will temporarily increase systemic blood pressure to normal range while fluid resuscitation and ischemia management is continuing and intravenous vasopressor medications are being prepared.

For intravenous administration, dopamine is the agent of choice in most acute situations. The initial dose in symptomatic hypotension is 5 μg/kg/min. The dopamine dose can be titrated upward until an adequate blood pressure is obtained. In critically ill patients, norepinephrine (Levophed) or epinephrine infusions may be required to obtain acceptable blood pressure.

In summary, nitroglycerin, beta-adrenergic, and calcium channel blocking agents reduce myocardial ischemia during coronary angioplasty through local decrement in myocardial oxygen consumption. Although these methods are effective, they may not consistently reduce ischemia enough to make them of significant value. Augmentation of collateral flow by these agents does not appear to be substantial. They are of value mostly for ameliorating patient symptomatology and decreasing epicardial vessel spasm.

Antegrade Hemoperfusion

Distal coronary perfusion during angioplasty uses autoperfusion and active (pump-driven) perfusion catheters to deliver blood or blood substitutes (Table 9-2).

Autoperfusion. Autoperfusion balloon catheters have multiple side holes along the shaft proximal and distal to the balloon and a central lumen that allows blood to flow pas-

* Serruys PW, van den Brand M, Brower RW, Hugenholtz PG: Regional cardioplegia and cardioprotection during transluminal angioplasty, which role for nifedipine? *Eur Heart J* 4(suppl C):115-121, 1983.

TABLE 9-2. Antegrade perfusion and support during angioplasty

Features	Autoperfusion	Active catheter hemoperfusion	IABP	CPS
Additional vascular access	No	Yes	Yes	Yes
Venous access	No	No	No	Yes
Pump necessary	No	Yes	Yes	Yes
Unique features	High-profile balloon; lower flow; requires adequate blood pressure	Hemolysis; thrombosis	CO, 20% to 30%; rhythm-dependent	CO 4 to 6 l/min; rhythm-independent
Potential duration	>4 hr (maximum 24 hr)	<4 hr	1 to 3 days	<6 hr
Ventricular unloading	No	No	Yes	Yes
Increased coronary perfusion	Yes	Yes	Yes	+/−

sively through the catheter. Distal coronary perfusion is related directly to arterial (perfusion) pressure. Coronary blood flow of 40 to 60 ml/min is provided only with near-normal (mean arterial pressure >75 mmHg) systemic blood pressure. Under these conditions, autoperfusion during prolonged balloon inflations appears to be adequate to maintain near-normal ventricular function. Under hypotensive conditions, however, inadequate perfusion may result. Vasopressors or intraaortic balloon pumping have been found helpful in maintaining blood flow through the catheter.

Active perfusion.   In both experimental and clinical studies, autologous blood pumped through a balloon catheter has demonstrated preservation of ventricular function and myocardial metabolism. Autologous blood for active perfusion systems is obtained via an oversized femoral arterial sheath, renal vein, or contralateral femoral artery. Active antegrade hemoperfusion has been used in high-risk, unstable patients and in those undergoing dilatation of vessels supplying substantial amounts of myocardium.

In an attempt to eliminate hemolysis and thrombosis, antegrade perfusion of an oxygen-carrying fluorocarbon (Fluosol-DA 20%, a moderate-viscosity emulsion of perfluorodecaline and perfluorotriprophylamine) has been used. It has a lower oxygen affinity than blood and requires hyperoxygenation at a P_{O2} of 600 mmHg to carry approximately one-third of oxygen-saturated blood concentration. Prolonged fluosol perfusion appears to be well tolerated but cannot be expected to reduce ischemia in all patients. This agent is no longer available clinically.

Mechanical Support Techniques

Intraaortic balloon pumping.   Intraaortic balloon pumping (IABP) is an important adjunct to diagnostic and interventional cardiac catheterization. Intraaortic balloon counterpulsation increases myocardial oxygen supply and decreases myocardial oxygen demand. Inflation at the onset of diastole (at the dicrotic *notch* on the central arterial pressure tracing) results in augmentation of diastolic pressure, which increases coronary artery and systemic perfusion. Deflation of the balloon just before systole (end diastole on the arterial pressure tracing) results in decreased ventricular afterload, which decreases myocardial oxygen consumption and increases cardiac output.

There appears to be a 20% to 30% increase in cardiac output in patients with low-output syndromes and a significant amount of afterload reduction as demonstrated in reduction of mitral regurgitation. Direct measurement of coronary blood flow during intraaortic balloon pumping demonstrated augmentation in nondiseased and postangioplasty vessels, but no increase in vessels distal to significant stenosis (Fig. 9-1).

Before a diagnostic cardiac catheterization or interventional procedure, the patient should be treated medically to optimize hemodynamics and reduce myocardial ischemia. In unstable patients, an IABP may be required before proceeding with the catheterization. During diagnostic cardiac catheterization or interventional procedures, hypotension (not responding to volume loading or IV vasopressors) and medically refractory angina are important indications for IABP placement.

Indications and contraindications for IABP are listed in the accompanying boxes on p. 332.

Insertion techniques. Before the percutaneous insertion of an intraaortic balloon, careful assessment of contraindications is required. A low abdominal aortogram will identify the course and extent of disease in the iliac and femoral vessels before the IABP insertion.

For high-risk procedures, anticipate IABP placement and recall that the puncture site should be 2 cm below the inguinal ligament, similar to or slightly more proximal than a standard femoral puncture for cardiac catheterization. A puncture lower than the prescribed site may introduce the balloon into a superficial femoral artery too small to accept the large IABP catheter.

The balloon is inserted into either groin using standing Seldinger technique as described in detail in *The Cardiac Catheterization Handbook.* Some manufacturers are making "sheathless" IABP balloon catheters, which are especially useful in the elderly and those with some peripheral vascular disease (PVD) that requires support. Fluoroscopic observation of the balloon inflated above the renal arteries confirms optimal placement.

Complications. Procedural complications of intraaortic balloon placement most commonly result from a low puncture site, perforation of the superficial femoral artery, or forceful

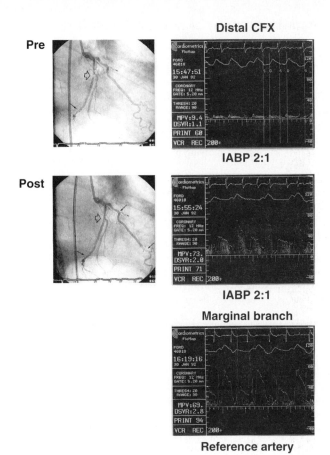

Fig. 9-1. Effect of intraaortic balloon pumping on coronary blood flow velocity before and after coronary angioplasty. *Upper left,* Angiogram in high-risk patient with unstable angina due to a severe circumflex stenosis (open arrow). The left anterior descending artery was previously occluded. A Doppler guidewire is passed and positioned in the distal vessel (small arrow). *Upper right,* Flow velocity during 2:1 IABP shows no augmentation of the low pre-PTCA blood flow. *Lower left,* Angiogram after successful PTCA. Arrows point to adjacent normal reference marginal branch. *Lower middle,* Flow velocity after PTCA is markedly increased and further augmented by IABP. The increases seen in the post-PTCA vessel are nearly identical to that in the reference vessel (lower right). (From Kern MJ, Aguirre F, Bach R, Donohue T, Segal J: Augmentation of coronary blood flow by intra-aortic balloon pumping in patients after coronary angioplasty, *Circulation* 87:500-511, 1993.)

Indications for Intraaortic Balloon Pump Counterpulsation for
High-Risk Angioplasty

After PTCA of a total occlusion
After rescue coronary angioplasty
After unsuccessful coronary angioplasty before surgery
After vessel closure following initially successful coronary
    angioplasty
Anterior infarctions, elevated left ventricular end diastolic pressure
    (LVEDP), or extensive wall motion abnormalities
Cardiogenic shock
Hemodynamic instability
Hypotension
Left main stenosis, unprotected or protected with moderately
    depressed LV function
Left ventricular dysfunction, moderate to severe
Single remaining patent artery
Ventricular tachycardia, intractable, due to myocardial ischemia

advancement of the catheter causing damage to the arterial
entry site. The most common complication of intraaortic balloon pumping, ischemia of the lower extremity, may occur
in 10% of patients. The use of smaller catheters and sheathless
insertion have reduced vascular complications. There remains
a 5% to 10% complication rate that does not appear affected
by the duration of balloon usage. Thirty percent of patients

Contraindications for Intraaortic Balloon Pump Counterpulsation for
High-Risk Angioplasty

Anatomic abnormality of femoral-iliac artery
Aortic dissection or aneurysm
Aortic regurgitation, moderate or severe
Atherosclerotic disease, iliac or aortic, impairing blood flow
Bleeding diathesis
Bypass grafting to femoral arteries or aorta
Patent ductus (augment the abnormal shunting)
Sepsis

who have symptomatic lower-extremity ischemia may require catheter removal. Ten percent of patients may require an additional vascular procedure. Other complications include acute aortic dissection and hemolysis and platelet destruction, particularly in prolonged use.

Despite the use of IABP during angioplasty in high-risk patients, there remains an in-hospital mortality of 6.2% to 19%, with a rate of vascular complications of 2.1% to 14%. The combination of IABP and a perfusion balloon is a particularly attractive physiologic combination in patients who appear to be at high risk.

Percutaneous cardiopulmonary support. Percutaneous cardiopulmonary support (CPS) is used in the catheterization laboratory as an adjunct to high-risk angioplasty to maintain adequate perfusion in hemodynamic catastrophes instead of, or in conjunction with, an intraaortic balloon pump, and for rescue of an unexpected catastrophe during diagnostic and interventional procedures. Angioplasty with percutaneously inserted cardiopulmonary bypass (PCPB) in high-risk patients, termed "supported angioplasty," was instituted prophylactically, before PTCA, allowing the expansion of angioplasty to include patients who formerly would not have been considered suitable candidates for the procedure. Patients with severely impaired left ventricular function, a large area of jeopardized myocardium supplied by the target vessel, or with the target vessel as the only patent vessel remaining were felt to be at extraordinarily high risk for hemodynamic collapse due to acute vessel closure or ischemia during the procedure. Early feasibility studies concluded that percutaneous bypass could be performed to support high-risk PTCA with a high likelihood of initial success and with an acceptable, though not insignificant, incidence of morbidity.

This high incidence of associated morbidity, however, makes the ability to identify prospectively those patients most likely to benefit from a supported procedure that much more important (see Table 9-3). Certain angiographic characteristics (>50% myocardium at risk, LVEF <25%, "last remaining patent vessel") identify patients at "manifest risk"; however, no prospective study has been published to assess the accuracy of this method. Based on these experiences with supported angioplasty, current indications and recommenda-

TABLE 9-3.   Circulatory support during angioplasty based on risk

Risk category	Patient characteristics	Strategy
Low	Single stenosis; normal or near-normal LV function	Usual
Complex	Multivessel disease; one or more complex lesions; moderate LV dysfunction	Usual
High	Target supplying >50% of myocardium; LVEF 15% to 25%	Antegrade perfusion; IABP; standby PCPB
Manifest	Only patent vessel; LVEF ≤15%; collapse during procedure	PCBP; Hemopump; IABP and antegrade perfusion

From Tommaso CL, Vogel RA: National Registry for Supported Angioplasty: results and follow-up of three years of supported and standby supported angioplasty in high-risk patients, *Cardiology* 84:238-244, 1994.

tions for the use of adjunctive supportive techniques during PTCA have been modified. Only extremely high-risk patients should be candidates for supported angioplasty. However, the use of CPS as an emergent tool in the catheterization laboratory for hemodynamically compromised patients has been successful. Considerations for use should include a priori decisions regarding outcome after leaving the catheterization laboratory.

Technique. The CPS system utilizes a centrifugal pump that provides negative pressure for venous outflow as well as positive pressure for arterial inflow. A flow probe, heat exchanger, and membrane oxygenator are all in series in the circuit. Two cannulae, venous and arterial, are inserted either percutaneously or by cutdown. The venous cannula is 16 to 20 French, 75 cm in length, and inserted over a tapered dilator. It is positioned with the distal end in the right atrium for venous blood withdrawal. The arterial cannula is 16 to 20 French, 32 cm in length, and is inserted into the femoral artery for retrograde aortic perfusion.

The cannula are relatively easily inserted by an experienced invasive cardiologist using the percutaneous technique. If a cutdown is employed, either a surgeon or a cardiologist proficient with this technique is required.

A separate arterial access is necessary to monitor blood pressure. During an operator's early experience, the procedure should be performed with a perfusionist and cardiac anesthesiologist in attendance.

For elective CPS insertion, iliac/femoral angiography is performed where the cannula will be inserted to ascertain patency of the vessel, and to facilitate access in the common femoral rather than the femoral profunda artery. Vessel tortuosity may interfere with insertion of the cannula and the flow rate. A single wall puncture is made in the femoral artery and vein. After the vein is punctured, sequentially enlarging dilators (8, 12, and 14 French) prepare the vessel for cannula insertion. The cannula and dilator assembly is inserted and positioned so that the distal end lies in the upper portion of the right atrium. An extra-stiff 0.038-in. guidewire will facilitate passage through a tortuous femoral system. An alternative to the sequential dilator method is the use of a 5- or 6-mm balloon catheter, a technique that may be faster.

As the inner dilator is removed from the venous cannula, the patient should be asked to perform a Valsalva maneuver or pressure should be applied to the abdomen to create positive pressure, filling the sheath with blood and avoiding an air embolism. The blood-filled sheath is then locked using the attached thumb clamp. The cannula and connector tubing are filled with saline by an assistant using a large syringe while the operator mates the tubing and sheath, taking care to eliminate any air in the circuit.

The arterial cannula is inserted in a similar manner. The artery is dilated subsequently with 8, 12, and 14 French dilators (or a 5- or 6-mm balloon); the cannula and dilator assembly is then inserted. The arterial cannula and connector are mated in a similar fashion as the venous system. A side port and stopcock allow the arterial system to be purged of air.

After the cannulae are inserted, 300 units/kg of heparin is administered for full anticoagulation. Activated clotting times are frequently measured (approximately every 20 min), with additional heparin administered to keep the activated clotting time >400 sec.

After the interventional procedure has been concluded, the patient is weaned from CPS by gradually reducing CPS flow while observing the patient's hemodynamic status. When flow reaches 0.5 L/min, the venous line is closed with the thumb clamp. At this time, if volume repletion is needed, fluids are infused via the arterial line. Once volume repletion is complete, the arterial line is clamped off. The recirculation line is then opened to prevent stasis in the circuit. If it is necessary to return to CPS, the recirculation line is closed with reinstitution of CPS. With this system, destruction of blood elements and activation of clotting factors by the oxygenator preclude having patients on CPS for more than 6 hour.

The large amount of fluid required for the priming circuit and connecting lines will result in a significant drop in the hematocrit during the procedure. Therefore, following the procedure, blood remaining in the circuit is retrieved using a cell saver and returned to the patient.

If the system was inserted percutaneously, the patient is transferred to a stretcher with a full metal base and positioned near the edge of the stretcher. The cannulae are withdrawn with hemostasis achieved manually. A C-clamp compression system is used to compress the vessels to the point where no bleeding is noted but where pulses are still present, either by palpitation or by Doppler. The patient can then be transported to the intensive-care unit for further monitoring. The C clamp is left in place for 6 hour or until the PTT has reached 70 sec. At this time, the C clamp can be gradually released, and if no further bleeding is noted, the patient is usually maintained at bed rest on the same stretcher for another 12 to 24 hour. Some operators keep the cannulae in for 4 to 6 hour after the procedure to allow for metabolism of heparin and then remove the cannulae and maintain hemostasis by manual compression (1 to 1.5 hour).

Standby CPS for high-risk coronary angioplasty. The elective use of CPS in high-risk PTCA patients may provide stable hemodynamics during the procedure. The indications for elective use of CPS are yet to be determined. In most high-risk PTCA patients (e.g., those with poor left ventricular function, dilatation of the only remaining vessel, dilatation of a territory supplying $\geq 50\%$ of the myocardium), standby CPS seems a reasonable approach. In this method, 5 French sheaths are placed into the contralateral femoral artery and vein. These small sheaths allow easy placement of the cannula, saving valuable time. Angiography is performed to document the patency of the iliac/femoral artery. Elective percutaneous CPS should not be attempted in patients with obstructive disease in the ilio-femoral system. The external circuit is primed and purged of air and is kept ready for immediate use should a hemodynamic catastrophe occur during angioplasty. It is important to remember that because CPS will not increase regional myocardial blood flow or alleviate myocardial ische-mia, acute coronary dissection or occlusion should be treated immediately with perfusion catheters, distal perfusion stent-ing, or emergency coronary artery bypass graft surgery.

The complications of percutaneous CPS are primarily vas-cular in nature: bleeding, thromboembolism, and pseudoan-eurysm formation. Complications specific to CPS (e.g., throm-bocytopenia, disseminated intravascular coagulation) are seen especially in patients where long-term support (>6 hour) was necessary.

Hemopump. Another support device that has been used only sporadically for support of high-risk angioplasty is the Hemopump (Johnson & Johnson Interventional Systems Company, Inc., Rancho Cordova, Calif.). The Hemopump is a miniaturized axial-flow pump which, in the 21 French size, is capable of full circulatory support and has been used in the treatment of cardiogenic shock. A 14 French catheter capa-ble of partial support, which may be inserted percutaneously, is under development.

Coronary sinus retroperfusion. Myocardial support can be achieved via the cardiac venous system. Synchronized retroperfusion of the coronary sinus involves the use of elec-trocardiographic synchronized retroperfusion of arterialized blood during diastole, allowing for normal physiologic drain-age during systole. Brachial or femoral artery blood is deliv-ered through a catheter placed in the coronary sinus. Diastolic autoinflation of a balloon catheter in the coronary sinus pro-duces a brief obstruction of the coronary sinus, which facili-tates the retroinjection of blood or pharmacologic agents. Syn-chronized retrograde perfusion reduces the onset of ischemia and may permit prolonged balloon inflations when necessary.

Pressure-controlled intermittent coronary sinus occlusion also involves a balloon placed into the coronary sinus. The balloon is inflated for a time to allow venous pressures to reach equilibrium. Deflation then occurs, allowing drainage, delivery of oxygen, and washing out of accumulated toxic materials. Coronary sinus retroperfusion techniques have been used in patients undergoing coronary bypass surgery and in high-risk angioplasty. Cannulation of the coronary sinus in some patients may be difficult. Clinical availability and practical application are limited.

MANAGEMENT OF ABRUPT VESSEL CLOSURE IN HIGH-RISK PATIENTS

Approximately 70% of abrupt closures occur while the patient is still in the cardiac catheterization laboratory, and the mechanism of vessel occlusion is due predominantly to dissection in association with intracoronary thrombus. Spasm plays a variable role. Treatment strategies therefore focus on management of these pathophysiologic mechanisms.

Pharmacologic Approach

Antiplatelet agents.   Aspirin, a relatively weak platelet antagonist, decreases the complications of coronary angioplasty that are especially important in the high-risk patient. The Montreal Heart Institute demonstrated an incidence of 1.6% in abrupt closure leading to myocardial infarction in patients treated with aspirin and dipyridamole versus 6.9% in those receiving placebo. A comparison of ticlopidine, aspirin and dipyridamole, and placebo found that the incidence of ischemic complications was 1.8%, 5.4%, and 13.6% respectively.

Heparin and antithrombin agents.   The importance of intravenous heparin therapy to the acute procedural outcome of PTCA has been well demonstrated. Studies in patients with unstable angina and acute myocardial infarction treated with thrombolysis show that hirudin and hirulog may have advantages over heparin as antithrombotic agents. Hirulog was shown to represent an effective alternative to heparin when performing coronary angioplasty in aspirin-pretreated patients. In patients with stable angina undergoing PTCA, myocardial infarction and/or emergency coronary bypass surgery occurred in 1.4% of hirudin-treated patients compared with 10.3% of heparin-treated patients (relative risk, 7.6; 95% confidence interval, 0.9, 75.6) without significant bleeding complications. Evidence is mounting that these agents may have beneficial effects in the setting of PTCA above their effect on the coagulation cascade by reducing platelet and fibrin deposition.* However, excessive bleeding may be associated with these new agents.

Vasodilators. Although refractory coronary vasospasm is rarely the sole cause of abrupt vessel closure, vasospasm should be treated with intracoronary nitroglycerine. Intracoronary nitroglycerine administered in doses of 100 to 200 μg is the most appropriate first course of action in the management of acute arterial occlusion. For vasospasm that is unresponsive to nitroglycerine, intracoronary administration of calcium channel blockers has been employed. The "noreflow" phenomenon, which is the severe impairment of antegrade flow associated with ischemia, without evidence of vessel dissection or thrombus formation, may be treated with intracoronary calcium channel blockers. "No reflow" treated with intracoronary verapamil (50 to 900 μg total dose) improved coronary blood flow in 89% of patients, whereas only 19% of patients with a mechanical obstruction to blood flow had improvement in coronary blood flow with verapamil.

Thrombolytic therapy. Conflicting data exist on the utility of intracoronary thrombolytic therapy in conjunction with repeat dilatation for the treatment of abrupt vessel closure. Angiographic success is reported to be between 65% and 90%. These studies reported on small numbers of patients with clinical success rates ranging from 48% to 90% using a variety of different agents (streptokinase, urokinase, or tissue plasminogen activator) in a variety of clinical settings (patients with stable, unstable, or acute ischemic syndromes). Thrombolytic therapy is probably best reserved for use in patients with abrupt vessel closure with angiographic, ultrasound, or angioscopic evidence of a significant thrombus that is unresponsive to redilation with conventional angioplasty.

Mechanical Treatment

Conventional balloon angioplasty approach. Repeat dilatation with a conventional balloon may successfully restore patency in 35% to 87% of cases, thereby avoiding emergency bypass surgery. This strategy may allow for a dissection flap

* Serruys PW, Herrman JR, Simon R, et al: A comparison of hirudin with heparin in the prevention of restenosis after coronary angioplasty, *N Engl J Med* 333:757-763, 1995.

to be "tacked up," thus restoring antegrade flow. A proposed algorithm of the management of abrupt or threatened closure during PTCA is shown in Fig. 9-2.

An improved salvage rate has been seen using prolonged balloon inflations. Although prolonged balloon inflations may

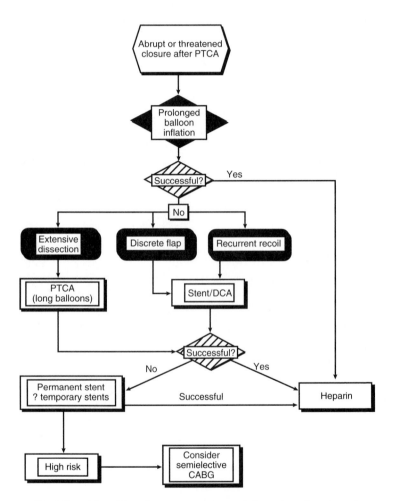

Fig. 9-2. Algorithm for management of abrupt or threatened closure during PTCA. DCA, Directional atherectomy. (From Popma JJ, Leon MB: *A lesion specific approach to New-Device angioplasty* in Topol EJ, editor. Textbook of Interventional Cardiology, ed 2, Philadelphia, 1994, W. B. Saunders, pp 973-985.)

allow improved vessel remodeling by further tacking up dissection flaps and compressing thrombus, ischemic effects generally limit the duration of balloon inflation. Autoperfusion catheters allow prolonged dilations with clinically improved tolerance for ischemia.

Angioplasty balloons greater than 20 mm in length have been employed to reduce dissection in the setting of a long coronary lesion and other high-risk subsets. While no comparative studies of this application have been performed, successful use has been reported.

Directional coronary atherectomy. Directional coronary atherectomy (DCA) has been used to remove obstructive intimal flaps and medial dissections and treat recurrent elastic recoil after conventional balloon angioplasty, and to provide larger lumens after inadequate PTCA and possibly remove thrombus. Vessel perforation is the greatest risk when directional coronary atherectomy is performed for abrupt vessel closure. Salvage atherectomy is probably not indicated in the setting of a long, deep dissection, because of the risk of perforation, and it has limited utility in small, tortuous, or calcified vessels because of the rigid device. The major technical limitation to salvage atherectomy is a need to exchange the smaller guiding catheter and sheath used for conventional balloon angioplasty for the larger equipment needed for atherectomy. Delivery of a 6 French AtheroCath using an 8 French guiding catheter with an 0.086-in. inner lumen, however, may be possible.

Stents. Stents have been the greatest development in the management of abrupt vessel closure and threatened vessel closure since the inception of PTCA. Stents secure dissection flaps by producing a radial scaffolding of the vessel lumen and preventing elastic recoil, improving vessel geometry. The incidence of in-hospital death, myocardial infarction, and need for bypass surgery in patients treated with stenting for abrupt or threatened vessel closure compare favorably to historical controls who were treated for abrupt vessel closure after angioplasty. This method should be available in every laboratory for treating high-risk patients.

MANAGEMENT OF ARRHYTHMIAS DURING CORONARY ANGIOPLASTY

The most important determinant of short- and long-term, neurologically intact survival after hemodynamic collapse is the interval from the onset of collapse to the restoration of effective, spontaneous circulatory function. This section reviews guidelines for arrhythmia treatment in high-risk patients. A full description of arrhythmia management during catheterization may be found in *The Cardiac Catheterization Handbook*. The guidelines discussed in the text that follows do not preclude other measures that may be indicated on the basis of the specific characteristics of the patient.

Serious arrhythmias (including ventricular fibrillation, ventricular tachycardia, supraventricular tachycardia, asystole, and heart block) occur in approximately 1% of catheterizations. In almost all instances, the arrhythmias can be managed successfully by prompt recognition and appropriate treatment. Arrhythmias may result from intracardiac catheter manipulation (e.g., right heart catheters), coronary artery contrast injections, or balloon catheter-induced myocardial ischemia.

Prompt recognition of arrhythmias requires satisfactory electrocardiographic monitoring and is essential in performing a safe high-risk PTCA. Problems with the electrocardiographic leads or equipment during the procedure must be remedied before continuing.

Components of Arrhythmia Management
Immediate modalities

Cough. When sustained hypotension is recognized before loss of consciousness (and cardiac arrest), forceful coughing may generate sufficient blood flow to the brain to maintain consciousness until definitive treatment can be initiated.

Precordial thump. A solitary precordial thump can be accomplished quickly and may terminate ventricular tachycardia, ventricular fibrillation, asystole, marked bradycardia with hemodynamic instability, or convert complete AV block to a more stable rhythm. It should not delay defibrillation in a patient without a blood pressure.

Defibrillation and cardioversion. Definitive electrical treatment has the highest priority of any treatment modality. During procedures, the defibrillator should be turned on and conductive jelly should be applied to the defibrillator paddles to minimize delays in treatment. If pulseless ventricular tachycardia or ventricular fibrillation occurs, defibrillation should be performed immediately.

Proper defibrillator technique, including paddle placement and the use of proper conducting material, is essential to success. The individuals using the paddles must make sure that the angioplasty operators and nurses are not touching the bed or the patient during defibrillation. Redraping and regowning may be required after defibrillation.

Continuing modalities

Standby transvenous pacing. The need for prophylactic pacemaker insertion is determined by the patient's risk of developing a bradyarrhythmia and the patient's ability to tolerate the arrhythmia if it occurs. Risk factors for the development of bradyarrhythmia include:

1. Preexisting right bundle branch block
2. Preexisting left bundle branch block during right heart catheterization
3. Heart block greater than first degree
4. Marked sinus bradycardia
5. Coronary artery angioplasty involving the (dominant) artery supplying the AV node

Flexible, balloon-tipped, flow-directed 5 and 6F pacemaker wires have the lowest risk for cardiac perforation.

Treatment of Specific Arrhythmias

Vasovagal reactions. Unexplained hypotension during PTCA may be the result of a vasodepressor vagal response without bradycardia. Vasovagal reactions, often preceded by slowing of heart rate before a drop in blood pressure occurs, respond dramatically to IV atropine (0.6 to 1.0 mg). Elevation of the legs is generally impractical during PTCA. Infusion of saline is helpful. Early signs include pallor, nausea, or yawning.

Bradycardia. Bradycardia (ventricular heart rate <60 beats/min) may be caused by ischemia, autonomic influences, or intrinsic cardiac conducting system disease. Atropine sulfate can be given for symptomatic bradycardia (a heart rate inappropriate for the hemodynamic state—e.g., a heart rate of <80 beats/min with hypotension). The initial dose is 0.6 to 1.0 mg. The dose may be repeated every 5 min to a maximal dose of 2 mg. Doses of less than 0.5 mg may induce vagotonic effects.

AV block. Junctional rhythm and second-degree AV block (type I) often do not require specific treatment, but will usually respond to atropine in doses as described above. If symptomatic bradycardia persists after a third dose of atropine, a transvenous pacemaker should be placed. An external pacemaker can be used in the symptomatic patient if atropine fails to maintain the patient until a transvenous pacemaker can be placed.

Second-degree AV block (type II) and third-degree AV block are treated with a temporary transvenous pacemaker even in the absence of symptoms. If bradycardia is associated with adverse hemodynamics or symptoms (e.g., hypotension, congestive heart failure, ischemia, infarction), atropine can be used to temporize the situation in divided doses up to 2 mg until the pacemaker can be inserted. If atropine fails, an external pacemaker can be used to maintain the patient until a transvenous pacemaker can be placed.

Ventricular fibrillation. If possible, intracardiac catheters should be repositioned or removed and defibrillation should be carried out immediately. Coronary access should be maintained if possible so that stenting or antegrade catheter hemoperfusion can be performed. It is unknown how defibrillation affects the coronary artery with a guidewire in place. A single precordial thump may be employed if it will not delay defibrillation. Guidelines for defibrillation and CPR are available in Appendix II.

Nonsustained ventricular tachycardia. Nonsustained ventricular tachycardia usually can be eliminated by repositioning or withdrawing intracardiac or coronary catheters. Frequent nonsustained ventricular tachycardia secondary to acute myocardial ischemia should be treated with periodic myocardial perfusion and lidocaine.

Sustained ventricular tachycardia. If sustained ventricular tachycardia persists after removing intracardiac catheters, management proceeds according to the stability of the patient. A single precordial thump may be employed by the operator before cardioversion. Hypotension due to sustained ventricular tachycardia is treated the same as ventricular fibrillation. In patients who are hemodynamically unstable (e.g., conditions of hypotension [systolic blood pressure <90 mm Hg], pulmonary edema, or unconsciousness), synchronized car-

dioversion with 50 J is performed. Synchronized cardioversion uses the largest R wave. If the QRS cannot be distinguished, use the unsynchronized mode.

If the arrhythmia is refractory, successive synchronized
attempts with 100, 200, and then 360 J are appropriate. If
cardioversion is unsuccessful, lidocaine should be administered, followed by bretylium. If these two drugs fail, an infusion of Pronestyl should be tried. Repeat synchronized cardioversion with 360 J after each dose of antiarrhythmic agent.

Antiarrhythmic agents for ventricular tachycardia. Lidocaine
is the drug of choice for the management of ventricular ectopy, including ventricular tachycardia and ventricular fibrillation. Lidocaine initially should be given as a bolus of 1 mg/
kg. Additional boluses of 0.5 mg/kg can be given subsequently (every 8 to 10 min) to a total dose of 3 mg/kg in the
arrest setting. In the non-arrest setting, the initial bolus should
be reduced by half if any of the following conditions is present: congestive heart failure, shock, hepatic dysfunction, or
age greater than 70 years. After a successful resuscitation, a
constant infusion of lidocaine at a rate of 2 to 4 mg/min
should be initiated.

Bretylium tosylate (5 mg/kg) is given as an IV bolus for
refractory ventricular fibrillation or refractory pulseless (or
hemodynamically unstable) ventricular tachycardia. For hemodynamically stable patients, 5 to 10 mg/kg of bretylium
tosylate should be diluted to 50 ml with 5% dextrose in water
and administered by slow IV infusion over 8 to 10 min to
reduce the acute hypotensive effects of the agent. Subsequently, a constant infusion can be initiated at a dose of 1 to
4 mg/min if bretylium has been successful during the resuscitation.

Procainamide requires a relatively long time to achieve
therapeutic levels. In the urgent situation, 1 g of procainamide
hydrochloride can be administered over 30 min. A constant
infusion rate (1 to 4 mg/min) is then administered and later
titrated to serum drug levels. In situations that are not urgent,
1 g should be given over at least 1 hour. The rate of drug
administration should be reduced or discontinued if hypotension is induced or if there is >50% prolongation of the QRS
complex or QT interval.

Note: Wide complex tachycardia of uncertain etiology (i.e.,
ventricular tachycardia versus paroxysmal supraventricular

tachycardia [PSVT] with aberrancy) should be treated as ventricular tachycardia until proven otherwise. Verapamil is contraindicated.

Asystole.   Asystole is usually the result of extensive myocardial ischemia. Asystole should be confirmed in two leads because it can be difficult to distinguish fine ventricular fibrillation from asystole. If the diagnosis is unclear, one should assume that fine ventricular fibrillation is present and treat accordingly. Right ventricular pacing should be instituted as quickly as possible. Atropine (1 mg) should be given and can be repeated in 5 min, if necessary. External pacing can be employed if right ventricular pacing cannot be established immediately. Metabolic abnormalities, including hyperkalemia or severe preexisting acidosis, may contribute to the genesis of the arrhythmia and may respond to the use of buffers. A solitary precordial thump may be employed.

Epinephrine, the catecholamine of choice for cardiac arrest, has vasoconstrictor alpha-adrenergic properties that make it superior to other alpha-adrenergic agents (methoxamine and phenylephrine), with comparable cardiac effects, but failure to increase central nervous system blood flow as much as epinephrine. The dose of epinephrine is 0.5 to 1 mg given at least every 5 min. During cardiac arrest, higher rather than lower doses may be more efficacious. If asystole is refractory to the above measures, emergency cardiopulmonary bypass should be considered.

Electromechanical dissociation.   Electromechanical dissociation (EMD) is a rhythm disturbance that is almost uniformly fatal unless the underlying cause can be identified and immediately treated. General treatment includes the use of epinephrine (1 mg) every 5 min. Bicarbonate may be considered. If EMD is refractory, emergency cardiopulmonary bypass may be considered.

Underlying causes of EMD include:
1. Hypovolemia, especially resulting from bleeding.
2. Pericardial tamponade, especially in patients with acute infarction, recent cardiac biopsy, recent endocardial pacer insertion, or uremia. If tamponade is suspected, blind pericardiocentesis is warranted.
3. Enhanced vagal tone in patients with ischemic heart disease. Consider this whenever the heart rate is inappropriate for the degree of hypotension. Atropine is required.

4. Massive pulmonary embolism.
5. Tension pneumothorax, especially in patients on ventilators or in patients with central venous access above the diaphragm. Fluoroscopy may be helpful if it is available immediately. If there is any suspicion of tension pneumothorax, the operator should carefully insert a needle attached to a glass syringe into the pleural space. If a tension pneumothorax is present, air under pressure will push the plunger out of the syringe.

Supraventricular arrhythmias. In cases of PSVT and atrial fibrillation, therapy depends on the hemodynamic stability of the patient. Specific treatment regimens are provided in Appendix II.

SUMMARY

Several strategies are available for limiting risk in the high-risk patient. Some involve complex technology, but others, such as the use of IABP and perfusion balloons, should be widely applicable and familiar to all interventional cardiologists. Table 9-3 lists patient characteristics and strategies for circulatory support during angioplasty based on risk.

SUGGESTED READINGS

Caldwell G, Millar G, Quinn E, Vincent R, Chamberlain DA: Simple mechanical methods for cardioversion: defence of the precordial thump and cough version, *Br Med J* 291:627-629, 1985.

Eisenberg MS, Hallstrom AP, Copass MK, et al.: Treatment of ventricular fibrillation: emergency medical technician defibrillation and paramedic services, *JAMA* 251:1723-1726, 1984.

Hartzler GO, Rutherford BD, McConahay DR, Johnson WL, Giorgi LV: "High-risk" percutaneous transluminal coronary angioplasty, *Am J Cardiol* 61:33G-37G, 1989.

Holmes DR, Holubkov R, Vietstra RE, et al.: Comparison of complications during percutaneous transluminal coronary angioplasty from 1977 to 1981 and from 1985 to 1986: the national heart, lung, and blood institute percutaneous transluminal coronary angioplasty registry, *J Am Coll Cardiol* 12:1149-1155, 1988.

Kahn JD, Rutherford BD, McConahay DR, et al.: Supported "high risk" coronary angioplasty using intraaortic balloon pump counterpulsation, *J Am Coll Cardiol* 15:1151-1155, 1990.

Kern MJ, Aguirre F, Bach R, Donohue T, Segal J: Augmentation of coronary blood flow by intra-aortic balloon pumping in patients after coronary angioplasty, *Circulation* 87:500-511, 1993.

Ohman EM, Califf RM, George DS, et al.: The use of intraaortic balloon pumping as an adjunct to reperfusion therapy in acute myocardial infarction. The Thrombolyses and Angioplasty in Myocardial Infarction (TAMI) Study Group, *Am Heart J* 1218:895-901, 1991.

Pennington DG, Merjavy JP, Codd JE, et al.: Extra-corporeal membrane oxygenation for patients with cardiogenic shock, *Circulation* 70:I-130-I-137, 1984.

Reichman RT, Joyo CI, Dombitsky WP, et al.: Improved patient survival after cardiac arrest using a cardiopulmonary support system, *Ann Thorac Surg* 498:101-105, 1990.

Ryan TJ, Faxon DP, Gunnar RM, et al.: Guidelines for percutaneous transluminal coronary angioplasty. A report of the American College of Cardiology/American Heart Association Task Force on assessment of diagnostic and therapeutic cardiovascular procedures, *Circulation* 78:486-502, 1988.

Shawl FA, Domanski MJ, Wish MH, Davis M: Percutaneous cardiopulmonary bypass support in the catheterization laboratory: technique and complications, *Am Heart J* 120:195-203, 1990.

Standards and guidelines for cardiopulmonary resuscitation (CPR) and emergency cardiac care (ECC), *JAMA* 255:2905-2914, 1986.

Stertzer SH, Myler RK, Insel H, Wallsh E, Rossi P: Percutaneous transluminal coronary angioplasty in left main stem coronary stenosis: a five year appraisal, *Int J Cardiol* 9:149-159, 1985.

Stueven HA, Tonsfeldt DJ, Thompson BM, Whitcomb J, Dastenson E, Aprahamian C: Atropine in asystole: human studies, *Ann Emerg Med* 13:815-817, 1984.

Tommaso CL: Management of high-risk coronary angioplasty, *Am J Cardiol* 64:E33-E37, 1989.

Vignola PA, Swaye PS, Gosselin AJ: Guidelines for effective and safe percutaneous intra-aortic balloon pump insertion and removal, *Am J Cardiol* 48:660-664, 1981.

Vogel RA, Shawl F, Tommaso C, et al.: Initial report of the National Registry of Elective Cardiopulmonary Bypass Supported Coronary Angioplasty, *J Am Coll Cardiol* 15:23-29, 1990.

Voudris V, Marco J, Morice M-C, Fajadet J, Royer T: "High-risk" percutaneous transluminal coronary angioplasty with preventive intra-aortic balloon counterpulsation, *Cathet Cardiovasc Diagn* 19:160-164, 1990.

Williams DO, Korr KS, Gewirtz H, Most AS: The effect of intraaortic balloon counterpulsation regional myocardial blood flow on oxygen consumption in the presence of coronary artery stenosis in patients with unstable angina, *Circulation* 66:593-597, 1982.

10

NONANGIOGRAPHIC CORONARY LESION ASSESSMENT

John McB. Hodgson, Morton J. Kern, Thomas J. Donohue, and Thomas L. Wolford

Angiography produces a two-dimensional luminogram of the coronary artery. Angiography cannot identify the plaque distribution, composition, extent, or the physiologic significance of lesions in the intermediately severe range (40% to 70% diameter narrowing). Quantitative arteriographic techniques have not improved the assessment of lesions beyond providing standardized measurements. Because of the limitations of angiography for coronary lesion assessment, three nonangiographic methods for lesion assessment have emerged:
1. Intravascular ultrasound imaging
2. Intravascular Doppler flow
3. Intravascular angioscopy
The advantages, disadvantages, and equipment specifications for each technique are summarized in Tables 10-1 and 10-2.

INTRAVASCULAR ULTRASOUND IMAGING

Contrast angiography has not been able to provide a clear picture of the disease process within the vascular wall. The development of intravascular ultrasound imaging (IVUS) has provided a new tool for assessing the atherosclerotic process and monitoring therapeutic interventions. Intracoronary ul-

349

TABLE 10-I. Specifications of intravascular diagnostic devices

Type of system (company)	Catheter size	Frequency (mH₃)	Resolution (μm at 2 mm)
Angioscopy			
Coronary angioscope (Baxter)	4.5F	—	50
Doppler			
FloWire (Cardiometrics)	0.018-in. guidewire	12 to 15	—
Ultrasound			
Mechanical (Cardiovascular Imaging Systems)	Peripheral 5F	20	750
	Intracardiac 10F	10 to 15	1500
	Coronary 4.3F	30	200 to 500
	Coronary 2.9F	20 to 30	200 to 500
	Coronary 3.1F sheath	20 to 30	
Phased array (Endosonics)	Coronary 3.5F	20	200 to 500
Mechanical (Boston Scientific)	Peripheral 4.8, 6.2F	12 to 20	1500
	Coronary 3.5F	20 to 30	

From Siegel RJ, Forrester J: Advantages and limitations of intravascular imaging devices in clinical applications, *ACC Curr J Rev*, p 80, March/April 1993.

TABLE 10-2.   Imaging technologies as adjuncts to endovascular intervention

Advantages	Disadvantages
Angioscopy	
Best method to identify thrombus	Requires blood displacement by constant flushing
Excellent detail of surface characteristics	Limited image acquisition time (>60 sec)
Forward viewing	Potential for vascular damage
Potential combination with angioplasty	Does not provide quantitative data
Doppler FloWire	
On-line assessment of coronary flow before, during, after interventions	Nonimaging modality
Easily combined with angioplasty device	Complexity in interpretation
Assesses significance of stenoses	
Assesses coronary flow reserve	
Small-diameter guidewire	
Intravascular ultrasound imaging	
Quantifies wall thickness	Needs miniaturization
Qualitative tissue characterization	Not forward viewing
Provides a 360° tomographic view	Potential for vascular damage
Potential combination with angioplasty	

Modified from Siegel RJ, et al.: Advantages and limitations of intravascular imaging devices in clinical applications. *ACC Curr J Rev,* p 77, March/April 1993.

trasound provides complementary information to angiography.

Although angiography will continue to provide important information with respect to diagnosis and guidance of therapy and interventions, it is no longer the "gold standard" for assessing atherosclerosis. The major reason for this is that IVUS allows clear delineation of the disease within the blood vessel wall, similar to information obtained with postmortem histology studies. Table 10-3 outlines the important differences between angiography and IVUS.

Improvement of IVUS image quality over the past few years has enabled interventionalists to strategize therapy according to lesion-specific criteria, assess optimization of ther-

TABLE 10-3.   Contrast between angiography and ultrasound

Angiography	Intracoronary ultrasound
Planar	Tomographic
Shadow of lumen	Direct lumen visualization
Wall not imaged	Visualizes wall structures with high resolution; detects minimal disease
Repeated injections needed	Continuous information
Magnification errors	Precise measurements
Provides global assessment	Provides localized details
Implies presence of plaque	Characterizes plaque
Lumen measures used for device selection	Assists in selection of device type and size based on plaque geometry, composition, degree of reference segment disease, plaque distribution, and degree of remodeling
Assesses gross luminal changes after intervention	Precisely defines lumen area after intervention; defines vessel recoil after intervention; defines dissections and closures

apy, and guide approaches during intervention according to specific goals. IVUS provides a precise image of coronary artery geometry and identifies morphologic features of coronary plaque. Although it has been suggested that appropriate coronary interventions can be selected based on IVUS, no physiologic information currently can be derived from intravascular ultrasound data. The present indications for IVUS are listed in the accompanying box.

Indications for IVUS

1. Assessment of lesion calcium
2. Vessel dimensions
3. Confirmation of atherosclerotic plaque
4. Stent deployment
5. Endothelial function research

Imaging Catheters

Intravascular ultrasound catheters utilize 20- to 40-MHz silicon piezoelectric crystals on a rotating internal cable or externally mounted on 2.9F to 5.0F monorail-style catheters and controlled electronically.

The two basic approaches to producing IVUS images are mechanical and solid-state electronic (Fig. 10-1). In the mechanical systems, the majority of studies have been performed using a rotating imaging core passed within an outer sheath. The imaging core is rotated via a flexible drive shaft in order to sweep the transducer continuously through a 360° arc in the vessel. Examples of such a design include the systems manufactured by CVIS/Boston Scientific, DuMed, and Hewlett Packard/Boston Scientific. An alternative mechanical design developed by DuMed uses a micromotor (1-mm diameter) packaged in the catheter tip to rotate the imaging element. Thus, although the transducer is rotated, a drive shaft is not

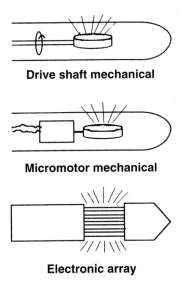

Drive shaft mechanical

Micromotor mechanical

Electronic array

Fig. 10-1. Three basic catheter designs for intravascular ultrasound. *Top*, Mechanically rotated transducer employing a drive shaft. *Middle*, Mechanically rotated transducer employing a micromotor. *Bottom*, Electronically switched array transducer. (From John McB. Hodgson, M.D.)

needed. The solid-state electronic design has been used by Endosonics. In this system, multiple ultrasound transducers are arranged circumferentially around the catheter tip and sequentially activated electronically to produce a 360° image. This system also reconstructs the image using techniques similar to CT or MRI scans. All systems have facilities for recording images on videotape, for analysis of dimensions and area, and for printing hard copy images.

The lumen, intima, media, and adventitial interfaces have relatively large differences in acoustic impedance, providing differential reflecting surfaces. A two-dimensional image can resolve the transverse structure of a coronary artery from the catheter axis perpendicular to the artery (Fig. 10-2).

Image Features

Regardless of the imaging system used, the images are presented in a tomographic real-time video format. The basic image features are described below from the center outward.

1. *Dead zone:* The black circular ring in the middle of the image is caused by the space occupied by the catheter.
2. *Artefact:* A "halo" artefact around the catheter usually encroaches onto lumen areas and therefore may affect analy-

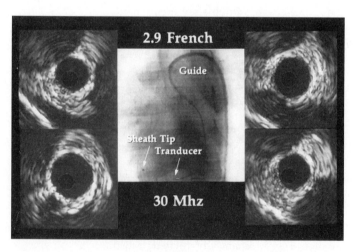

Fig. 10-2.   Normal arterial structure by IVUS. Single-layer appearance in young patients. Trilaminar appearance in older patients.

sis. It may also encroach onto the signals transmitted from the vessel wall. These artefacts are related to either the imaging sheath or to a property of ultrasonic imaging termed "ringdown" (reflected reverberations).

3. *Lumen:* The dark, echolucent area surrounding the catheter artefact signal is the lumen.

4. *Inner layer:* In a normal artery, the intima is often too thin to be seen reliably. The thin inner echogenic layer surrounding the lumen usually represents the internal elastic lamina. In a diseased coronary artery, the atheromatous intima is seen as a thick echogenic layer surrounding the lumen. In vessels with mild to moderate atherosclerosis, a thin echodense layer at the intima–media interface can be seen, correlating histologically to the internal elastic lamina. This may be obscured in severely diseased atherosclerotic arteries.

5. *Middle hypoechoic layer:* The media, packed with smooth muscle cells and a few elastin fibers, appears as a relatively echolucent area. The external elastic lamina may sometimes be seen as an echodense layer at the media–adventitia interface.

6. *Outer echogenic layer:* The adventitia is seen as an echodense layer surrounding the hypoechoic media. The adventitia shows increased echodensity due to both the inhomogeneous histologic structures and the high elastin and collagen content. This structure has the most intense echoes in normal arteries. Echoes that are more intense than the adventitia are therefore abnormal. In this region, perivascular structures may also be observed (i.e., veins and pericardium).

Image Display and Interpretation

Alternative display formats include sagittal or three-dimensional (3-D). In sagittal images a series of individual tomograms has been combined and then "sliced" lengthwise. This presents a format similar to the familiar angiographic appearance. A 3-D representation can also be constructed from the image set used in sagittal images.

It is important that both the physician who will be handling the catheter and the technical support staff understand basic image interpretation. Normal vessels appear as circular, featureless lumens with a single echodense surrounding structure. The thickness of normal endothelium and intima is usually below the resolving power of the ultrasound system (<100 μm, Fig. 10-3A). When disease is present, the inner echodense reflection becomes thicker, and often a three-layered appearance is apparent. This inner layer represents fibrous hyperplasia and the internal elastic lamina. The media is echolucent, thus giving the appearance of 3 layers (Fig. 10-3B). Accumulation of plaque can be extensive and may result in marked narrowing of the lumen (Fig. 10-3C). Finally, calcification is often present and appears as very strong echoes with an acoustic "shadow." This shadow results from nearly complete reflection of the incident ultrasound signals and is

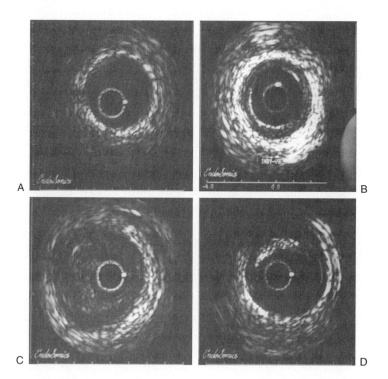

Fig. 10-3. IVUS images for various types of coronary arterial disease. **A,** Normal vessel. **B,** Mild atherosclerosis. **C,** Soft atheroma. **D,** Calcified atheroma. (From John McB. Hodgson, M.D.)

highly characteristic of calcium (Fig. 10-3D). Vascular remodeling may result in expansion of the adventitia in areas of plaque accumulation. When initially viewing images it is important to search for the echolucent (black) band, which usually retains a circular shape at the edge of the adventitia. Once this is identified, structures internal to this band are part of the arterial wall or atheroma. Structures outside this band are in the adventitia or periadventitia.

In human coronary arteries, intravascular ultrasound provides two characteristic normal artery patterns. Young arteries usually have a monolayered appearance with circular geometry. Older coronary arteries often show a three-layered image with a characteristic lucent band defining the medial boundaries. Inner luminal areas of plaque have been correlated with histopathologic vessel structure. Lumen size and wall thickness validation studies by histology have been excellent. The dimensions of the individual vessel layers and overall wall thickness are less accurate than measurements of lumen area by angiography or histology. In normal vessels, angiographic coronary diameters have a close correlation to ultrasound diameters ($r = 0.86$ to 0.88), depending on the degree of perpendicular alignment of the intravascular catheter. The correlation of angiography and two-dimensional image dimensions after angioplasty is highly variable, depending on the degree of vessel disruption.

One should also watch closely for artefacts due to air within the catheter, or malrotation of the drive shaft or the guidewire. Thorough knowledge of the types of artefact possible with the specific system is important.

Imaging Technique and Catheterization Laboratory Setup

Integration of IVUS into the laboratory is critical for the widespread use of the technology. Although the systems are portable, moving them into and out of the catheterization suite can be a frustrating experience. To minimize the problems associated with this process, it is important for several members of the support staff to take specialized training and assume responsibility for the equipment. We have found that the following preparations make use of IVUS most efficient:

1. Specialized support staff familiar with operation of the equipment and image interpretation

2. A hard-wired ancillary video monitor on the angiographic monitor boom for display of the IVUS images to the physician operator
3. Hard-wired fluoroscopic image output to the IVUS machine
4. An ample supply of super VHS videotapes and premade IVUS report worksheets, kept with the machine
5. A lapel microphone to be attached to the physician operator, allowing "voiceover" on the IVUS images being recorded (critical to later interpretation)
6. Maintenance of a time log during the procedure that is keyed to the IVUS time code (facilitates later video review)
7. Use of an automated pullback device, which standardizes the procedure to prevent too rapid scanning and eliminate much of the physician operator effect on image quality
8. A system of maintenance for IVUS-related records and videotapes
9. An image review station that is separate from the IVUS machine itself

Although many IVUS examinations are performed in conjunction with interventional procedures, diagnostic studies are also performed frequently. For these cases, appropriate guide catheters, guidewires, and hemostatic valves are necessary. It is also important to ensure full anticoagulation with heparin before beginning IVUS imaging. Heparin may be reversed with protamine following scanning if desired.

IVUS Catheter Technique

Standard angioplasty catheter positioning techniques with guiding catheters, guidewires, and heparin administration are employed. An intracoronary ultrasound catheter can be positioned over an angioplasty guidewire distal to the lesion using a monorail guidewire method. After device positioning, IVUS images are recorded at specific locations within the vessel and during slow catheter pullback up to the normal proximal segments. Documentation of each intravascular ultrasound catheter position is facilitated by simultaneous angiographic recording. In addition, careful audio annotation of the position should also be recorded on tape.

Intravascular Ultrasound Morphologic Plaque (Fig. 10-4)

Plaque composition.   In general, plaque may be classified as "soft" or "hard" based on whether the echodensity is less than or similar to the adventitia.

1. Soft plaque: More than 80% of the plaque area in an integrated pullback throughout the lesion is composed of thickened intimal echoes with homogeneous echo density less than that seen in adventitia.
2. Fibrous plaque: More than 80% of plaque in an integrated pullback throughout the lesion is composed of thick and dense echo involving the intimal leading edge with homogeneous echo density greater than or equal to that seen for adventitia.
3. Calcified plaque: Bright echoes within a plaque demonstrate acoustic shadowing and occupying >90% of the vessel wall circumference in at least one cross-sectional image of the lesion. The extent of calcification, defined as the presence of any hyperechogenic structure that shadows

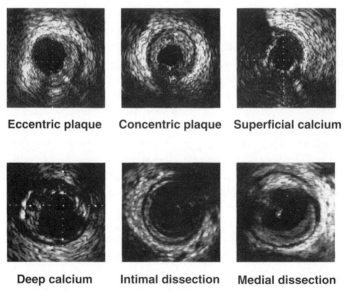

| Eccentric plaque | Concentric plaque | Superficial calcium |

| Deep calcium | Intimal dissection | Medial dissection |

Fig. 10-4.   IVUS images illustrating plaque morphology.

underlying ultrasound anatomy, is reported in degree of circumference in which shadowing is present. Calcium is also classified as deep or superficial.

4. Mixed plaque: Bright echoes with acoustic shadowing encompass <90% of the vessel wall circumference, or a mixture of soft and fibrous plaque with each component occupying <80% of the plaque area in an integrated pullback through the lesion.

5. Subintimal thickening involving reference vessel segments is defined as a concentric prominent leading edge echo and a widened subintimal echolucent zone with combined thickness >500 μm.

Further classification of soft lesions includes the presence of very lucent regions representing lipid deposits or plaque hemorrhage. Thrombus also appears soft but has a distinctive mobile pattern when viewed in real time. Hard lesions may be predominantly fibrotic or contain calcium. Calcium may be characterized as superficial (near the lumen) or deep. Such classification has implications for selection of interventional strategies.

Plaque morphology

Location. Plaque may be described as concentric or eccentric, with or without ulceration. In describing a nonconcentric plaque, its location is noted in relation to a clock, that is, "plaque is present, extending from the 8 o'clock position to the 11 o'clock position, with calcium deposits seen at 9 o'clock."

Intimal flap/dissection. This is seen as a linear structure with or without a free edge. True and false channels can also be visualized. This characteristic motion of the intimal flap may also be seen within the lumen. Radiographic contrast injection can assist in defining the lumen and indicating whether there is communication of the lumen with an echo-free area below a flap.

Thrombus. Fresh thrombus is a low to moderately echogenic or granular mass that occupies part of the lumen and adjoins the adjacent wall; often it is mobile and has an irregular border. Edge definition is possible with contrast injection.

Aneurysm. Aneurysmal areas are expanded, thin-walled structures adjoining the lumen. They can be mistaken for branches, which appear similar.

Side branches. Side branches appear as "buds" with a loss of the internal band.

Dimensional Measurements (Fig. 10-5)

One of the major advantages of IVUS is its ability to provide precise measurements. Several studies have analyzed the accuracy of the ultrasound images in measuring lumen size and wall thickness. Correlations with histologic measurements have been uniformly high, although measurements of the dimensions of the layers and overall wall thickness have been reported to be less accurate than lumen area determinations. The lumen–intima and media–adventitia interfaces are generally accurate using ultrasound scanning; both interfaces show a relatively large increase in acoustic impedance as the beam passes through the layers. The intima–media interface may also provide a significant change in impedance, particularly in the presence of a prominent internal elastic lamina. At this interface, however, there is a "trailing-edge" effect that can result in the spreading or blooming of the intimal image. The net result is that the transition is obscured, the intima appears thicker than by histologic determination, and the media appears correspondingly thinner. However, wall thickness combined in intima and media corresponds closely to the histological dimensions.

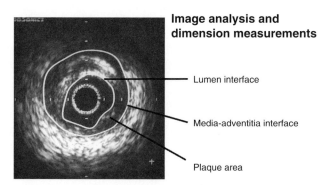

Image analysis and dimension measurements

— Lumen interface

— Media-adventitia interface

Plaque area

Fig. 10-5. Ultrasound-derived measurements are obtained from planimetry of lumen interface and media–adventitial interface edges. (From John McB. Hodgson, M.D.)

All ultrasound measurements are performed on end-diastolic images, unless specified otherwise. Artery lumen dimensions are quantitated from images of proximal, distal, or reference vessel segments and within the target lesion(s) or stent. The following measurements are routinely obtained.

Lumen and vessel diameters.   Minimal, maximal, and mean lumen and vessel diameters may be obtained.

Percent diameter stenosis.   Percent diameter stenosis is mean total vessel area diameter minus mean lumen diameter divided by mean total vessel diameter.

Total vessel area.   Total vessel area is integrated area central to the medial adventitia border. The vessel cross-sectional area is the area confined within the external elastic lamina or the media–adventitia interface.

Lumen area.   The lumen area is the integrated area central to the leading-edge echo. The area is confined within the lumen–intima interface. If the catheter is tangential, the lumen area is overestimated.

Wall area (intima and media).   Wall area equals total area minus lumen area. In abnormal vessels, this is the plaque area.

Percent area stenosis.   Percent area stenosis equals total vessel area minus lumen area divided by total vessel area:

$$\text{Percent plaque area} = \left(\frac{\text{total area} - \text{lumen area}}{\text{total area}} \right) \times 100$$

Indices of irregularity

1. The circular shape factor (CSF), an index of vessel eccentricity, is calculated from vessel diameter (d), cross-sectional area (CSA), and perimeter (P). The perimeter for a perfect circle of this diameter is determined as

$$P = \pi * d$$

This calculated perimeter is compared to the actual measured perimeter (by planimetry) of the vessel lumen. The circular shape factor is defined as

$$\text{CSF} = \frac{(\text{calculated perimeter})^2}{\text{observed perimeter}}$$

A value of 1.0 is a perfect circular lumen. Vessels with increasing eccentricity have values progressively smaller than 1.0.

2. A lesion eccentricity index (L_{ECC}) is calculated by lumen dimensions:

$$L_{ECC} = \frac{\text{maximum diameter}}{\text{minimum diameter}}$$

Plaque thickness measurements

1. Maximum thickness of any visible echogenic intimal leading edge.
2. Minimum thickness of any visible echogenic intimal leading edge.
3. Mean thickness of the intimal leading edge, determined by planimetry of the inner and outer borders of the intimal leading edge. For each border (inner and outer), the mean diameter is calculated as

$$d = 2 * \sqrt{\frac{\text{CSA}}{\pi}}$$

The mean thickness is defined as

$$\text{Mean thickness} = \frac{1}{2} * \frac{\text{outer diameter}}{\text{inner mean diameter}}$$

Plaque distribution.   Plaque distribution is classified into three categories:

1. *Concentric plaque.* Maximum plaque thickness (leading-edge plus sonolucent zone) <1.3 times minimum plaque thickness.
2. *Moderately eccentric plaque:* Maximum plaque thickness (leading edge plus sonolucent zone) 1.3 to 1.7 times minimum plaque thickness.
3. *Severely eccentric plaque:* Maximum plaque thickness (leading edge plus sonolucent zone) >1.7 times minimum plaque thickness.

Safety of IVUS

Among 2207 intracoronary ultrasound studies in a large review of multicenter results 505 (23%) were performed in heart transplant recipients and 1702 (77%) in nontransplant patients. There were no complications in 2034 patients (92.2%). In 87 patients (3.9%), complications occurred but were judged by the operator to be "not related" to IVUS. Vasospasm occurred during IVUS imaging in 63 patients (2.9%). Complications other than spasm were judged to have a "certain relation" to IVUS in 9 patients (0.4%), including acute procedural events in 6 (3 acute occlusions, 1 embolism, 1 dissection, and 1 thrombus) and major events in 3 patients (2 occlusions and 1 dissection, all resulting in myocardial infarction). Complications with "uncertain relation" to IVUS occurred in 14 patients (0.6%), including acute procedural events in 9 (5 acute occlusions, 3 dissections, and 1 arrhythmia) and major events in 5 patients (2 myocardial infarctions and 3 emergency coronary artery bypass surgeries). Acute procedural or major complications judged to be associated with IVUS (uncertain relation or certain relation to IVUS) were compared in different patient groups. The complication rate was higher in patients with unstable angina or acute myocardial infarction (2.1% events) as compared with patients with stable angina pectoris and asymptomatic patients (0.8% and 0.4%, respectively; p < .01). Complications were also more frequent in patients undergoing interventions (1.9%) as compared with transplant and nontransplant patients undergoing diagnostic IVUS imaging (0% and 0.6%, respectively; p < .001). Adverse events were few, and no association was detected between these events and the size or type of IVUS catheter used.

IVUS is associated with, but not necessarily the direct cause of, a minor acute clinical risk. Vessel spasm is the most frequent event that occurs during IVUS. Other complications occur predominantly in patients with acute coronary syndromes and during guidance for intervention.

Diagnostic Applications

Diagnosis of angiographically questionable stenoses.
Intracoronary ultrasound is useful for planning in patients for whom the presence of significant plaque is questionable on routine angiography. It is also indicated if a variation exists between angiography and clinical presentation, as in those patients with a question of a left main stenosis or ischemia in the presence of an otherwise "normal" angiogram. The disparity between IVUS and angiography has been well described. For defining discrete mild stenoses, IVUS is more accurate than angiography in identifying lumen area, and possibly more importantly, the degree of vessel remodeling. At one center, 112 ambiguous lesions were assessed for possi-

ble intervention, no revascularization was performed in 52%, and 13 patients were found to have significant unsuspected left main stenoses requiring coronary artery bypass surgery. Intermediately severe lesions should be assessed physiologically before intervention.

Diagnosis of allograft vasculopathy.   Intravascular ultrasound has been an excellent means to diagnose and quantitate cardiac transplant vasculopathy. Routine annual angiographic studies often reveal "normal" vessels in the transplant patient, whereas IVUS studies of the same cohort reveal diffuse intimal hyperplasia.

Progression and regression of coronary atherosclerosis. Because of the limitations of angiography in defining wall structure and pathology, IVUS use for quantifying and qualitatively appraising extent and progression of atherosclerosis may be especially helpful for regression trials with primary or secondary intervention. Several studies to assess atheroma progression and regression after randomization to a lipid-lowering regimen (diet and/or medication, exercise, and stress reduction) or "regular care" are now under way. All patients will have angiography and IVUS evaluation at baseline and will be reevaluated at 6 to 12 months. Serial assessments of the progression of intimal proliferation in cardiac transplant patients with angiography and IVUS have documented accelerated vasculopathy occurring most actively within the first year following transplant.

Evaluation of vasomotor tone.   Intracoronary ultrasound yields a beat-to-beat analysis of vascular compliance (systolic-to-diastolic lumen area ratio). Additionally, the effects of vasoactive substances can be monitored directly and continuously during IVUS imaging. These unique advantages allow study of the early effects of atherosclerosis and/or intervention on vessel compliance and also allow evaluation of endothelial function in patients with varying degrees of atherosclerosis.

Interventional applications

Device selection and strategical planning. Interrogation of the reference segments, as well as defining the morphological characteristics of the suspect lesion, is a suggested way to determine the most appropriate device for intervention. For example, if an arc of superficial calcium is present, a strategy using rotational atherectomy to remove this layer has been advocated. The lesion with of deeper calcium and superficial soft or mixed plaque components is amenable to directional coronary atherectomy (DCA), PTCA, or stent placement, depending on the location of the stenosis. Lesion eccentricity may also favor DCA or stent placement. In one single-center study, the initial interventional strategy was altered after IVUS imaging in 44% of patients. Outcome studies to determine whether IVUS-based decisions are clinically important for these strategies are in progress.

Device sizing during coronary intervention. Ultrasound is employed in special institutions for selecting device size in all patients undergoing DCA or stent placement. This allows the appropriate device to be used at the outset of the procedure as well as providing information regarding eccentricity of the atheroma and plaque composition. A multicenter pilot study has recently explored aggressive PTCA balloon sizing based on IVUS-defined adventitial vessel size. Preliminary results suggest that such a strategy may be useful for improving minimal lumen diameters (MLD) without excess complications.

Assessing interventional end points. Angiographic and IVUS quantitative measurements are similar in healthy arteries, but discrepancies between these two modalities become significant when the lumen is distorted by the presence of an atheromatous plaque or dissections. Intracoronary ultrasound can therefore be employed following an interventional procedure to identify and quantify plaque removal with DCA, vessel stretching and plaque fissuring with PTCA, plaque obliteration with rotational atherectomy or laser excision, and adequate deployment of coronary stents (Fig. 10-6). Optimizing the residual lumen diameters with IVUS confirmation assists in achieving a final result in keeping with the "bigger is better" theory and may therefore decrease the risk of restenosis.

Assessing complications. Following coronary interventions, vessel stretching, plaque redistribution and shifting, plaque removal, plaque fissuring, and dissections can be clearly outlined by IVUS. The morphologic characteristics as well as specific dissection patterns following intervention have

Arterial segments

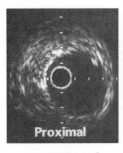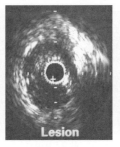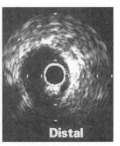

Proximal	Lesion	Distal
LA: 9.36 mm²	2.32 mm²	4.69 mm²
MLD: 3.45 mm	1.72 mm	2.44 mm

A   3.0/2.5 tapered balloon was selected

Initial stent assessment

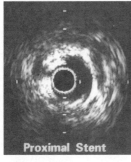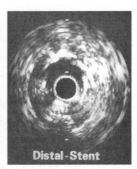

Proximal Stent	Distal-Stent
LA: 5.47 mm	LA: 5.03 mm
(90% target: 8.4 mm²)	(90% target: 4.22 mm²)

B

Fig. 10-6. **A,** Initial IVUS evaluation showing the proximal, lesion, and distal segments. The lumen areas (LA) and minimal lumen diameters (MLD) are shown. Based on the tapering nature of this vessel, a tapered balloon was selected for stent deployment. **B,** After initial inflation at 12 atm, the lumen areas within the stent do not meet criteria for discharge without anticoagulation (90% of the reference segment). **C,** After repeat dilation at 16 atm, the lumen areas and minimal lumen diameters are enlarged and the implantation is completed. (From John McB. Hodgson, M.D.)

Final stent assessment

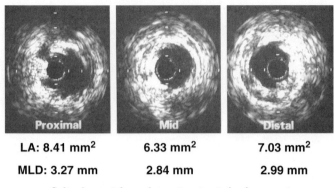

| LA: 8.41 mm² | 6.33 mm² | 7.03 mm² |
| MLD: 3.27 mm | 2.84 mm | 2.99 mm |

Criteria met for adequate stent deployment

C

Fig. 10-6. (*Continued*).

shown that dissections are dependent on differential plaque types, usually occurring at the edge of calcified segments.

Predicting restenosis. Several clinical trials are analyzing the importance of IVUS findings following interventional procedures for predicting restenosis. The presence or absence of calcium detected by IVUS, the type of dissection following an intervention, and the clinical presentation all correlate with restenosis. Additionally, IVUS has redefined restenosis; recent data suggest that a large proportion of patients have chronic remodeling as a major contributor to restenosis. This may explain why therapies aimed only at intimal proliferation have been unsuccessful in reducing restenosis.

Influence of IVUS beyond angioplasty. Published data from recent clinical studies reveal that incorporating IVUS data after an angiographically successful procedure will often convince operators to change strategies and move toward a larger lumen diameter (see the box). This strategy may translate into a decrease in the predicted restenosis rate according to the Baim and Kuntz model. Thus, using IVUS, an additional 12% to 42% increase in lumen cross-sectional area can be anticipated. This appears to be true not only for stenting, but also for DCA and PTCA. If these improvements are sustained, decreases in restenosis should be expected.

Intravascular Ultrasound Imaging During
Coronary Interventions

1. Angioplasty
   a. Plaque distribution
   b. Vessel size
   c. Extent of calcium
   d. Calculate percent stenosis
2. Atherectomy
   a. Plaque distribution
   b. Composition of plaque
   c. Direct atherectomy device
   d. Assess posttreatment result
3. Stents
   a. Vessel size
   b. Expansion of stent

Summary

Intracoronary ultrasound is an important adjunctive technique for the diagnosis and treatment of arterial diseases, especially coronary atherosclerosis in the catheterization laboratory. Application of this technology to specific patient subsets can be expected to result in improved outcomes at lower overall expense.

INTRACORONARY DOPPLER FLOW VELOCITY
Background

Intracoronary Doppler flow velocity provides an objective, physiologic measurement of coronary blood flow on which to base treatment decisions, and is especially important for angiographic findings of intermediate or indeterminate severity.

In the past, Doppler flow velocity was not incorporated into routine practice because of the need to use large catheters, measurements limited to only proximal regions, the necessity to exchange the Doppler catheter for an interventional device, and difficulty in ascertaining optimal signals with the zero cross Doppler technique. The Doppler guidewire (Cardiometrics, Inc., Mountain View, Calif.) has overcome catheter limitations, making it suitable for routine clinical use. Coronary flow velocity can be measured distal to a coronary steno-sis, does not interfere with normal blood flow, can be used as a primary interventional guidewire, and can monitor flow following angioplasty. Spectral Doppler signal analysis im-proves operator confidence in measurement accuracy. During diagnostic angiography, translesional flow can determine the hemodynamic significance of an intermediately severe (40% to 70%) angiographic lesion for interventional decision mak-ing. During multivessel angioplasty, secondary lesions can be assessed before undergoing additional interventions. The clinical applications of intracoronary flow velocity measure-ments are summarized in Table 10-4.

The Doppler Flow Wire

The Doppler angioplasty guidewire (FloWire, Cardiomet-rics, Inc., Mountain View, Calif.) is a 175-cm-long, 0.014-0.018-in.-diameter, flexible, steerable guidewire with a piezo-electric ultrasound transducer integrated into the tip (Fig. 10-7A). The forward-directed ultrasound beam diverges in a 27° arc from the long axis (measured to the −6-dB round-trip points of the ultrasound beam pattern). A pulse repetition frequency of >40 kHz, pulse duration of +0.83 msec, and sampling delay of 6.5 msec are standard for clinical us-

---

TABLE 10-4.   Clinical uses of intravascular doppler coronary flow velocity

1. Intermediate (40% to 70%) lesion assessment
2. Angioplasty
   End point
   Monitoring complications
   Assessing additional lesions
   Collateral flow
   Stent
   Atherectomy
3. Coronary vasodilatory reserve
   Syndrome X
   Transplant coronary arteriopathy
   Saphenous vein graft, internal mammary artery
4. Coronary research
   Pharmacologic studies
   Intraaortic balloon pumping
   Coronary physiology of vascular disease
   Thallium correlations

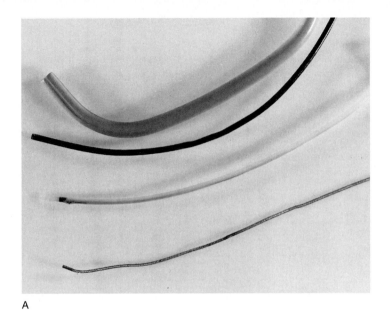

A

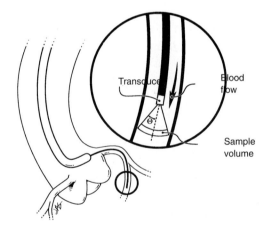

B

Fig. 10-7. A, Doppler catheters (top 3) and 0.018-in. Doppler guidewire. (From Kern MJ, Anderson HV, editors: A symposium: the clinical applications of the intracoronary Doppler guidewire flow velocity in patients: understanding blood flow beyond the coronary stenosis, *Am J Cardiol* 71:1D-86D, 1993.) **B,** Diagram of Doppler guidewire positioned through angiographic catheter. The sample volume and beam angle (ϕ) permit accurate velocity measurements. (From Ofili EO, Kern MJ, Labovitz AJ, et al: Analysis of coronary blood flow velocity dynamics in angiographically normal and stenosed arteries before and after endolumen enlargement by angioplasty, *J Am Coll Cardiol* 21:308-316, 1993.)

age. The system is coupled to a real-time spectrum analyzer, a videocassette recorder, and a video page printer. The quadrature/Doppler audio signals are processed by the spectrum analyzer using on-line fast-Fourier transformation to provide a scrolling gray-scale spectral display. The frequency response of the system calculates approximately 90 spectra/sec. Simultaneous electrocardiographic and arterial pressure are also input to the video display. Doppler guidewire velocity demonstrated excellent correlation with electromagnetic flow velocity and volumetric flow in straight and curved tubed models as well as in in-vivo testing using a circumflex canine coronary artery. The Doppler guidewire measures phasic flow velocity patterns and tracks linearly with flow rates in most small, straight coronary arteries.

The timing of the sending and receiving velocity allows the flow wire to measure blood flow velocities from moving red cells in a sample area 5 mm ($\times$ 2 mm) from the tip of the wire, a distance far enough away that the blood velocity is not affected by the wake of the wire (Fig. 10-7B). The returning signal is transmitted, in real time, to the display console and is seen on a gray-scale spectral scrolling display of all velocities of the red blood cells within the sample volume. The key parameters are derived from the automatically tracked peak blood velocities within the sample area, making the parameter values less position sensitive. As long as the sample area accurately tracks the peak velocity in the center of the artery, the key parameters will remain positionally insensitive and reliable. The fundamentals and artefacts of flow velocity measurements have been described in detail elsewhere (see Suggested Readings).

Coronary Flow Velocity Signal Analysis

Flow velocity data are printed on an integrated video page printer, which provides computerized parameters of intracoronary flow velocity, including maximal peak velocity (MPV) and mean or average peak velocity (APV) diastolic and systolic velocities, diastolic and systolic velocity integrals (DVI) (obtained by planimetry of the total area under the peak instantaneous velocity profile), mean total velocities, and the total velocity integral (Fig. 10-8). These automatic parameters were validated using a custom software program and manual

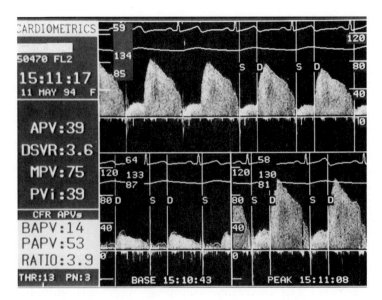

Fig. 10-8.   Example of flow velocity signals for the measurement of coronary vasodilatory flow reserve. Flow panel is
divided into upper and lower. The upper panel is a continuous
display in real time of the flow spectra. A normal phasic pattern
is seen shortly after hyperemia. The ECG and aortic pressure
are displayed on top of the flow signals. The numbers in the
upper left corner box are the heart rate, systolic pressure, and
diastolic pressure. The lower panel is divided into left and right
for the storage of the basal and hyperemic signals, respectively.
Codes at the left side of the figure are the values for the
flow parameters (of top panel, far right), APV, average peak
velocity; DSVR, diastolic–systolic velocity ratio; MPV, maximal peak velocity; Pvi, peak velocity integral; RATIO, coronary
flow reserve. BAPV and PAPV are the base and hyperemic
APV, respectively.

tracing of the spectral peak Doppler velocity signal on a digital computer.

Technique

Intravenous heparin (5000- to 10,000-unit bolus) is required
before inserting the Doppler guidewire. After diagnostic angiography or during angioplasty, the Doppler guidewire is
passed through a standard angioplasty Y connector attached

to either a 6F or 8F guiding catheter. The guidewire is then advanced into the artery. Baseline flow velocity data are obtained at least 1 cm proximal to the lesion. The wire is then advanced at least 5 to 10 artery-diameter lengths (>2 cm) beyond the stenosis, avoiding placement in any side branches. Distal flow velocity data are then obtained. Continuous flow velocity profiles, along with simultaneous electrocardiogram and aortic pressure, are displayed on the video monitor.

Coronary flow velocity reserve is computed as the quotient of hyperemic/basal mean flow velocity. Coronary hyperemia is induced by intracoronary adenosine (6 to 8 μg in the right coronary artery and 12 to 18 μg in the left coronary artery).

Although earlier studies report a coronary vasodilatory reserve ratio of 3.5 to 5 in normal patients, in our and other laboratories, lower values are more commonly observed in patients with chest pain and angiographically normal arteries (normal 2.7 $\pm$ 0.6). In transplanted hearts with angiographic normal arteries, coronary vasodilatory reserve ratios are usually higher (3.1 $\pm$ 0.6). It should be noted that in arteries with severe coronary lesions, proximally measured flow velocity can produce nearly normal hyperemia due to augmentation of branch vessel flow. For significant stenoses, distal flow velocity reserve is always impaired (<2.0).

The Doppler guidewire can be used as the primary wire during routine angioplasty in >85% of attempts. The Doppler flow wire (as well as other guidewires) may have difficulty traversing vessels that are severely angled or that have highly complex lesions. When velocity data are desired beyond a stenosis in the highly tortuous artery, a routine soft, torqueable 0.012- to 0.014-in. guidewire advanced through a 2.7F Tracker catheter can be used. The target lesion is crossed with the smaller guidewire; the Tracker catheter is advanced distally; the 0.014-in. wire is then exchanged for the 0.018-in. Doppler wire, and the Tracker catheter is withdrawn. Velocity data can then be easily acquired. This method also provides a means to measure a translesional pressure gradient through the tracking catheter. The setup time and measurement for the flow wire system is usually 10-15 min.

Influence of a Stenosis on Normal Coronary Flow Velocity

For coronary vessel diameters >2.0 mm, normal artery flow velocity is maintained within 15% from proximal to distal regions. In normal coronary vessels, the proximal to distal velocity ratio is nearly 1. In most epicardial coronary vessels, there is no significant decline in distal blood flow velocity, since the blood flow volume and epicardial conduit cross-sectional area both are reduced over the course of the vessel. A marked decrement in distal flow relative to proximal flow is seen with hemodynamically significant lesions and is predicated on a branched-tube model, wherein flow is diverted away from the branch with a high resistance (stenosis) to branches with lower resistances (normal branches). A proximal-to-distal blood flow velocity ratio >1.7 (i.e., distal velocity reduced) is associated with a translesional gradient >30 mmHg, lesions that usually warrant intervention. The proximal–distal flow ratio will not apply in conduits without branches, wherein the continuity equation mandates equality of flow at all points along the circuit. A proximal–distal flow ratio is not useful for very proximal lesions, left internal mammary artery (LIMA), or bypass graft conduits (SVG). The transstenotic velocity (P/D) ratio is not useful for predicting stenosis severity in ostial lesions, coronary conduits (SVG or LIMA), diffusely diseased vessels, or those vessels with serial stenoses.

Normal flow criteria.   A hierarchy of flow velocity findings describing normal flow characteristics is identified below.

1. Poststenotic coronary vasodilatory reserve >2.0
2. Diastolic-systolic velocity ratio (DSVR) >1.5
3. Proximal–distal ratio <1.7.

When coronary vasodilatory reserve is abnormal and the proximal–distal ratio and diastolic–systolic velocity ratio are normal or unavailable, a translesional pressure gradient during hyperemia can be measured to confirm a lesion-specific impairment of coronary flow reserve. A normal pressure gradient obtained with a Tracker catheter (2.7F) is <20 mmHg in our laboratory. The ratio of distal coronary to aortic pressure during hyperemia is called the fractional flow reserve of the myocardium. A value of >0.75 corresponds to negative stress testing (see Fractional Flow Reserve below).

The comparison of poststenotic flow reserve >2.0 with myocardial perfusion stress imaging has demonstrated a high correlation with normal perfusion scintigraphy. High sensitivity, specificity, and predictive accuracy are reported for both perfusion sestamibi and thallium-201 imaging with distal coronary flow reserve.

Hemodynamically significant lesion flow criteria. Criteria of lesion significance for flow velocity findings distal to severe coronary stenoses are illustrated in Fig. 10-9. The four criteria are:

1. Decrease in mean velocity, usually <20 cm/sec.
2. Mean proximal–distal flow velocity ratio >1.7.
3. Impaired phasic pattern of coronary flow (DSVR <1.5). A normal DSVR is usually >1.8 for the left coronary artery. This value may vary normally among vessels, but a DSVR <1.4 is common in severe lesions.
4. Impaired distal coronary hyperemia, coronary flow reserve <2.0.

Flow velocity criteria for successful angioplasty. Criteria of flow velocity for successful angioplasty are:

1. Distal mean velocity is increased (usually >20 to 30 cm/sec).
2. Phasic pattern of flow is normalized (DSVR >1.5).
3. Coronary flow reserve is improved, >2.0. An inadequate lumen or microvascular impairment may yield lower coronary flow reserve. Use a reference vessel coronary flow reserve to compare.

Clinical Applications

Monitoring coronary blood flow during PTCA. Flow velocity during angioplasty demonstrates physiologic responses to coronary occlusion, recanalization, and potential flow-limiting complications. In a complicated or high-risk case, a brief monitoring period after angioplasty to identify potential for vessel closure has obvious benefits. Interruption of unstable flow with conversion to a stable postprocedure flow pattern reduces morbidity related to an out-of-laboratory acute vessel closure and reduces the need for a repeat procedure, angioplasty catheters, or stent placement. Early warning signs of an adverse outcome derived from flow trend monitoring can potentially save the cost of repeat angioplasty or bypass surgery.

Abnormal cyclical flow variations due to dissection, thrombus, or vasospasm may be seen using the mean velocity trend plot. Cyclical flow variations have been associated with early thrombus formation and abrupt closure. Flow velocity changes often precede angiographic signs of vessel occlusion.

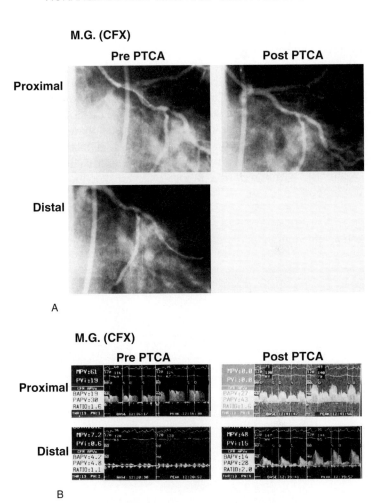

Fig. 10-9. **A,** Cinegrams from an angioplasty of a circumflex marginal branch with measurements of flow velocity. Position of FloWire is shown proximal (*top left*) and distal (*bottom left*) to the stenosis. Angiographic result after PTCA is shown on top right panel. **B,** Flow velocity recordings before PTCA (left panels). Proximal flow reserve is impaired at 1.6 (normal, >2.0), with abnormal phasic pattern. Flow is even more disturbed in the poststenotic distal region, with nearly no flow. After PTCA (*right panels*), both distal and proximal flow improve with distal CFR = 2.0 and return of normal phasic pattern.

Monitoring flow can also reduce total contrast volume when assessing stability of angioplasty results. Figure 10-10 illustrates flow trend monitoring after PTCA.

Assessing lesions of intermediate angiographic severity. High interobserver and intraobserver variability in judging the angiographic severity of coronary lesions, especially for lesions of >40% and <70% to <80% diameter, requires physiologic stress testing to establish clinical significance. Direct assessment by translesional velocity measurement in the catheterization laboratory can also be used to

41-year-old woman, acute anterior MI

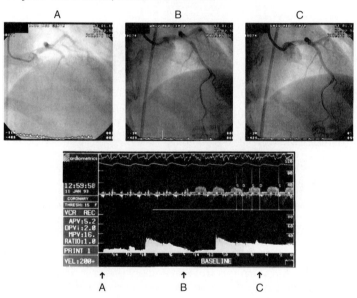

Fig. 10-10.   Flow velocity trend monitoring during PTCA for acute myocardial infarction demonstrates two patterns of flow after PTCA. **A,** Initial dilation flow is followed by **B,** unstable flow. **B** has continuous downward trend and led to abrupt closure, which responded with a stable flow pattern (**C**) after longer high-pressure balloon inflations. (From Kern MJ, Aguirre FV, Donohue TJ, Bach RG, Caracciolo EA, Flynn MS: Coronary flow velocity monitoring after angioplasty associated with abrupt reocclusion, *Am Heart J* 127:436-438, 1994.)

establish the physiologic significance of intermediate stenoses.

The clinical outcome of the prospective deferment of angioplasty of intermediate stenoses based on normal flow criteria is excellent. Of 88 patients with 100 lesions 40% to 70% diameter stenosis over a mean of 10 ± 5 months, the cardiac event rates were 4, 6, 0, and 2 patients requiring repeat angioplasty, coronary artery bypass surgery, myocardial infarction, or death, respectively. Of the 10 patients having angioplasty or coronary artery bypass surgery, only 6 had lesion progression, with 4 being new stenoses requiring intervention for nontarget arteries. In a comparative angioplasty patient cohort undergoing similar Doppler flow measurements over the same period, 26% of patients required angioplasty or coronary artery bypass surgery, compared to 12% of the deferred group. Angioplasty should be performed based on objective evidence of flow limitation responsible for the clinical syndrome.

Multivessel PTCA.   In patients with multivessel disease undergoing culprit vessel angioplasty, additional coronary stenoses of intermediate severity may occur in 15% to 25% of cases. Lesion assessment for the secondary stenoses may obviate the necessity of a staged coronary angioplasty procedure, saving the cost of further hospital days, myocardial stress perfusion imaging, and a repeat coronary angioplasty procedure.

Collateral flow velocity.   During coronary balloon occlusion, flow velocity often falls rapidly to near zero. However, persistent antegrade or new retrograde flow suggests collateral supply to the epicardial location (Fig. 10-11). The presence of retrograde collateral flow velocity occurs in 10% to 15% of cases and may be a useful indicator of the patient's potential tolerance for prolonged balloon occlusions.

In patients with angiographically visible epicardial collateral pathways, the total flow velocity (10 to 15 units) is higher than the velocity measured from intramyocardial pathways (5 to 10 units). Acutely recruitable collateral flow velocity is the lowest (3 to 7 units). Collateral flow velocity integrals were similar among the Rentrop angiographic grades of collateral filling. Three predominant patterns of coronary collateral blood flow velocity (monophasic, biphasic, bidirectional) can

Collateral flow reversal during balloon occlusion

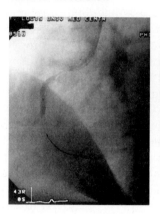 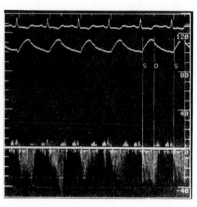

Fig. 10-11. Collateral flow velocity reversal can be observed during balloon occlusion. *Left panel,* PTCA balloon occluding artery with FloWire in distal segment. *Right panel,* inverted flow velocity signal indicates retrograde flow coming toward the tip of the FloWire. These signals disappear after successful PTCA.

be seen. Epicardial (grade 3) collaterals generally had predominantly biphasic collateral flow patterns; intramyocardial (grade 2) collaterals were evenly distributed between monophasic and biphasic flow patterns; and acutely recruitable (grades 0 and 1) collaterals were the only categories with a significant percentage of bidirectional flow patterns.

The majority of collateral flow in the ipsilateral receiving vessel occurs during systole. The measurement of coronary collateral flow velocity provides a unique means to study the effects of pharmacologic or mechanical interventions on human collateral blood flow velocity.

Summary

The goal of coronary interventions in most patients is the relief of ischemic symptoms and myocardial dysfunction through the restoration of coronary blood flow. Translesional flow velocity techniques, which can be used both for the diagnosis of flow limiting coronary stenosis and for the assessment of procedural end points, are superior to angiography (and IVUS) alone. Direct measurement of coronary blood in awake subjects in the catheterization laboratory now permits objective determinations of results on a physiologic basis.

TRANSLESIONAL PRESSURE MEASUREMENTS

Indications

Although translesional pressure measurements are not used routinely, this information has value for lesion assessment before or after angioplasty, especially when questionable angiographic results or coronary flow reserve data are obtained (Fig. 10-12).

Equipment

No guidewire pressure systems are currently available in the United States. The smallest fluid-filled catheter for coronary pressure gradients is a 2.7F Tracker catheter (Target Therapeutics) with a 2.2F tip and an inner lumen of 0.020 mm. The following equipment is required to measure pressures across a stenosis:

1. Two pressure manifolds, transducers, and pressure-tubing Y connector

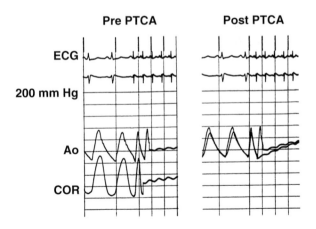

Fig. 10-12. Translesional pressure gradients measured before PTCA of severe lesion (*left*) using a 2.7F pressure catheter shows a gradient of 50 mmHg. After PTCA (*right*), pressure gradient is zero. Ao, Aortic pressure; cor, coronary pressure distal to stenosis.

2. Hemodynamic monitor and recorder
3. Small-diameter (<2.7F, e.g., Tracker, Cook) catheter or pressure guidewire
4. Guide catheter >6F

Technique

Proximal pressure.   The guiding catheter measures aortic pressure proximal to the coronary stenosis.

Distal pressure.   The small pressure catheter (or pressure wire, when available) measures distal artery pressure beyond the lesion.

1. Using angioplasty technique, the pressure catheter is advanced through the guide catheter over a 0.014-in. to 0.018-in. angioplasty guidewire, exactly as for a balloon angioplasty.
2. The pressure catheter is positioned distal to the stenosis.
3. The guidewire is removed and both catheters are flushed.
4. The two pressures are recorded simultaneously.
5. The distal pressure can then be observed at baseline (and during hyperemia, see Fractional Flow Reserve, below). The pressure catheter is then pulled back proximal to the stenosis and then into the guide catheter.
6. A small difference between the two pressures measured proximal to the lesion is called the intrinsic gradient of the system and is subtracted from the transstenotic pressure gradient, the proximal–distal mean pressure. An example of a pressure gradient measurement before and after PTCA is shown in Fig. 10-12.

Clinical Significance of Pressure Gradients

The risk of abrupt closure and restenosis increases with high residual pressure gradients. A persistent postprocedure pressure gradient, especially if the angiographic result is suboptimal, is an indication for further balloon inflations (either prolonged inflations or upsizing of the balloon) or stent. A pressure gradient of <15 mmHg has been considered a successful postangioplasty result. Using a Tracker catheter, a translesional gradient of 15 to 20 mmHg is considered satisfactory for intermediate stenoses in our laboratory. The evaluation of pressure gradients is valuable only if a reliable pressure tracing can be obtained. The reliability of pressure gradients is questioned when one is dealing with small vessels (<2.5 mm diameter), acute artery bends, or multiple lesions in a vessel. Resting pressure gradients do not correlate well to ischemic test results.

Coronary Reserve Derived from Pressure Measurements

As proposed by Pijls et al.,* pressure measurements during hyperemia are another means to determine coronary flow reserve.

Rationale. When blood flows from the proximal to the distal part of the normal epicardial coronary artery, virtually no energy is lost and, therefore, the pressure remains constant throughout the conduit. In the case of epicardial coronary narrowing, potential energy is transformed into kinetic energy and heat when blood traverses the lesion. The resultant pressure drop reflects the total loss of energy. To maintain resting myocardial perfusion at a constant level, a decrease in myocardial resistance compensates for the pressure loss due to the epicardial narrowing. Arteriolar resistance decreases to increase the flow. The decrease in myocardial resistance reserve is proportional to the transstenotic pressure gradient and hence the latter represents an index of the physiologic consequences of a given coronary narrowing on the myocardium.

Because coronary flow occurs predominantly during diastole, the pressure drop across mild to moderate lesions may be present exclusively during diastole. The separate contributions of systolic and diastolic gradients to the mean gradient can be assessed only by a good phasic pressure tracing. In humans without coronary artery disease, Doppler flow velocity has shown that the systolic component of coronary blood flow represents approximately 15% to 40% of total coronary blood flow. The mean transstenotic pressure gradient of the whole cardiac cycle (rather than just the diastolic gradient) should be considered.

Concept of fractional flow reserve. The relationship between pressure gradient and myocardial blood flow during

* Pijls NHJ, van Son AM, Kirkeeide RL, De Bruyne B, Gould KL: Experimental basis of determining maximum coronary, myocardial, and collateral blood flow by pressure measurements for assessing functional stenosis severity before and after percutaneous transluminal coronary angioplasty, *Circulation* 87:1354-1367, 1993.

maximal arteriolar vasodilation represents the fractional flow reserve, which is defined as the ratio of hyperemic flow in the presence of an epicardial coronary stenosis to normal (maximal) hyperemic flow in the same artery without the stenosis. The maximal blood flow in the presence of a stenosis is expressed as a fraction of its normal expected value if there was no lesion. A fractional flow reserve can be derived (see the box) separately for the myocardium, for the epicardial coronary artery, and for the collaterals, based on several assumptions regarding translesional pressure measured during

Calculations of Myocardial, Coronary, and Collateral Fraction Flow Reserve from Pressure Measurements Taken During Maximal Arterial Vasodilation

Myocardial fraction flow reserve (FFRmyo):

$$\text{FFRmyo} = 1 - \frac{\Delta P}{P_a - P_v}$$

$$= \frac{P_c - P_v}{P_a - P_v}$$

$$= \frac{P_c}{P_a}$$

Coronary fractional flow reserve (FFRcor):

$$\text{FFRcor} = 1 - \Delta P(P_a - P_w)$$

Collateral fractional flow reserve (FFRcoll):

$$\text{FFRcoll} = \text{FFRmyo} - \text{FFRcor}$$

Note: All measurements are made during hyperemia except P_w. P_a, Mean aortic pressure; P_c, distal coronary pressure; ΔP, mean translesional pressure gradient; P_v, mean right atrial pressure; P_w, mean coronary wedge pressure or distal coronary pressure during balloon inflation.
From: Pijls NHJ, van Son AM, Kirkeeide RL, De Bruyne B, Gould KL: Experimental basis of determining maximum coronary, myocardial, and collateral blood flow by pressure measurements for assessing functional stenosis severity before and after percutaneous transluminal coronary angioplasty, *Circulation* 87:1354-1367, 1993.

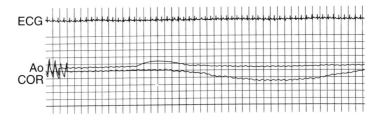

Fig. 10-13. Fractional flow reserve (FFRmyo) can be derived from pressure tracings obtained during maximal hyperemia. This example shows basal and hyperemic pressure responses with distal coronary pressure (cor) falling from 100 to 70 mmHg at peak hyperemia. Aortic pressure (Ao) remains at 110 mmHg. FFRmyo = P_{cor}/P_{ao} = 70/100 = 0.70. Normal is >0.75. P_{cor}, Distal coronary pressure; Pao, aortic pressure during hyperemia. Pressure scale, 20 mmHg/division.

maximal hyperemia. Figure 10-13 illustrates data to derive FFRmyo.

Clinical applications.   A clinical correlation of pressure data and exercise-induced ischemia has been reported.* The values for sensitivity and specificity for the three variables that most accurately predict an abnormal ECG test were 0.66 for FFRmyo, 31 mmHg for maximal hyperemic pressure gradient, and 12 mmHg for resting pressure gradient. These data establish threshold values for pressure gradients with ECG signs of myocardial ischemia and permit clinicians to use these data for decision making. In addition, these data support the concept that stenosis physiology is better reflected by hyperemic than by resting pressure gradient measurements.

PERCUTANEOUS CORONARY ANGIOSCOPY

Percutaneous coronary angioscopy can be used as an adjunct to angiography to visualize intracoronary surfaces during diagnostic angiography and interventional procedures. The nonquantitative video images of endoluminal topography

* From de Bruyne B, Bartunek J, Sys SU, Heyndrickx GR: Relation between myocardial fractional flow reserve calculated from coronary pressure measurements and exercise-induced myocardial ischemia, *Circulation* 92:39-46, 1995.

identify color, distribution, and surface textures but do not provide physiologic information. Percutaneous angioscopy data have been reported during percutaneous coronary angioplasty, thrombolysis, and coronary laser angioplasty.

Indications

Angioscopy is used to differentiate thrombus from arterial dissection. It can also visualize stent struts protruding into the lumen.

Equipment

A coronary angioscope consists of two components, a video imaging chain and a fiber-optic delivery catheter. The arterial image is transmitted through the fiber-optic image bundle to a videotape recorder and a monitor. Angioscopy systems employ a high-resolution color video camera to display the artery imaging on a color monitor. The image is magnified after exposure to an imaging sensor within the video camera.

Currently available percutaneous angioscopes are steerable and can maintain a blood-free field. A soft, atraumatic balloon on the distal tip of the angioscope is inflated when imaging is performed and deflated to allow return of coronary blood flow. Clear saline flush solution is delivered through the distal tip of the angioscope when the occlusion balloon is inflated. Saline displaces a small amount of blood to provide a clear view of the coronary lumen.

A monorail angioscope (Imagecath, Baxter Edwards, Irvine, Calif.) is a catheter within a catheter (Fig. 10-14). The inner catheter contains 3000 image fibers and is guided within the coronary artery over a 0.014-in. angioplasty guidewire. The outer catheter measures 4.5F in diameter and has a separate lumen for inflating and deflating an occlusion balloon located at its distal tip with a 1:1 mix of saline and radiographic contrast. Warm saline is infused through the lumen of the delivery catheter distal to the occlusion balloon to create a blood-free field of view. Both the inner and outer catheters are guided by the same angioplasty guidewire through a monorail design, facilitating rapid exchange. A conventional coronary angioplasty guiding catheter is used to deliver the angioscope to the coronary artery ostium.

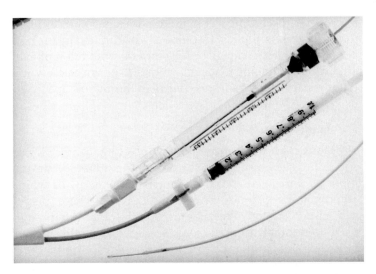

Fig. 10-14.   Percutaneous coronary angioscope by Baxter, Inc. *Bottom,* Imaging bundle inside the infusion catheter with the latex balloon metal marker band. *Middle,* Occluding balloon inflation syringe. *Top,* Calibrated Y connection to advance imaging bundle during saline infusion.

Technique

Before introducing the angioscope, a white reflector is used to color balance the video image.

1. Using standard angioplasty guidewire technique, the angioscope is introduced into the coronary artery with the fiber-optic tip and occluding balloon situated proximal to the target lesion.
2. Warm saline is infused (10 ml/min).
3. Gradual inflation of occluding balloon is performed until the artery is visualized.
4. The fiber-optic bundle can be advanced over the guidewire to record video images.
5. After 60 sec, the balloon is deflated and the vessel perfused with blood.
6. Steps 2 through 5 are repeated for more visualization.

The operator must be able to position the inflated balloon of the angioscope proximal to the lesion in order to image it properly, excluding very proximal lesions and lesions in tortuous vessels. Optical resolution is still limited by the number of pixels in the image bundle and the resolution of available video technology. Visualization of specific areas within the coronary artery requires control of the angioscope tip and use of a wide-angle angioscope lens.

Angioscope Data

Plaque color and lumenal topography (Fig. 10-15).   Uchida and colleagues, using several different angioscope devices, reported narrowed coronary lumens with yellow or whitish atheromatous plaques before angioplasty. These plaques had either smooth surfaces or spiral folds. After angioplasty, endothelial exfoliations, scattered thrombi, bellowslike folds, longitudinal clefts, and plaque rupture that were

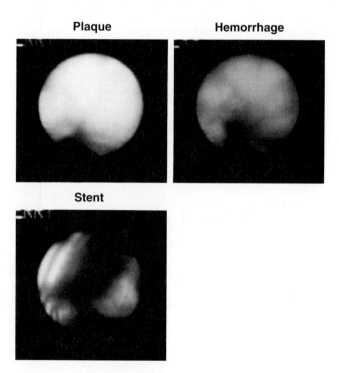

Fig. 10-15.   Angioscopic images.

not visible angiographically were easily appreciated by angioscopy.

By depicting both color and texture, angioscopy can distinguish white or yellow plaque in the vessel lumen from red thrombus. However, "white" thrombus and white tissue elements are difficult to differentiate from plaque structure. The distinguishing feature of white intraluminal masses is shape and texture. Tissue fragments or dissection flaps usually demonstrate angular, sharp edges, whereas white thrombi (platelet aggregates and fibrin strands) are globular, with indistinct margins.

Thrombus.   Angioscopy can differentiate intracoronary thrombus from dissection better than angiography. Angioscopic thrombus is defined as a red solid material within and adherent to the vascular lumen, which persists despite saline flushing. Angiographic thrombi, in contrast, are defined as discrete or mobile filling defects, surrounded by contrast, at the site of the lesion. There is no known association of angioscopic intracoronary thrombi with patient age, sex, or minimal lumen diameter measurements of the reference segment or the lesion, before or after angioplasty. There is an increased frequency of angioscopically detected intracoronary thrombi in the angiographically more complex type B (B1 and B2) and C lesions when compared with type A lesions in patients with unstable angina undergoing coronary angioplasty. Circumferential visualization of the target lesion can be accomplished in >75% of patients using a balloon-tipped, steerable angioscope. Angioscopy can diagnose thrombus in 50% of patients, compared to 10% of patients by angiography before coronary angioplasty. After angioplasty, 95% of patients had thrombus detected by angioscopy, compared to 10% with angiographically defined thrombus. The clinical role of angioscopically defined thrombus and dissection as contributors in abrupt reocclusion and restenosis has not yet been clinically defined.

Safety

The outcome of coronary angioscopy in patients after angioplasty has been satisfactory. The few complications reported with early angioscopy procedures were related to occlusion balloon rupture or leakage, or ischemia related to prolonged coronary occlusion.

SUGGESTED READINGS

Bach RG, Kern MJ, Bell C, Donohue T, Aguirre F: Clinical application of coronary flow velocity for stent placement during coronary angioplasty, *Am Heart J* 125:873-877, 1993.

Braden GA, Herrington DM, Downes TR, et al.: Qualitative and quantitative contrasts in the mechanisms of lumen enlargement by coronary balloon angioplasty and directional coronary atherectomy, *J Am Coll Cardiol* 23:40-48, 1994.

Cacchione JG, Reddy K, Richards F, Sheehan H, Hodgson JM: Combined intravascular ultrasound/angioplasty balloon catheter: initial use during PTCA, *Cathet Cardiovasc Diagn* 24:99-101, 1991.

De Bruyne B, Bartunek J, Sys SU, Heyndrickx GR: Relationship between myocardial fractional flow reserve calculated from coronary pressure measurement and exercise-induced myocardial ischemia, *Circulation* 92:39-46, 1995.

Di Mario C, de Feyter PJ, Slager CJ, de Jaegere P, Roelandt JRTC, Serruys PW: Intracoronary blood flow velocity and transstenotic pressure gradient using sensor-tip pressure and Doppler guidewires, *Cathet Cardiovasc Diagn* 28:311-319, 1993.

Donohue TJ, Kern MJ, Aguirre FV, et al.: Assessing the hemodynamic significance of coronary artery stenoses: analysis of translesional pressure-flow velocity relations in patients, *J Am Coll Cardiol* 22:449-458, 1993.

Doucette JW, Corl PD, Payne HM, et al.: Validation of a Doppler guide wire for intravascular measurement of coronary artery flow velocity, *Circulation* 85:1899-1911, 1992.

Eichhorn EJ, Grayburn PA, Willard JE, et al.: Spontaneous alterations in coronary blood flow velocity before and after coronary angioplasty in patients with severe angina, *J Am Coll Cardiol* 17:43-52, 1991.

Hall P, Colombo A, Almagor Y, et al.: Preliminary experience with intravascular ultrasound guided Palmaz-Schatz coronary stenting: acute and short-term results on a consecutive series of patients, *J Interven Cardiol* 7:141-159, 1994.

Hausman D, Erbel R, Alibelli-Chermarin MJ, et al.: The safety of intracoronary ultrasound: a multicenter survey of 2207 examinations, *Circulation* 91:623-630, 1995.

Hodgson JMcB, Reddy KG, Randeep S, et al.: Intracoronary ultrasound imaging: correlation of plaque morphology with angiography: clinical syndrome and procedural results in patients undergoing coronary angioplasty, *J Am Coll Cardiol* 21:35-44, 1993.

Hodgson JMcB, Sheehan HM, editors: *Atlas of intravascular ultrasound,* New York, 1994, Raven Press.

Isner JM, Rosenfield K, Losordo DW, et al.: Combination balloon-ultrasound imaging catheter for percutaneous transluminal angioplasty: validation of imaging, analysis of recoil, and identification of plaque fracture, *Circulation* 84:739-754, 1991.

Joye JD, Schulman DS, Lasorda D, Farah T, Donohue BC, Reichek N: Intracoronary Doppler guide wire versus stress single-photon emission computed tomographic thallium-201 imaging in assessment of intermediate coronary stenoses, *J Am Coll Cardiol* 24:940-947, 1994.

Kern MJ, Aguirre FV, Bach RG, Caracciolo EA, Donohue TJ: Translesional pressure-flow velocity assessment in patients, *Cathet Cardiovasc Diagn* 31:49-60, 1994.

Kern MJ, Aguirre FV, Bach RG, Caracciolo EA, Donohue TJ, Labovitz AJ: Fundamentals of translesional pressure-flow velocity measurements, *Cathet Cardiovasc Diagn* 31:137-143, 1994.

Kern MJ, Donohue TJ, Aguirre FV, et al.: Clinical outcome of deferring angioplasty in patients with normal translesional pressure and flow velocity measurements, *J Am Coll Cardiol* 25:178-187, 1995.

Kern MJ, Aguirre F, Bach R, Donohue T, Siegel R, Segal J: Augmentation of coronary blood flow by intra-aortic balloon pumping in patients after coronary angioplasty, *Circulation* 87:500-511, 1993.

Kern MJ, Bach RG, Donohue TJ, et al.: Clinical utility of continuous coronary flow velocity monitoring during interventional studies, *Cathet Cardiovasc Diagn* 29:81, 1993.

Kern MJ, Donohue T, Bach R, Aguirre F, Bell C: Monitoring cyclical coronary blood flow alterations following coronary angioplasty for stent restenosis using a Doppler guidewire, *Am Heart J* 125:1159-1160, 1993.

Kern MJ, Donohue TJ, Bach RG, Aguirre FV, Caracciolo EA, Ofili EO: Quantitating coronary collateral flow velocity in patients during coronary angioplasty using a Doppler guidewire, *Am J Cardiol* 71(14):34D-40D, 1993.

Kimura BJ, Fitzgerald PJ, Sudhir K, et al.: Guidance of directional coronary atherectomy by intracoronary ultrasound imaging, *Am Heart J* 124(5):1365-1369, 1992.

Konishi T, Inden M, Nakano T: Clinical experience of percutaneous coronary angioscopy in cases with coronary artery disease, *Angiology* 1:18-23, 1989.

Mallery JA, Tobis JM, Griffith J, et al.: Assessment of normal and atherosclerotic arterial wall thickness with an intravascular ultrasound imaging catheter, *Am Heart J* 119:1392-1400, 1990.

Miller DD, Donohue TJ, Younis LT, et al.: Correlation of pharmacologic 99mTc-sestamibi myocardial perfusion imaging with post-stenotic coronary flow reserve in patients with angiographically intermediate coronary artery stenoses, *Circulation* 89:2150-2160, 1994.

Nakamura S, Colombo A, Gaglione A, et al.: Intracoronary ultrasound observations during stent implantation, *Circulation* 89:2026-2034, 1994.

Nishimura RA, Edwards WD, Warnes CA, et al.: Intravascular ultrasound imaging: in vitro validation and pathologic correlation, *J Am Coll Cardiol* 16:145-154, 1990.

Nissen SE, Gurley JC: Application of intravascular ultrasound for detection and quantitation of coronary atherosclerosis, *Int J Cardiac Imaging* 6(3–4):165-177, 1991.

Ofili E, Kern MJ, Tatineni S, et al.: Detection of coronary collateral flow by a Doppler-tipped guidewire during coronary angioplasty, *Am Heart J* 122:221-225, 1991.

Ofili EO, Kern MJ, Labovitz AJ, et al.: Analysis of coronary blood flow velocity dynamics in angiographically normal and stenosed arteries before and after endoluminal enlargement by angioplasty, *J Am Coll Cardiol* 21:308-316, 1993.

Pinto FJ, St. Goar FG, Gao SZ, et al.: Immediate and one-year safety of intracoronary ultrasonic imaging: evaluation with serial quantitative angiography, *Circulation* 88:1709-1714, 1993.

Potkin BN, Bortorelli AL, Gessert JM, et al.: Coronary artery imaging with intravascular high-frequency ultrasound, *Circulation* 81:1575-1585, 1990.

Reddy KG, Nair RN, Sheehan HM, et al.: Evidence that selective endothelial dysfunction may occur in the absence of angiographic or ultrasound atherosclerosis in patients with risk factors for atherosclerosis, *J Am Coll Cardiol* 23:833-843, 1994.

Segal J, Kern MJ, Scott NA, et al.: Alterations of phasic coronary artery flow velocity in man during percutaneous coronary angioplasty, *J Am Coll Cardiol* 20:276-286, 1992.

St. Goar FG, Pinto FJ, Alderman EL, et al.: Intracoronary ultrasound in cardiac transplant recipients: in vivo evidence of "angiographically silent" intimal thickening, *Circulation* 85:979-987, 1992.

Straur B: The significance of coronary reserve in clinical heart disease, *J Am Coll Cardiol* 15:775-783, 1990.

Tobis JM, Mallery J, Mahon D, et al.: Intravascular ultrasound imaging of human coronary arteries in vivo: analysis of tissue characteristics with comparison to in vitro histological specimens, *Circulation* 83:913-926, 1991.

Uchida Y, Tomaru T, Nakamura F, Furuse A, Fujimore Y, Hasegawa K: Percutaneous coronary angioscopy in patients with ischemic heart disease, *Am Heart J* 114:1216-1222, 1987.

Wilson RF, Wyche K, Christensen BV, Zimmer S, Laxson DD: Effects of adenosine on human coronary arterial circulation, *Circulation* 82:1595-1606, 1990.

Wilson RF, Johnson MJ, Talman CL, et al.: The effect of coronary angioplasty on coronary flow reserve, *Circulation* 76:873-885, 1988.

Yock PG, Fitzgerald PJ, Linker DT, et al.: Intravascular ultrasound guidance for catheter-based coronary interventions, *J Am Coll Cardiol* 17:39B-45B, 1991.

Younis L, Kern MJ, Bach R, et al.: Postprocedural normalization of coronary flow dynamics following successful atherectomy, PTCA and stenting: analysis of intracoronary spectral Doppler (abstr), *J Am Coll Cardiol* 21:79A, 1993.

11

PERIPHERAL AND CEREBRAL VASCULAR CATHETERIZATION AND ANGIOPLASTY TECHNIQUES

Morton J. Kern and Camillo R. Gomez

Cardiologists are often confronted with patients who have peripheral vascular disease that requires assessment and intervention. Despite versatile coronary angioplasty equipment, the performance of peripheral vascular interventions requires not only skill and experience but also judgment in the management of peripheral vascular disease, which may not be familiar to the cardiac interventionalist.

The goal of peripheral vascular angioplasty should be to increase quality of patient life and provide cost-effective treatment for claudication, renal vascular hypertension, and potentially, cerebral ischemia. Cardiologists who perform peripheral vascular interventions should acquaint themselves with the pathophysiology of peripheral atherosclerosis, renal vascular hypertension, and outcome of interventions regarding limb salvage. The management of asymptomatic patients with peripheral arterial disease presents a difficult challenge for the interventionalist. Given the limitations of angiography, objective evidence of significant flow impairment should ac-

393

company treatment, to demonstrate benefit and balance the risk of complications. Symptomatic vascular disease should be assessed in the context of medical and surgical options, appropriateness of angioplasty, or surgery, and in consultation with a vascular surgeon. Indications and contraindications for peripheral vascular angioplasty are shown in the accompanying box.

PERIPHERAL VASCULAR ANGIOPLASTY PROCEDURE
Preprocedure Medications

1. Aspirin, 325 mg PO the night before and the morning of the procedure
2. Alternatively, aspirin (325 mg bid) and dipyridamole (75 mg tid) up to 3 days before the procedure

Antegrade Femoral Artery Access

Antegrade femoral artery access is technically more difficult and has higher complication rates related to hemorrhage and dissection than does retrograde femoral access. Needle entry into the common femoral artery should be caudal to the ingui-

---

Peripheral Vascular Angioplasty

INDICATIONS

1. Intermittent claudication
2. Rest pain in extremity
3. Nonhealing ulcer or gangrene
4. Inflow augmentation before distal surgical bypass
5. Graft anastomotic stenoses
6. Limb salvage

CONTRAINDICATIONS

Absolute

1. Medically unstable patient
2. Hemodynamically insignificant lesion (see below)

Relative

1. Long-segment iliac (>4-cm) or superficial femoral (>10-cm) stenoses or occlusion
2. Lesions in critical limbing-saving collateral vessels

nal ligament, since a higher puncture location may result in intraperitoneal bleeding and difficult postprocedural hemostasis. Potentially life-threatening hemorrhage has been reported for punctures above the inguinal ligament. Assess satisfactory antegrade femoral access with iliofemoral arteriography. This image, which delineates the course of the inferior epigastric artery and the inferior edge of the inguinal ligament, will provide confirmation for device positioning. The arterial puncture must be made proximal to the femoral bifurcation of the profundus and superficial femoral arteries. The appropriate skin entry site will be several centimeters above (cephalad to) the inguinal crease. This location may be difficult to identify in obese individuals.

After placing the femoral sheath, the operator must successfully maneuver the guidewire into the superficial femoral rather than the profunda femoral artery. This task may be difficult in some individuals. Thirty-degree anterior oblique rotation may provide satisfactory visualization of the common femoral bifurcation and better identify the origins of the profunda and superficial femoral arteries.

Alternative vascular access routes include the axillary and popliteal arteries. These routes are rarely required and are associated with higher complication rates of hematoma, peripheral nerve damage, and venous compression. Stroke has been associated with the axillary approach.

Procedural Steps

1. Access vessel via an antegrade or contralateral approach. Give 10,000 IV heparin. Use of sheath techniques facilitates multiple catheter exchanges.
2. Assess stenosis angiographically. Digital subtraction angiography using cine digital cardiac imaging (DCI) techniques is suitable.
3. Measure pressure gradient across stenosis. A 20 mmHg gradient between peak-to-peak systolic pressure (or mean pressure) at rest is significant.
4. Select angioplasty balloon catheter and other equipment based on lesion characteristics.
   a. Use balloon diameter equal to vessel diameter. Table 11-1 lists common dimensions of major peripheral angioplasty balloon diameters.

TABLE 11-1.   Common balloon diameters for peripheral arteries

Artery	Balloon diameter (mm)
Common or external iliac artery	6 to 10
Common or superficial femoral artery	4 to 6
Popliteal artery	3 to 5
Distal artery (below trifurcation)	>4
Renal artery	4 to 8

   b. Use high-pressure polyethylene balloons (diameter 4 to 12 mm for 2-cm to 10-cm lengths).
   c. Use coronary balloon catheters with increased flexibility to traverse bends, distal lesions, or to approach the contralateral side.
   d. Balloon and catheter options:
      (1) Low-profile balloon (Schwarten, ACS)
      (2) Ultrathin (Meditech, uses 0.016-in. to 0.018-in. guidewires)
      (3) Tracker catheter 18 or 25 (helpful to identify lesion location in distal segments and infuse thrombolytic agents)
      (4) Balloon-on-a-wire
5. Lesion dilatation
   a. Cross lesion with guidewire through the guide catheter. The guidewire should be floppy and have a straight tip (e.g., Wholey wire) in order to prevent vessel wall perforation. Use movable core J-tip, high-torque floppy guidewires or coronary guidewires as alternatives. Guidewires are different from those used in the coronary circulation. Operators should be familiar with the several types of guidewires listed in the accompanying box.
   b. Exchange the guide catheter for an angioplasty balloon catheter or advance the balloon catheter through the guide catheter. Metallic markers on the balloon catheter should straddle the lesion.
   c. Inflate balloon (4 to 10 atm for high-pressure balloon) for 30 to 45 sec.
   d. Deflate balloon catheter.
   e. Remove balloon catheter, leaving guidewire across the stenosis to assess the vessel after it has been dilated.

Guidewires for Peripheral Vascular Angioplasty

1. Fixed-core guidewires (Benson wire)
2. Teflon-coated guidewires (LT and LLT)
3. Amplatz super-stiff guidewires (Meditech)
4. Ross and exchange wires (Cook)
5. Movable-core wires
6. Torque-control wire (Wholey wire, ACS)
7. Magic wire (Meditech)
8. Cad wire (ACS)
9. Tapered torque wire (Meditech)
10. Glide wires (hydrophilic-coated wires, Terumo, Meditech)
11. SOS wire (injectable infusion, hollow-core guidewire)

f. Repeat angiogram to check result. Post-angioplasty result is often seen as a hazy area or dissection.
g. Remeasure pressure gradient.
h. If angiographic result and post-angioplasty pressure gradient are acceptable, the procedure is completed. Otherwise, the original or a larger balloon is reintroduced across the stenotic segment over the guidewire. Angioplasty is repeated until satisfactory results are obtained.

Special Considerations

Bifurcation lesions.   Angioplasty at the aorto-iliac bifurcation may require simultaneous two-balloon inflation ("kissing balloon") technique (see Chapter 5).

Vessel perforation.   If a guidewire or other angioplasty equipment produces a perforation, stop the procedure. Reverse the heparin with protamine. Some clinicians recommend a 10-day to 2-week recuperation period before attempting another angioplasty.

Vasospasm.   For prophylactic treatment of vasospasm, give intraarterial nitroglycerin (100 to 200 μg). This method is especially important if there is decreased blood flow or small vessels.

If vasospasm occurs, give intraarterial nitroglycerin (100 to 200 μg) or intraarterial lidocaine (50 mg).

Complications

Serious complications	3.0%
Death	0.4%
Acute thrombus occluding arterial lumen	2.0%
Puncture-site hematoma	5.0%
Requiring surgical intervention	1.0%
Distal embolization	0.6% to 4.6%
Clinically significant emboli	0% to 2.3%
Subintimal passage of guidewire	0.3% to 2.0%
Vessel perforation	1.0%
Vasospasm	2.0%
Pseudoaneurysm	0.3%

Management of Complications

Percutaneous balloon angioplasty has complications common to other interventional procedures. Although complications such as contrast-induced acute renal failure, arterial perforation, tear, rupture, flow-limiting dissection, particulate embolization, or acute thrombosis may not always produce clinical sequelae, these events require physician recognition and understanding leading to necessary action or intervention.

Major complications at the angioplasty site or distal vessel bed include vessel occlusion, embolization (cholesterol, particulate, air, or thrombus), perforation or rupture, retroperitoneal bleeding, femoral pseudoaneurysm, AV fistula formation, acute renal failure, cardiorespiratory arrest, sepsis, acute myocardial infarction, stroke, severe hypertension or hypotension, guidewire or balloon catheter breakage, compartmental syndrome of lower limb, emergency surgery, and limb loss.

Minor complications include guidewire vessel perforation, device breakage requiring extrication without problems, brachial or groin hematoma, and lower-limb swelling.

An approach to the treatment of complications involves one or more of the following options: (1) no treatment; (2) postponement of other treatment; (3) nonoperative treatments (e.g., blood transfusions, diuretics, or aspiration of embolism); (4) operative treatment, either an anticipated or salvage procedure.

Emergency surgery usually involves arterial repair, thrombectomy, embolectomy, hematoma evacuation, fasciotomy, or bypass, whereas complementary surgical procedures might be planned as adjunctive to a successful interventional procedure.

Medications for postprocedure management

1. Continue aspirin, 325 mg, or persantine, 75 mg tid × 24 to 48 hr, or both. Long-term therapy is of unproven benefit.
2. IV heparin may be given for 24 to 48 hr if low blood flow occurs distal to the angioplasty site.

Doppler studies and ankle or brachial indices to document improvement (see Tables 11-2 and 11-3). Noninvasive evaluation by duplex ultrasound provides direct real-time imaging of lesions with simultaneous Doppler measurements to determine the hemodynamic significance of the femoral, popliteal, posterior tibial, and anterior tibial (dorsalis pedis) arteries and assists in further localizing the lesions. Criteria for severity of a peripheral artery stenosis are based on the pressure index and Doppler spectrum data (Tables 11-2 and 11-3). These noninvasive data will determine the suitability of angioplasty for a given stenosis.

Clinical Results (Table 11-4)

Expected outcomes after peripheral vascular angioplasty in general have

1. Initial success rates reportedly >90%
2. Lower patency rates in vessels with poor distal runoff

TABLE 11-2. Correlation of ankle-brachial index (ABI) with clinical presentation and severity of obstructive lesions

ABI	Symptoms	Disease severity
0.90-1.30	Asymptomatic	No hemodynamically significant lesions
0.60-0.90	Claudication	Single segment stenosis or occlusion
0.30-0.60	Claudication	Multiple segment disease
0.15-0.30	Resting pain	Multiple segment total occlusions
<0.15	Impending tissue loss	Multiple segment total occlusions
>1.30	Indeterminate	Medial wall calcification; nondiagnostic

From Freed M, Grines C, Safian R, editors: *The new manual of interventional cardiology,* Birmingham, Michigan, 1996, Physician's Press.

TABLE 11-3.   Doppler velocity spectrum diagnostic criteria for grading severity of stenosis

Diameter stenosis	Spectrum characteristics
Normal-<20%	No increase in Vp relative to proximal arterial segment; minimal spectral broadening
20-49%	>30% increase in Vp relative to proximal arterial segment; Vp < 125 cm/sec; spectral broadening throughout pulse cycle
50-75%	>100% increase in Vp relative to proximal arterial segment; Vp > 125 cm/sec; spectral broadening throughout pulse cycle
>75%	Spectrum similar to 50-75% stenosis, but with diastolic velocity >100 cm/sec

Vp, Peak systolic velocity.
From Freed M, Grines C, Safian R, editors: *The new manual of interventional cardiology*, Birmingham, Michigan, 1996, Physician's Press.

3. Lower patency rates for long (>30 to 40 cm) stenoses or occlusions
4. Success rates for limb salvage similar to claudication, but long-term patency rates 5% to 10% lower
5. Lower success and long-term patency rates in diabetic patients
   In comparison to surgical revascularization:

   Overall incidence of complications:
   Aorto-femoral bypass graft   11%
   Femoropopliteal bypass graft   7%
   Serious complications   1% to 4%
   Surgical mortality of aorto-iliac and   2% to 6%
      femoral bypass procedures

RENAL ARTERY BALLOON ANGIOPLASTY

Renal artery angioplasty is the treatment of choice for patients with renal vascular hypertension. Younger hypertensive populations tend to have a low incidence (0.5%) of significant renal artery stenosis compared to older populations with more extensive multisystem vascular disease and a much higher incidence of renal artery stenosis. Some investigators have found renal artery stenosis in up to 30% of patients with abdominal or peripheral vascular disease. Vetrovec et al. observed a 16% to 18% incidence of significant renal artery stenosis in patients with hypertension undergoing diagnostic

TABLE 11-4. Results of lower extremity PTA for claudication

| Patency rate (%) | | | | | |
Site	Initial success (%)	1 year	3 years	5 years	7 years
Aorta	94	80	70	—	—
Common iliac artery					
Stenosis	95-98	80-98	70-95	60-90	90
Occlusion	90	72	56	48	—
External iliac and femoropopliteal					
Stenosis	90	75-89	62-80	53	—
Occlusion	87	63	46-75	36	—
Common femoral artery	78	58	37	—	—
Profunda femoris artery	46	23	—	—	—
Femoropopliteal					
Stenosis	81-92	81	61-77	70	60
Occlusion	92	82	68	—	—
Popliteal and calf vessels	81-89	89	—	—	—
Bypass grafts	78	78	52	—	—

From Kandarpa K: *Handbook of cardiovascular and interventional radiologic procedures.* Little, Brown and Company, Boston, 1989, p 48.

cardiac catheterization, whereas the incidence of renal artery stenosis was even greater (40%) in patients with renal insufficiency. Hypertensive patients who develop renal failure during captopril therapy should be considered for workup of renal artery stenosis. Renal artery stenosis producing hypertension in a young female patient is a likely treatable cause. Renal artery stenosis should be considered in renal transplant patients who develop progressive hypertension.

The indications and contraindications to renal artery angioplasty are shown in the accompanying box.

Renal Artery Angioplasty

INDICATIONS
1. Renovascular hypertension caused by atherosclerotic or
   fibromuscular narrowing of renal artery after:
   a. Failed medical therapy
   b. Increased renal vein renin on side of arterial disease
2. Renal transplant artery stenosis
3. Renal artery or vein bypass graft stenosis
4. Renal insufficiency with >50% artery stenosis

CONTRAINDICATIONS
1. Unstable medical condition
2. Borderline lesion (<50% stenosis or no pressure gradient, or
   without elevated lateralized renin level)
3. Long stenosis segment (>2 cm) or total occlusion
4. Aortic plaque extending into renal artery

Screening for Renal Vascular Hypertension

1. Urography and radionuclide renal flow scans have been
   used but are generally unreliable, especially in cases of
   bilateral disease.
2. Selective vein renin may likewise be of little value in
   identifying patients who are suitable for renal vascular angioplasty.
3. Intravenous renal digital subtraction arteriography can
   be performed on an outpatient basis.
4. Intraarterial digital angiography at the time of diagnostic coronary angiography is a simple, easy, and low-risk
   screening procedure.
5. Digital subtraction aortography also can identify renal
   artery abnormalities before selective injection, if required.

Renal Angiography

Screening abdominal aortography during cardiac catheterization is safe and requires minimal time and radiographic contrast. A pigtail catheter placed at the level of L1 will visualize
most renal artery origins. Slightly lower positioning reduces
filling of abdominal visceral vessels, which often overlap visu-

alization of the renal arteries. An anterior-posterior (AP), or preferably a 20° left anterior oblique (LAO), 15° caudal, projection best identifies the renal ostia. A contrast injection of 20 to 30 cc/sec is sufficient to opacify the renal arteries. If one or both arteries are not well visualized, selective angiography can be performed using a right Judkins or internal mammary artery coronary catheter. Do not "scrape" the aorta during entry of the renal artery, to avoid precipitating the atheroembolic syndrome. Studies have demonstrated minimal risk of complications because, even in the setting of renal insufficiency, the additional injection of 20 cc/sec of dye does not appear to increase renal failure significantly.

Functional Testing

After identification of renal artery stenosis, a technetium-99 renal blood flow scan may aid in assessing relative renal blood flow to each kidney. This test will identify a small atretic kidney with a totally occluded vessel, which may be suitable for nephrectomy as an alternative to angioplasty. Decisions regarding intervention with angioplasty or surgery for renal artery stenosis are based on the functional significance of the stenosis and the potential to improve the clinical syndrome (see box on p. 402). Radioisotope renal flow scans provide a method of assessing functional effects of renal artery stenosis. These, however, are somewhat time consuming and delay decision making regarding therapy. Recently, some investigators have utilized the vascular Doppler guidewire to assess the physiologic significance of a lesion (Table 11-3). When passing the Doppler guidewire through the area of stenosis, high-velocity signals can be seen because of increased stenosis flow. Following successful dilatation, the high-velocity signals are abolished. This technique has the potential to provide a rapid, in-laboratory method of estimating the functional significance of an observed stenosis. Further evaluation may be necessary.

Angioplasty Technique

Approach to renal artery

1. Femoral arterial access; sheath and guiding catheter inserted. Initial angiograms are performed.

2. Brachial or axillary arterial approach for down-pointing renal artery origin. In some cases, the inferior approach to the renal artery may not be possible due to the acute angle with the aorta. In these cases, left axillary or brachial access and approach are selected using headhunter-style catheters for renal artery engagement. This approach should be utilized only by operators who are fully experienced in peripheral angiography with these difficult catheters (Fig. 11-1).
3. Heparin, 5000 to 10,000 units IV, and 100 to 200 μg intraarterial nitroglycerin.

Guiding catheter selection. The renal artery is cannulated with a selective guide catheter for angioplasty backup support. Common guide catheters include Simmons, Shepherd's crook, Cobra, and Levin catheters (Fig. 11-2).

Guiding angiography. Conventional arteriography is performed. Hand injection of 7 to 10 ml of contrast is usually sufficient, especially for digital imaging techniques (Fig. 11-3).

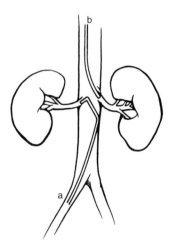

Fig. 11-1. Caudal angulation of the proximal arteries demonstrates an advantage of the brachial approach using a brachial guiding catheter denoted by the letter b. A femoral guiding catheter (a) may be used for a downward angulation in some cases. The femoral approach is the more common approach. (From Topol EJ, editor: *Textbook of interventional cardiology,* Philadelphia, 1994, W. B. Saunders, p 562.)

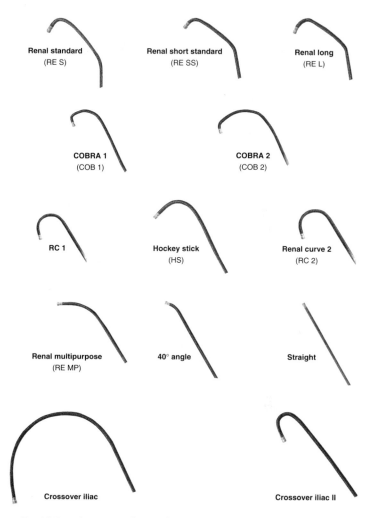

Fig. 11-2. Angiographic catheters used in peripheral vascular interventions. (From Schneider Co., Europe.)

Balloon catheter selection. A balloon catheter of the short-est acceptable length is selected based on vessel diameter imme-diately proximal to the stenosis. A magnification factor of 20% based on the arteriogram can be expected to result in a larger balloon selection with slight overdilatation of the renal artery. Overdilatation should be limited to avoid complications of dis-section, occlusion, or rupture of the renal artery.

Guidewire and balloon catheter techniques. A guide-wire is inserted across the stenosis and the balloon is ad-vanced over the guidewire. Before crossing the stenosis, nitro-glycerin is administered intraarterially. The balloon is positioned across the stenosis and appropriate inflation is performed for 30 to 60 sec at 4 to 6 atm, until the waist of the balloon is eliminated. The guidewire is left across the

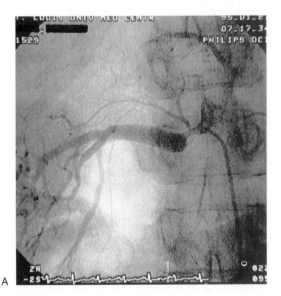

A

Fig. 11-3. **A,** Typical angiogram of a renal artery stenosis in the downward position approached with femoral technique. **B,** Intravascular Doppler guidewire flow velocity measure-ments in angiographic normal renal arteries. Doppler flow spectrum similar to external Doppler measurements but lo-cated precisely within the region of highest interest to avoid false-positive results. (From J.G. Mudd Catheterization Labo-ratory, St. Louis University, St. Louis, Missouri.)

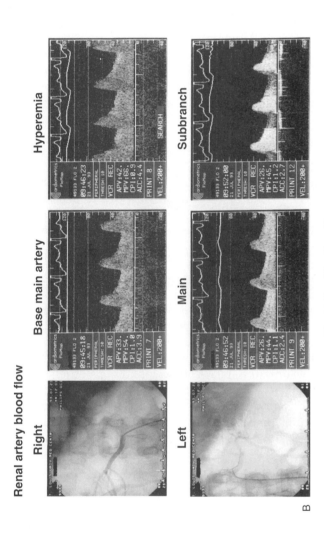

Fig. 11-3. (Continued).

lesion. The balloon is removed and repeat arteriography is performed.

Pressure gradient measurements.   Pressure gradients or velocity data (Fig. 11-3B) can be measured as described for peripheral vascular angioplasty.

Special considerations.   Distal lesions of smaller segmental branches, possibly involving branch points, may require dilation. Many of the smaller segments are prone to vasospasm requiring intraarterial nitroglycerin. Small angioplasty-size balloons can be used to approach these vessels of 2 to 5 mm in diameter. Bifurcating renal artery branches should be managed in a fashion similar to coronary branch points (see Chapter 8, Difficult Angioplasty).

Postprocedural management.   Blood pressure should be monitored for the first 24 hr because of the possibility of transient hypertension after intervention. Nitroprusside infusion may be required to control blood pressure. Patients are treated with aspirin (325 mg daily) and dipyridamole (75 mg tid) for up to 2 months after the procedure.

Expected results.   Criteria for successful dilation are similar to those for coronary angioplasty with <30% residual stenosis. Initial success rates for renal artery angioplasty range from 80% to 97% with long-term favorable results in 75% to 90% of patients. A mortality rate of <1% is commonly associated with this procedure. Emergency vascular bypass or nephrectomy precipitated by complications of renal angioplasty range from 0.9% to 2.5% of patients.

The outcome for dilatation for hypertension is somewhat unpredictable in older patients, who often have chronic hypertension. However, some reduction in blood pressure occurs in most patients, particularly in those with recent exacerbation of their hypertension. Most patients with renal insufficiency show some improvement in clinical factors of renal failure, congestive heart failure, and high blood pressure.

Late complications.   Back pain or flank pain persisting after angioplasty may indicate segmental renal embolization of infarction. Infarctions appear as peripheral wedge-shaped defects on postangioplasty nephrogram during the venous phase. Severe flank pain may indicate renal artery rupture appearing as localized contrast extravasation on the postangioplasty arteriogram. This complication generally can be managed conservatively by prolonged inflation such as is employed for coronary dissections using reperfusion balloons.

Renal artery stent placement. Renal artery stenting is an effective treatment for renovascular hypertension. The initial angiographic restenosis rates are encouraging when compared to balloon angioplasty. Stent placement appears to be an attractive alternative to surgical revascularization in some patients. Balloon angioplasty of renal artery ostial lesions has a poor long-term outcome because these lesions are composed primarily of plaque in the wall of the aorta, which does not respond well to balloon dilation. For this reason, renal artery stents are preferred for ostial lesions, restenosis lesions, and those following a suboptimal angiographic result.

White et al.* report angiographic success by quantitative angiography of 95/97 (98%) lesions. Complications of stent placement included subacute thrombosis (1%), emergency surgery (0), death (0), contrast nephropathy (1%), and access-site complications (5%). Angiographic follow-up in a mean of 7.6 months revealed restenosis (>50% diameter narrowing) in 26% stented vessels.

INTRAVASCULAR ULTRASOUND GUIDANCE FOR PERIPHERAL VASCULAR INTERVENTIONS

Intravascular ultrasound (IVUS) imaging catheters provide adjunctive information regarding the distribution and composition of atherosclerotic disease encountered in peripheral vascular interventions. A detailed description of the technique for use in the coronary circulation applies here and can be found in Chapter 10. Although clinical outcome has not been dramatically improved by assessing these lesions by intravascular ultrasound (IVUS), complex procedures may require more precise lesion assessment for selection of stents, rotablation, atherectomy, and balloon angioplasty for interventions.

Intravascular ultrasound provides useful information with regard to specific vascular characteristics, such as:
1. Lumen diameter of cross-sectional area
2. Wall thickness

* From White CJ, Ramee SR, Collins TJ, et al: Guiding catheter assisted renal artery angioplasty, *Cathet Cardiovasc Diagn* 23:10, 1991.

3. Lesion length, shape, and volume
4. Eccentric versus concentric plaque placement
5. Lesion type—calcific versus fibrous
   In the postinterventional period, intravascular ultrasound can identify the extent of dissection, intimal flaps, the presence of ulceration, and the presence and volume of intravascular thrombus.
   Intravascular ultrasound may assist at several clinical decision points.
1. Selection of appropriate balloon size and lesion composition
2. Selection of device or stent sizing based on normal artery reference diameter
3. Establishing the presence of thrombus and whether to continue or initiate anticoagulation or intravascular thrombolytic therapy
4. Identification of dissection to establish the need for stenting
5. Determination of severity of residual stenosis for selection of larger balloon, high-pressure balloon, or stent placement
6. Guidance in decision making for atherectomy or rotablation (Fig. 11-4). If the postprocedure lumen has residual plaque, further directional atherectomy or a larger burr diameter rotablator may be employed. However, the crite-

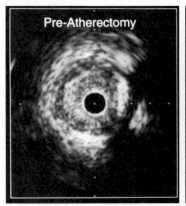 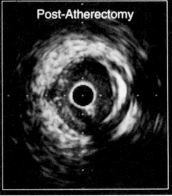

Fig. 11-4.   Intravascular ultrasound imaging before and after directional atherectomy. (From J.G. Mudd Catheterization Laboratory, St. Louis University, St. Louis, Missouri.)

ria for IVUS-determined end points are not specified and at this time are subjective without physiologic correlations. For stent deployment, gauging the precise arterial diameter proximal and distal to a stenosis to attain a 0.7 ratio of distal arterial diameter for stent placement and identification of appropriate stent expansion is associated with reduced abrupt closure rates.

CEREBRAL CATHETERIZATION AND INTERVENTIONAL TECHNIQUES

Cerebral angiography was introduced in 1927 by Egas Moniz, a Portuguese neurologist, as a technique for neurologic diagnosis. Since then, the role of cerebral catheterization and angiography has changed significantly with the development of less invasive techniques, particularly neurovascular ultrasonography, computed tomography, and magnetic resonance imaging. Nevertheless, there are still situations in which the data provided by angiography cannot be replaced by any other diagnostic method. Because of its invasive nature and inherent risk (even though small), cerebral catheterization must always be weighed against its potential complications. Although it is most commonly performed by radiologists, neurologists, and cardiologists have recently become involved in the performance of cerebral catheterizations. This section is intended as a practical resource for individuals with previous experience in basic vascular catheterization techniques.

Indications

Although the technique of performing cerebral catheterization and angiography is relatively simple and can be mastered by most experienced angiographers, the decisions related to when the procedure is indicated, when the indications outweigh the potential complications, what type of clinically relevant information is being sought, what vessels need to be studied in any one patient, and what impact the acquired information will have on the care of the patient are complex. In general, the cognitive aspects of cerebral angiography (including decisions that invariably need to be made during the performance of the procedure) require a deeper understanding of cerebrovascular disorders, their pathogenesis, clinical evolution, natural history, outcome, and treatment options, as well as the management of complications that can result from the procedure.

Diagnostic cerebral angiography is of significant utility in almost any cerebrovascular disorder, as well as in the management of certain neoplastic conditions. The box below lists applications of cerebral catheterization and angiography.

Contraindications

The contraindications for cerebral catheterization are relative, and similar to those for other types of angiography. They include renal dysfunction, fever and infections, acute gastrointestinal bleeding (particularly if heparinization will be carried out), allergy to iodine (including contrast agents and fish), and bleeding diathesis. In addition, other conditions that may increase the risk associated with the procedure include a history of migraine (currently controversial) and a recent cerebral infarction.

Complications

As with any other invasive technique, experience and meticulous attention to detail are factors that will minimize the risks of the procedure. Unfortunately, complications may occur even in the best of cases. The angiographer must be prepared to correct them whenever possible. The complications of cerebral catheterization are related to the length of the procedure, the experience of the angiographer, the amount of contrast

---

Applications of Cerebral Catheterization and Angiography

Assessment of vascular etiologic factors, surgical candidacy, and
vascular supply in:
  Ischemic stroke (cerebral infarction)
  Transient ischemic attack
  Subarachnoid hemorrhage
  Arteriovenous malformations
  Documenting saccular aneurysms
  Documenting and treating vasospasm
  Tumors
Planning therapy for all proposed interventions

agent utilized, and the severity of the cerebrovascular disorder being investigated.

The complications of cerebral catheterization may be divided into neurologic and nonneurologic complications.

Neurologic complications.   The incidence of neurologic complications from diagnostic cerebral catheterization averages <1%, and includes cerebral infarction, transient ischemic attack, and arterial laceration. The reasons for the development of neurologic complications are not completely defined, but are likely related to clots forming in the catheter or guidewire, to dislodgment by the catheter or guidewire of atheromatous material from plaques, or to vasospasm induced by the direct contact of the catheter with the vascular wall or by the injection of contrast.

Nonneurologic complications.   The nonneurologic complications are similar to those in other types of angiography, and include hematomas and pseudoaneurysms, infections, azotemia (renal and prerenal), and contrast allergic reactions. In addition, there is a small risk of fatal complications during cerebral angiography (approximately 1 in 20,000).

Technique

Patient preparation.   Cerebral catheterization and angiography begins when the angiographer first discusses the procedure with the patient, examines him or her, and reviews the medical history, medication record, and results of ancillary studies. The angiographer must establish rapport with the patient before the catheterization. The development of such a relationship with the patient, as well as with the family, facilitates full disclosure of the technical aspects of the test, existing and potential risks, and the possible complications. The discussion must include clear statements about benefit:risk ratio and the importance of the procedure in the overall care of the patient. Important questions should be answered: What is the purpose of the procedure? What are the potential problems and risks? How can these be minimized? What is the minimal study that will answer the clinically relevant questions being asked? How should the preprocedure care be orchestrated?

The preprocedure assessment of the patient includes an estimation of neurologic status, fluid and electrolyte status, renal function, peripheral vascular disease (particularly involving the lower-extremity arteries), and cardiopulmonary function. Preprocedure orders should include specific instructions about fluid administration and handling of medications. Patients are maintained without any oral intake through the night prior to the procedure, or for as long as possible when the procedure is being planned for later in the same day. Concurrently during the period of lack of oral intake, isotonic crystalloid solutions (0.9% NaCl or lactated Ringer) are administered intravenously at rates of 100 to 125 cc/hr. Essential medications that cannot be administered parenterally may be given orally with small amounts of water. IV heparin should be stopped when the patient is called to the catheterization laboratory, if not contraindicated.

In-laboratory preparation.   Once in the catheterization suite, intravenous premedication with 25 mg of diphenhydramine HCl (Benadryl) and 3 mg of Diazepam (Valium) is given. These medications may alter the baseline neurologic examination. It is possible to reverse the sedative effects of Diazepam with 0.2 to 0.5 mg of flumazenil (Romazicon) given intravenously. This medication is capable of inducing seizures in patients with abnormal neurologic function (particularly if related to cerebral ischemia). For this reason, it has been our practice to use other sedating agents in cases where a lengthy procedure is anticipated. Opiates are preferred because, in addition to sedation, they alleviate some of the discomfort that makes patients restless. Morphine sulfate is the most widely used of these agents, usually in incremental doses of 2 mg, up to 6 to 8 mg in any 1-hr period. Fentanyl (Sublimaze) is now preferred because it has a more rapid onset of action than morphine, and does not produce histamine release with its consequent vasoactive effects. The drug should be administered intravenously at doses of 25 to 50 mg, following the same precautions as are required for morphine administration. Their effects can be readily reversed with 0.4 to 1 mg of intravenous naloxone (Narcan).

Management during the procedure

Optimal blood pressure.   Specific clinical situations, the most common of which is elevated blood pressure, must be properly addressed. It is important for angiographers who are not familiar with the care of cerebrovascular patients to realize that the response of the cerebral circulation to elevations of systemic blood pressure is quite different from that of the heart. During the catheterization of patients suffering acute brain ischemia (either in relation to acute cerebral infarction or in the context of vasospasm), blood pressure levels higher than those commonly seen in a cardiac catheterization laboratory are required to perfuse the ischemic brain tissue. It is not unusual for these patients to require a state of hypervolemia (i.e., large-volume infusions of crystalloid or colloid solutions) and hypertension (i.e., vasopressor agents). The optimal blood pressure for patients suffering brain ischemia is unknown, and it is likely to be different according to the vessel occluded, the degree of collateral circulation, the temporal profile of the ischemic process, and the status of the cerebral autoregulation.

In general, however, the patient who is asymptomatic at the time of the elective procedure may have his or her blood pressure reduced to levels which are compatible with the general guidelines noted elsewhere in this book. In patients with acute brain ischemia, or those who are at risk for developing cerebral ischemia (e.g., vasospasm), the mean arterial blood pressure should not be below 115 to 120 torr. In case the mean arterial blood pressure requires reduction (e.g., concomitant congestive heart failure), it is important to choose the medication to be used carefully. Ideally, a short-acting, easily titrated, intravenous agent should be the first choice. Various antihypertensive agents may produce adverse effects in patients with neurologic disorders, the most common being the induction of cerebral vasodilation with its consequent steal of flow from ischemic areas or increased intracranial pressure due to increased cerebral blood volume. For this reason, the most widely used intravenous antihypertensive drugs, namely, nitroprusside (Nipride), nitroglycerin (Nitrol), and nicardipine (Cardene), are not as popular as other agents, such as labetalol (Normodyne), enalaprilat (Vasotec IV), or trimethaphan (Arfonad). Sublingual nifedipine (Procardia) should never be used in patients with unstable brain ischemia.

Intravascular volume status. Another difference between the care of patients with cardiac dysfunction and those with unstable cerebral ischemia is their fluid management. As noted earlier, the cerebral circulation (particularly the collateral microcirculation) performs more efficiently under conditions of euvolemia and hypervolemia. The state of hydration instituted before the procedure must be maintained throughout its performance. In view of the potent diuretic effect of some of the contrast agents, the level of hydration required in patients with brain ischemia is critical, and may be difficult to stabilize safely in patients with preload-sensitive cardiac dysfunction.

Managing cerebral ischemia. A special problem is presented by the stable patient who develops signs of acute brain ischemia sometime during an elective catheterization. Rapid assessment of the patient should identify the vascular territory that has been rendered ischemic. In order to document the occlusive site, immediate angiographic imaging should be performed, allowing a determination of the most appropriate therapeutic course to follow.

Postprocedure care. Once the procedure is concluded, postcatheterization orders should be written. In addition to basic orders related to the care of the puncture site, specific instructions about fluid administration, periodic neurologic assessments, and monitoring of renal function during the following 12 hr should be included. For patients who required anticoagulation before the procedure, the orders should also specify when and how to resume intravenous heparin. The angiographer should speak with family members about the results of the procedure as soon as possible.

Equipment and Instrumentation

The majority of the equipment available in most modern cardiac catheterization laboratories is suitable for the performance of cerebral catheterization and angiography. The cineangiography should include digital subtraction capabilities, particularly for the acquisition of intracranial images. The choice of contrast agent for cerebral angiography is a matter of personal preference. In general, nonionic, low-osmolar contrast media are the most widely used. A description of the most commonly utilized contrast agents can be found elsewhere in this book.

The great majority of cerebral angiograms can also be performed using catheters already available for coronary angiography. Aortic arch injections are routinely undertaken using pigtail catheters (preferably made out of Teflon) with multiple side holes, most commonly of 5 or 6 French sizes (Fig. 11-5). Selective catheterization of the innominate, left common carotid, and left subclavian arteries is easily accomplished using a right Judkins-style coronary catheter, most commonly a 6F JR4. This catheter can also be used to engage the ostia of the vertebral arteries. If a more straight tip is desired, an alternative is to use a right coronary vein bypass graft catheter (type I). However, angiographers who will be performing cerebral catheterizations should also be familiar with the various catheters designed specifically for this type of procedure (Fig. 11-6). The most widely used are the Hincks-style catheters (so-called "headhunters") and, of these, the No. 1 (H1H) is the easiest to manipulate and use for selective injections. The Hincks-style No. 3 has a shape similar to the left Amplatz-style coronary catheters, and can be used to negotiate tortuous and elongated great vessels. The Bentson-style No. 1 catheter

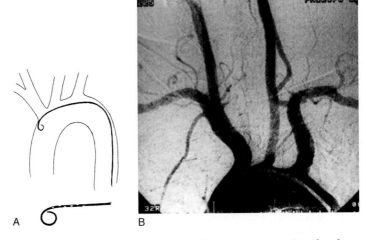

Fig. 11-5.   Technique for aortic arch imaging. **A,** A pigtail catheter is positioned in the root of the aortic arch. (From Johnsrude IS, Jackson DC, Dunnick MR: *A practical approach to angiography,* ed 2, Boston, 1987, Little, Brown.) **B,** Imaging is acquired in the LAO plane, with the patient's head rotated slightly to the right. (Angiogram from Cardiac Catheterization Laboratory, St. Louis University, St. Louis, Missouri.)

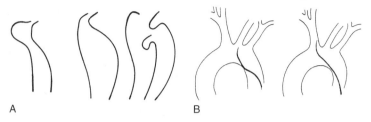

Fig. 11-6. **A,** Most common catheters used for cerebral angiography, from left to right: Hincks No. 3 and No. 1; Bentson No. 1 and No. 3; and Newton No. 1, No. 2, and No. 5. **B,** Technique for selective catheterization of the large vessels using the Hincks No. 1 catheter. (From Johnsrude IS, Jackson DC, Dunnick NR: *A practical approach to angiography,* ed 2, Boston, 1987, Little, Brown.)

is also selected because of its straighter configuration, which facilitates injections when the internal carotid arteries are selectively catheterized. In addition, there is a vertebral-style catheter, with a softer primary curve, well suited for vertebral artery studies. Finally, Newton-style catheters (particularly No. 2 and No. 5) are also useful in the catheterization of cerebral blood vessels.

For interventional procedures, the guide catheters utilized must show a balance between the flexibility necessary to negotiate the curves and bends commonly found in the proximal cerebral vasculature and the torqueability required for manipulation of the catheter. These two characteristics are somewhat mutually exclusive, and different catheters may be needed under different circumstances. The two most important guide catheters available for the performance of interventional cerebral procedures are the Target 38 catheter (Target Therapeutics, Fremont, Calif.) and the Royal Flush catheters (Cook, Inc., Bloomington, Ind.). The former has the advantage of being manufactured by the same company that provides the most popular microcatheters available, the Tracker 18 and Tracker 10, and has a wide range of products to fit this system of catheters.

Supraselective catheterization of the intracranial arteries can be performed using microcatheters that can be either flow-directed or steerable, each of them with its own advantages and disadvantages (Fig. 11-7). The flow-directed micro-

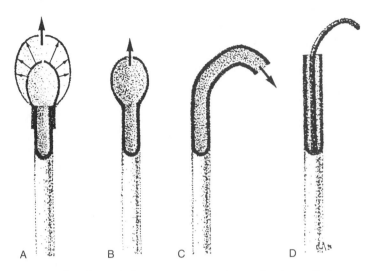

Fig. 11-7.   Tips of the most commonly used microcatheters, both flow-guided and steerable. **A** and **B** have calibrated-leak balloons that make them flow-sensitive. **C** and **D** require the use of a micro guidewire. (From Rufenacht DA, Latchaw RE: Principles and methodology of intracranial endovascular access, *Neuroimaging Clinics,* 2(2):251-268, 1992.)

catheters (e.g., Magic, Balt/Target Therapeutics, Fremont, Calif.) are usually manufactured so that the proximal shaft is stiffer than the very soft silastic distal segment. This progressive suppleness allows more distal, faster, and more comfortable placement of the catheter. The risk of vessel perforation using this type of microcatheter is virtually none, but, on the other hand, their lumen size is limited (tips vary between 1.5 and 3.3 French). They are maneuvered using saline or contrast agent flushes, in order to propel the microcatheter forward, and the use of guidewires is discouraged. Alternatively, steerable microcatheters with sizes that vary between 2.5 and 2.7 French at the tip are placed over floppy microguidewires (e.g., Seeker-10 or Dasher-14, Target Therapeutics, Fremont, Calif.), that vary in size from 0.010 in. to 0.018 in. The most commonly used microcatheters are the Tracker 10 and the Tracker 18.

In addition to the commonly available angioplasty catheters for extracranial cerebrovascular angioplasty, microcatheters tipped with nondetachable balloons are also available for intracranial angioplasty. A variety of latex and silicone balloons are available, the most popular being the silicone balloons (Stealth, Target Therapeutics, Fremont, Calif.). Among the available balloons, low-pressure, highly compliant, elliptically shaped silicone balloons (ITC-NDSB, Interventional Therapeutics Corp., San Francisco, Calif.) are becoming increasingly popular, mainly because their configuration limits the amount of radial pressure during balloon inflation and they are therefore safer for intracranial angioplasty.

Among other transluminal devices of interest in this field are the occlusion materials (e.g., embolic agents such as polyvinyl alcohol or gelfoam), coils (e.g., Dacron coils or Guglielmi detachable coils), and stents. The majority of these are useful in the management of arteriovenous malformations and aneurysms, and an extensive technical discussion of them is beyond the scope of this chapter. Their usefulness will be discussed in the context of their clinical applications.

Image Acquisition Technique

In most cases, the cerebral angiogram should begin with an aortic arch injection and imaging of the aorta and the most proximal portions of the cerebral arteries (Fig. 11-8). The main

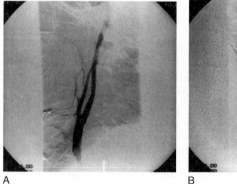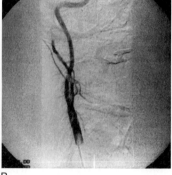

A   B

Fig. 11-8.   Lateral (A) and anteroposterior (B) views of the common carotid artery bifurcation. (From J.G. Mudd Catheterization Laboratory, St. Louis University, St. Louis, Missouri.)

purpose of this part of the study is to uncover abnormalities (e.g., atheromatous plaques) that are capable of producing the precipitating symptoms. Furthermore, imaging of the origin of these vessels helps in planning the method of selective catheterization, not only in the presence of pathologic findings, but also in the context of anomalous vessel origin. After placing a pigtail catheter in the ascending aorta, 30 cc of contrast agent are delivered using a power injector, commonly set for a rate of 20 to 30 cc/sec, using 600 to 900 psi (Table 11-5). Image acquisition is undertaken in the LAO plane and with the head of the patient turned partially to the right, having set the imaging field to include vascular structures between the origin of the great vessels and the bifurcation point of the common carotid arteries. It is sometimes necessary to repeat the injection with the head of the patient facing forward and using a right anterior oblique (RAO) projection in order to better visualize abnormalities of the great vessels.

Regarding nomenclature, the first proximal branch of the aorta is the innominate artery (brachiocephalic trunk), which, in turn, gives origin to the right common carotid and right subclavian arteries (Fig. 11-9). Distal to the innominate artery, the left carotid and left subclavian arteries commonly arise directly from the aortic arch. Numerous variations of the origin of these vessels can be found, their frequency ranging from 0.5% to 16%, depending on the specific anomaly. Their importance relates not only to their impact on the procedure itself, but also on the pathogenesis of the patient's symptoms.

After the arch injection, the pigtail catheter is replaced by another catheter chosen for selective angiography. Using the aortic arch images as a guide, the tip of the catheter is positioned at the point of origin of the target vessel. A simple

TABLE 11-5. Techniques for cerebral angiography

Vessel	Volume (cc)	Rate (cc/sec)	Projections
Aortic arch	30	20 to 30	LAO; RAO
Common carotid	8 to 10	8 to 10	AP; lateral (LAT)
Internal carotid	8 to 10	8 to 10	AP; LAT or Caldwell
Vertebral	6 to 8	6 to 8	AP; Townes; LAT

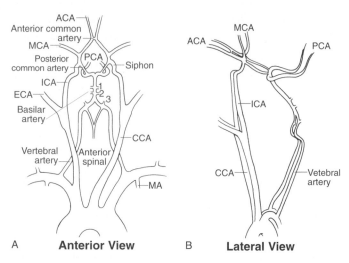

Fig. 11-9.   Diagram of the cerebral vascular anatomy. ACA, Anterior cerebral artery; ICA, internal carotid artery; ECA, external carotid artery; CCA, common carotid artery; MA, mammary artery. (From J.G. Mudd Catheterization Laboratory, St. Louis University, St. Louis, Missouri.)

clockwise turning of the catheter (approximately 90° to 180°) is usually sufficient to engage the ostia of the great vessels. At this point, a guidewire is used to advance the catheter further or, in cases where the innominate artery is being catheterized, to engage the right common carotid or subclavian artery.

Selective catheterization of either of the two carotid arteries is followed by image acquisition during contrast injection. Because of the size of the imaging field, the images are commonly divided into two groups, cervical and intracranial. The cervical images should allow optimal visualization of the common carotid bifurcation, as well as the portion of the internal carotid artery included between its origin and the base of the skull. At least two images, obtained in perpendicular planes (i.e., anteroposterior and lateral) are necessary for the appropriate assessment of this vascular system (Fig. 11-10). Following the acquisition of cervical images, and in the absence of atheromatous changes, the catheter is advanced over a guidewire into the internal carotid artery in order to

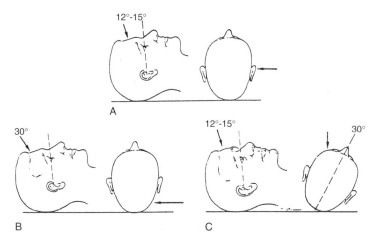

Fig. 11-10.   Proper positioning of the patient during acquisition of anteroposterior angiographic images of the intracranial portion of the carotid circulation. An angle of 12° to 15° cephalad is ideal for visualization of the middle cerebral artery (Caldwell view, **A**). A more pronounced angle (30°) is used when imaging the vertebrobasilar system (Townes view, **B**). An angle of 30° away from the x-ray tube will provide a transorbital view (**C**). (From Johnsrude IS, Jackson DC, Dunnick NR: *A practical approach to angiography,* ed 2, Boston, 1987, Little, Brown.)

obtain images of the intracranial vasculature. Again, a minimum of two perpendicular views is necessary for diagnostic purposes, and the images must include the portion of the internal carotid that was not imaged during the acquisition of cervical images, as well as its intracranial branches. The anteroposterior view is usually obtained by having the x-ray beam oriented cranially, at a 12° to 15° angle with the orbitomeatal line (Figs. 11-11 and 11-12). This angle superimposes the superior rim of the orbits on the superior ridge of the petrous bone (Caldwell view). To obtain an adequate lateral view, care must be taken to superimpose the external auditory canals during fluoroscopy, and to position the focal spot of the x-ray tube over the pituitary fossa. Most commonly, 8 to 10 cc of contrast medium are injected, either manually or using the power injector (Table 11-5). It is impor-

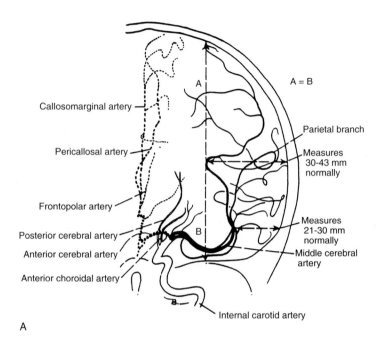

Fig. 11-11.   Anteroposterior view of the intracranial portion of the internal carotid artery and its branches (Caldwell view). Normal dimensions are shown in **A**. (From Johnsrude IS, Jackson DC, Dunnick NR: *A practical approach to angiography,* ed 2, Boston, 1987, Little, Brown.) An example is shown in **B**. (Example from J. G. Mudd Cardiac Catheterization Laboratory, St. Louis University, St. Louis, Missouri.)

tant to remember that when cineangiography is being performed, imaging should be carried out throughout the entire cycle, including arterial, arteriolar, capillary, venous, and sinusal phases. This procedure may yield exposure times that are generally longer than those used in coronary angiography.

Angiographic imaging of the vertebrobasilar circulation is accomplished by means of selective catheterization of each vertebral artery. A total of 6 to 8 cc of contrast material are injected, either manually or by means of a power injector (Table 11-5). As with carotid artery imaging, at least two perpendicular cervical and intracranial views must be obtained. The anteroposterior intracranial views should be acquired with the x-ray beam oriented cranially, at an angle of

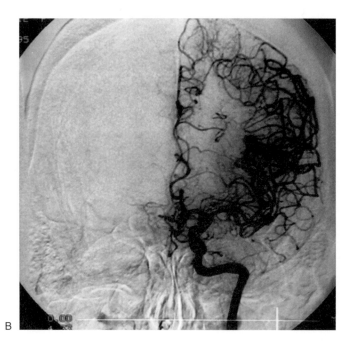

B

Fig. 11-11. (*Continued*).

approximately 30° from the orbitomeatal line (Fig. 11-13). An easy method of setting the anteroposterior images is to align the foramen magnum's anterior border with the planum sphenoidale (Towne's view). The lateral views should be set using a method similar to that used to set the carotid artery lateral views, with only a minor variation: The focal spot of the x-ray tube should be aligned with the point where the fourth ventricle would normally be located. Again, the two external auditory canals should be superimposed on one another to assure the true laterality of the image.

Nonangiographic Vascular Evaluation

The potential application of a variety of therapeutic techniques to the management of patients with cerebrovascular disorders, together with the inherent limitations of angiography as a diagnostic tool have kindled the interest of several groups of investigators in the development of endovascular techniques to provide information that is not accessible by conventional angiography. The limitations of angiography

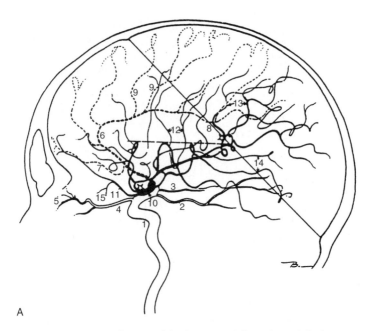

A

Fig. 11-12.   Lateral view of the intracranial portion of the internal carotid artery and its branches. Normal dimensions are shown in **A**. The most important arteries shown are the internal carotid (1), posterior cerebral (2), anterior choroidal (3), ophthalmic (4), and anterior cerebral (6). The remainder are branches of these. (From Johnsrude IS, Jackson DC, Dunnick NR: *A practical approach to angiography,* ed 2, Boston, 1987, Little, Brown.) An example of this type of image is shown in **B**. (Example from J. G. Mudd Cardiac Catheterization Laboratory, St. Louis University, St. Louis, Missouri.)

are widely known. The technique provides only "luminographic" images of the endothelial surface, without fully considering the vascular wall and its composition and without conveying any physiologic information. Furthermore, angiographic vessel overlap is commonly observed when imaging branching regions and intracranial vessels.

Advances in diagnostic technology have continued to be introduced in the mature field of coronary angiography and interventional catheterization. Indeed, a more physiologic approach to the invasive assessment of coronary atheromatous

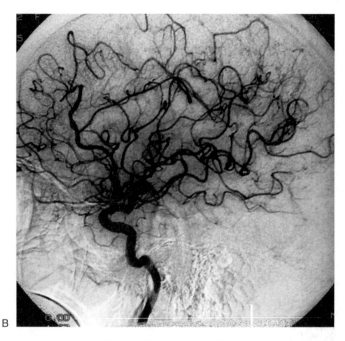

Fig. 11-12.   (*Continued*).

Neurointerventional Procedures Either Available or Under Investigation

Intraarterial thrombolysis
  Internal carotid artery
  Middle cerebral artery
  Basilar artery
  Central retinal artery
Therapeutic vascular occlusion
Embolization
Detachable coils
Detachable balloons
Percutaneous angioplasty balloons
Stents
Laser
Ultrasound ablation

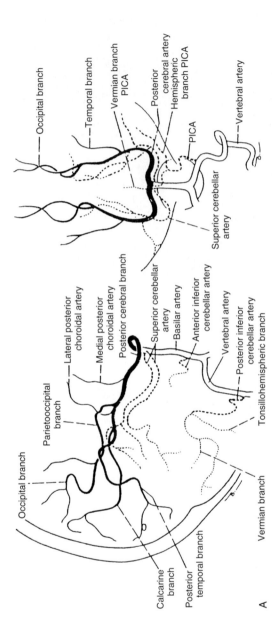

Fig. 11-13. **A,** Diagram of vertebrobasilar systems. (From Johnsrude IS, Jackson DC, Dunnick NR: *A practical approach to angiography*, ed 2, Boston, 1987, Little, Brown.) Lateral (**B**) and anteroposterior (**C**) views of the vertebrobasilar circulation. The anteroposterior view is obtained using a Towne's projection. The patient shown here has a basilar artery stenosis. (Angiograms from J. G. Mudd Cardiac Catheterization Laboratory, St. Louis University, St. Louis, Missouri.)

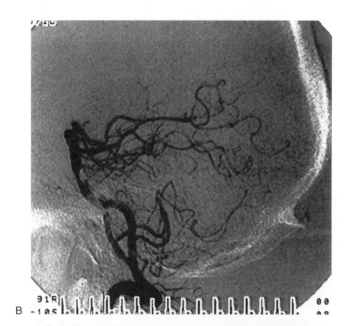

B

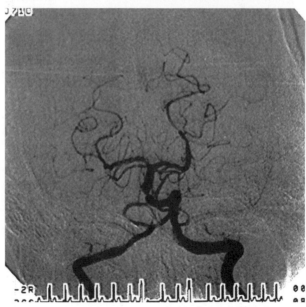

C

Fig. 11-13. (*Continued*).

plaques has resulted in the increasing application of non-angiographic endovascular techniques to the selection of patients for coronary angioplasty, stenting, or other forms of revascularization.

Rationale for Endovascular Physiologic Assessment. The ability of any stenotic lesion to induce cerebral ischemia is dependent on two major inherent characteristics: the embologenic properties of its surface, and its flow-reducing effect (i.e., its hemodynamic significance). The embologenic properties of the plaque surface, although partly related to the degree of narrowing that the plaque causes, depend mostly on an independent set of vessel characteristics such as surface irregularity and endothelial integrity. The hemodynamic significance of an atherosclerotic plaque is related directly to the degree of lumen and blood flow reduction that it causes. Until recently, however, the evaluation of neurologic patients for revascularization has traditionally been based on a purely anatomic concept: the percentage of stenosis, as estimated by diameter narrowing. Because of the inadequacies of extrapolating hemodynamic information from angiographically obtained stenosis measurements, a more direct and physiologic assessment of the flow-reducing characteristic of atheromatous plaques is required.

Translesional pressure gradient measurements. Using a coaxial system of small, flexible catheters delivered over guidewires, it is possible to measure blood pressures at points proximal and distal to lesions located anywhere in the large arteries of the cerebral circulation, thus determining the translesional pressure gradient. The identification of pressure reductions across stenotic cerebrovascular lesions, coupled with an assessment of the distal resistance responses, as described below, provides a better indicator of the hemodynamic compromise of the cerebral territory under study, regardless of the angiographic appearance of the narrowing (Fig. 11-14). Translesional pressure gradients can also discriminate between lesions that are angiographically similar but whose hemodynamic characteristics are significantly different. This approach may also help define the limitations of revascularization procedures such as angioplasty, and further qualify the use of endarterectomy.

Intravascular Doppler measurements and assessment of cerebrovascular blood flow reserve. Invasive techniques using catheters and guidewires specially designed for the performance of endovascular Doppler measurements have been used to assess the hemodynamic characteristics of the coronary circulation. In spite of the availability of noninvasive neurovascular ultrasound techniques, intravascular Doppler measurement provides additional information about flow characteristics at specific points in the cerebral vasculature and under specific circumstances. The advantages of intravascular Doppler over noninvasive Doppler techniques include the fact that there are portions of the cerebral arterial system that may not be reached with other methods (e.g., the petrous segment of the internal carotid artery). Also, in approximately 15% of the population, the transcranial Doppler ultrasound beam cannot effectively cross the skull and allow assessment of the circle of Willis. Furthermore, an externally placed ultrasound transducer used during monitoring of endovascular procedures is somewhat cumbersome and may be impractical. Finally, using intravascular Doppler, the localization of the ultrasound sample volume is extremely precise because the device can be positioned fluoroscopically. Concurrent measurement of vascular diameter using angiographic techniques allows the determination of hemodynamic variables that have not yet been explored (e.g., cerebrovascular impedance).

The most interesting aspect of the intravascular Doppler method is that it provides a practical means for the physiologic assessment of the vascular bed supplied by the artery in question, as well as its state of reactivity. Based on the relationship between flow and pressure in the brain circulation, it is obvious that downward changes in pressure will result in comparable changes in flow unless proportional reductions in resistance also take place. Such changes in resistance are part of the mechanism of autoregulation and, as with any other physiologic process, can compensate for reductions in pressure only up to a certain limit, beyond which flow will progressively decrease. The intraarterial administration of short-acting arterial vasodilators is normally followed by downstream arteriolar dilation, decreased distal resistance, and increased blood flow velocity, particularly during diastole. The same maneuver in a hemodynamically compromised vascular territory will result in little or no change, underscoring the lack of cerebrovascular reserve capacity of this territory. Combined with the translesional pressure gradient measurements described (Fig. 11-14), this technique adds to the evaluation of patients with brain ischemia, in some instances helping to identify subpopulations with different risks for stroke.

C.N., L ICA stenosis

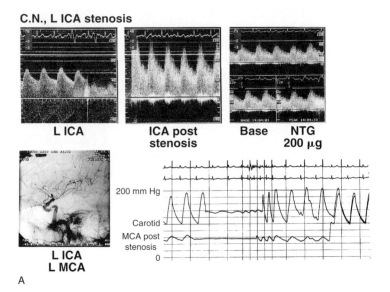

A

Fig. 11-14.   Examples of translesional pressure gradient measurements, intravascular Doppler, and cerebrovascular reserve assessment. **A,** The patient has a 50% diameter stenosis of the internal carotid artery siphon by angiography (*bottom left*), but a translesional pressure gradient of 80 torr (*bottom right*). Intravascular Doppler guidewire flow velocity in the left internal carotid artery (LICA, *top left*) and at the point of stenosis (*top middle*) show the mean blood flow velocity increases to >100 cm/sec. The administration of intraarterial nitroglycerin fails to produce cerebral vasodilation (*top right*). **B,** *Top,* Cerebral angiography in a patient with a 50% ICA siphon lesion similar to patient A. Lower 3 angiographic images show position of guidewire and tracker catheter. *Bottom,* Pressure and flow velocity did not demonstrate a significant gradient or abnormal increases in flow velocity across this stenosis. (From J.G. Mudd Catheterization Laboratory, St. Louis University, St. Louis, Missouri.)

G.B., 47-year-old woman

**Left middle
cerebral artery**

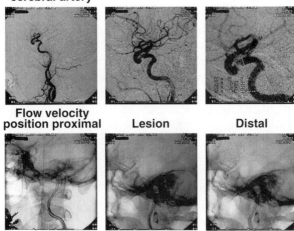

**Flow velocity
position proximal**   **Lesion**   **Distal**

G.B., 47-year-old woman, proximal MCA

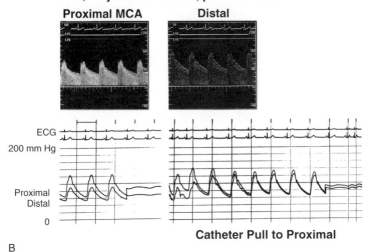

B

Fig. 11-14. (*Continued*).

Two-dimensional intravascular ultrasound. Recent technologic advances utilizing vascular catheters with specially fitted rotating ultrasound crystals provide tomographic 360° views of the vascular wall. This technology has been applied in the evaluation and management of patients with peripheral or coronary insufficiency. The assessment of the cerebral blood vessels by IVUS has unique importance in the determination of the cerebrovascular endothelial status in regions that are not accessible by conventional ultrasound imaging. Endothelial integrity and plaque surface compositions represent important variables in the consideration of nonsurgical revascularization techniques such as angioplasty. IVUS may direct the decision of what type of interventional procedure to use in which patient—for example, balloon versus laser angioplasty. In addition, IVUS provides immediate intraoperative assessment of the effects of these procedures on the arterial structures, and the opportunity to discover aspects about nonatherosclerotic vascular disorders, such as the vascular wall morphology of spontaneous dissections (Fig. 11-15).

Cerebral angioscopy. The identification of intraluminal thrombus by angiography is poor. In recent years, the development of ultrathin fiber-optic endoscopic systems has allowed the direct visualization of the endothelial surface of the coronary and peripheral arteries. Although the application to the cerebral blood vessels is still limited, angioscopes as thin as 500 μm can be used for direct in-vivo examination of the endovascular environment in which interventional techniques are being carried out. From the diagnostic point of view, angioscopy may provide immediate feedback about the effect of PTA on the endothelial surface, and may serve to guide certain therapeutic procedures such as occlusion of carotid cavernous fistulas. Angioscopy is the least explored of all the nonangiographic techniques described, but it has the greatest potential for rendering surface morphology and details of thrombi.

CURRENT AND FUTURE INTERVENTIONAL CEREBRAL CATHETERIZATION PROCEDURES

Cerebral catheterization is more than a diagnostic technique; it also represents a vehicle for percutaneous transluminal

W.J., 57-year-old man

Left common carotid	Left external carotid
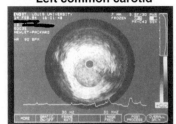	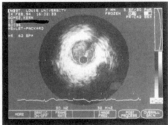
Left bifurcation	**Left common carotid**
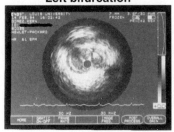	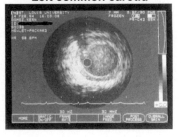

Fig. 11-15.   Intravascular ultrasound images of a patient with internal carotid artery occlusion following dissection. Note the remarkably thickened media, suggestive of a connective tissue abnormality. (From J.G. Mudd Catheterization Laboratory, St. Louis University, St. Louis, Missouri.)

therapeutic techniques. The major interventional procedures that are either currently available or being studied are listed in the box on p. 427. They will be discussed briefly, with an emphasis on their role in the care of patients with cerebrovascular disorders.

Intraarterial Thrombolysis

Intraarterial thrombolysis, an invasive therapeutic technique, continues to be evaluated in major multicenter trials. A favorable correlation between the expected natural course of the stroke and the typical angiographic findings of vascular occlusion will identify its clinical role. Contraindications to thrombolysis include impaired hemostasis, aneurysms, or arteriovenous malformations, radiographic evidence of a recent cerebral hemorrhage or hemorrhagic infarction, pregnancy, or surgery within 10 days preceding the stroke. At present, the most important clinical scenarios in the evaluation of intraarterial fibrinolysis include basilar artery occlusion, middle cerebral artery occlusion, internal carotid artery occlusion, and central retinal artery occlusion.

The most serious complication of intraarterial thrombolysis is intracerebral hemorrhage. Certain factors increase the risk for the development of this particular problem. In the vertebrobasilar circulation, once computed tomography (CT) shows evidence of brainstem infarction, hemorrhage is more likely to occur. In the carotid territory, if treatment is delayed beyond 6 hr, the risk of hemorrhage is also increased. Minor hemorrhagic complications such as those occurring at the site of the arterial puncture are usually handled without major problems. It is important to note that, even in those patients developing intracerebral hemorrhage, neurologic worsening does not necessarily occur as a result of it.

Therapeutic Vascular Occlusion

The use of materials that can be injected intraarterially to occlude specific vascular structures is an area of major clinical and research interest. The most important use is in the occlusion of vascular malformations, aneurysms, and tumors. The most appropriate occluding agent is selected based on the specific circumstances. The most commonly used occlusive materials belong to one of the following categories: particulate agents (i.e., polyvinyl alcohol, gelfoam powder, collagen, dura, and autologous clot), adhesive glue (i.e., isobutyl cyanoacrylate, and, more recently, N-butyl cyanoacrylate), and detachable coils. From the vascular neurologist's point of view, the latter are perhaps the most interesting type of agent because of their application to the management of saccular aneurysms. Coils are made of materials that are highly thrombogenic and therefore lead to rapid occlusion of the structures within which they are deployed. Of particular interest is the Guglielmi coil, which is used for the endovascular occlusion of saccular aneurysms. It works by causing thrombosis and occlusion of the aneurysms by electrolysis. In addition, detachable balloons are also useful in the occlusion of specific vascular pathologic conditions, most importantly carotid cavernous fistulas.

Percutaneous Angioplasty Techniques

More than 400 cases of balloon angioplasty of the cerebral vessels have been reported in the literature. The revascularization success rate has been encouraging (>85%), but the reported complication rates vary between 3% for extracranial vessels and up to 30% for intracranial vessels. It is important to note that balloon angioplasty is designed to change the flow-reducing characteristics of the lesion, not its emboligenic properties. In fact, endothelial surface disruption and plaque fracture commonly follow angioplasty, theoretically increasing the emboligenic properties of the treated lesions. However, distal embolization is not as serious a problem as it had been thought, and emboli are better tolerated by the brain than was previously suspected. Nevertheless, because of these considerations, alternative methods of angioplasty must be considered. A technique that causes the least amount of endothelial disruption while leading to sufficient improvement of flow across the lesions would be ideal. Along these lines, other techniques currently being studied are stents (Fig. 11-16), laser, and ultrasound angioplasty.

TRAINING STANDARDS FOR PERIPHERAL ANGIOPLASTY
Body of Knowledge

As described by the AHA/ACC Committee on Peripheral Vascular Disease, physicians should have extensive clinical training in the diagnosis and treatment of patients with peripheral vascular disease. The body of knowledge necessary includes the anatomy, natural history, and clinical manifestations of peripheral vascular disease; noninvasive assessment of peripheral vascular disease; indications and contraindications for angioplasty; risks and benefits of angioplasty; recognition of complications; alternative therapies; principles of thrombolytic techniques; and technical aspects and usage of x-ray equipment needed for diagnostic peripheral angiography and percutaneous transluminal angioplasty.

Basic Training

A basic training requirement must be met by each physician applicant and should include at least one of the following:
1. American Board of Radiology eligibility or certification

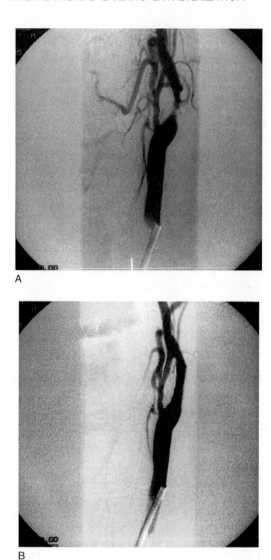

Fig. 11-16.   Example of carotid artery angioplasty and stenting.
A, The patient had an atheromatous lesion that narrowed the
internal carotid artery by more than 90% and that was
responsible for a mild cerebral infarction. **B,** Following angioplasty and stent placement, the vessel is clearly patent. (From
G. Roubin, University of Alabama, Birmingham, Alabama.)

2. American Board of Internal Medicine eligibility or certification with additional completion of a fellowship in vascular medicine or American Board of Internal Medicine certification with additional eligibility or certification in cardiovascular medicine
3. American Board of Surgery eligibility or certification with additional completion of a general vascular surgery residency

Specific Procedural Training and Experience

Specific training or experience in peripheral diagnostic angiography and peripheral percutaneous transluminal angioplasty is required. This may be obtained through one of the following.

Qualification by training. An applicant may qualify by completing a training program that includes extensive experience in diagnostic angiography and percutaneous transluminal angioplasty of peripheral vessels. At a minimum, this experience must include performance of 100 diagnostic peripheral angiograms and 50 renal or peripheral percutaneous transluminal angioplasties, and for at least half of these procedures the applicant must be the primary operator. In addition, the applicant should have training and experience in the use of thrombolytic therapy in peripheral arteries, having participated in at least 10 such cases. These requirements are normally met during a formal subspecialty training program of at least 1 year's duration, completed after at least one of the basic training requirements listed in the previous section has been met. However, they may be met in part or in total during initial residency or fellowship. In all instances, complete and detailed documentation of the aforementioned procedural training should be available.

Qualification by experience. An applicant may qualify by having extensive previous experience in peripheral angiographic diagnosis and percutaneous transluminal angioplasty with acceptable complication and success rates. This experience must include performance of a minimum of 100 diagnostic angiograms and 50 percutaneous transluminal angioplasties of the peripheral arteries, and the applicant must be the primary operator for at least half of these procedures. The applicant should have experience in the use of thrombolytic therapy in peripheral arteries, having participated in at least 10 such cases. The applicant should be able to present documentation of results and complications, and confirmation of these data may be requested from the institution where the experience was gained.

Qualification by apprenticeship. These physicians must be prepared to demonstrate knowledge of the principles of diagnosis and therapy of peripheral and visceral vascular disease, as outlined under "Body of Knowledge." Clear understanding of the methods of diagnostic angiography must be demonstrated, including knowledge of appropriate radiographic equipment, catheters and catheter techniques, and radiation safety associated with diagnostic and interventional procedures. The apprenticeship should be thoroughly documented and should include each of the following as a minimum.

1. Documented performance of 100 diagnostic peripheral angiograms, 50 peripheral percutaneous transluminal angioplasty procedures, and 10 peripheral arterial thrombolysis procedures under the direct supervision of a qualified physician preceptor. The applicant must have been the primary operator for at least half of these procedures. The requirement for diagnostic angiograms may be met in part by the previous experience of the operator if appropriate records are submitted (as outlined under "Qualification by Experience").
2. Observation of the applicant performing at least 10 peripheral percutaneous transluminal angioplasties by a person already qualified by these standards.
3. Attendance at postgraduate courses for a total of at least 50 Category 1 Continuing Medical Education credits in diagnostic peripheral angiography and percutaneous peripheral vascular interventional techniques.

Maintenance of privileges. Maintenance of percutaneous transluminal angioplasty privileges requires ongoing experience in performing these procedures, with acceptable success and complication rates. The determination of a minimum number of procedures per year is at the discretion of the credentials or clinical privileges committee of each hospital. Whether or not a minimum number is specified, maintenance of privileges is also dependent on the physician's active participation in the institution's quality improvement program that monitors indications, success rates, and complications. These data may be used within the individual institution in considering renewal of clinical privileges. All physicians performing these procedures must participate in the quality improvement program and will be evaluated using the same criteria.

Physicians who were granted privileges before the implementation of this standard should not necessarily have their status altered if they do not meet the qualifications outlined in this statement. However, if they do not meet the qualifications, they should acquire the necessary training or experience to do so within 3 years. They must also participate in the institution's quality improvement program and will be evaluated using the same standards for indications, success rates, and complications.

SUGGESTED READINGS

Alexandrov AV, Bladin CF, Maggisano R, Norris JW: Measuring carotid stenosis. Time for a reappraisal, *Stroke* 24:1292-1296, 1993.

Cardella JF, Casarella WJ, DeWeese JA, et al.: Optimal resources for the examination and endovascular treatment of the peripheral and visceral vascular systems: AHA intercouncil report on peripheral and visceral angiographic and interventional laboratories, *Circulation* 89:1481-1493, 1994.

Colapinto RF, Stronell RD, Johnston WK: Transluminal angioplasty of complete iliac obstruction, *Am J Radiol* 146:859-862, 1986.

Gomez CR: Carotid plaque morphology and the risk for stroke, *Stroke* 21(1):148-151, 1995.

Gomez CR: Is "carotid stenosis" an obsolete concept? *J Neuroimaging* (in press).

Greenfield AJ: Percutaneous transluminal angioplasty of the femoral, popliteal and tibial vessels. In Athanasoulis CA, et al., editors: *Interventional radiology*, Philadelphia, 1982, W.B. Saunders.

Guglielmi G, Vinuela F, Sepetka I, Macellari V: Electrothrombosis of saccular aneurysms via endovascular approach. Part I: electrochemical basis, technique, and experimental results. *J Neurosurg* 75:1-7, 1991.

Harding MB, Smith LR, Himmelstein SI, et al.: Renal artery stenosis: prevalence and associated risk factors in patients undergoing routine cardiac catheterization, *J Am Soc Nephrol* 2:1608-1616, 1992.

Higashida RT, Tsai FY, Halbach VV, Dowd CF, Hieshima GB: Cerebral percutaneous transluminal angioplasty, *Heart Disease and Stroke* 2:497-502, 1993.

Kandarpa K: *Handbook of cardiovascular and interventional radiologic procedures,* Boston, 1989, Little, Brown.

Katzen BT, Van Breda A: Transluminal angioplasty of the iliac arteries, *Semin Intervent Radiol* 2:196-205, 1985.

Kaufman SL, Barth KH, Kadir S, et al.: Hemodynamic measurements in the evaluation and follow-up of transluminal angioplasty of the iliac and femoral arteries, *Radiology* 142:329-336, 1982.

Kern MJ, Anderson HV, editors: A symposium—the clinical application of intracoronary Doppler guidewire flow velocity in patients. Understanding blood flow beyond the coronary stenosis, *Am J Cardiol* 11:1D-86D, 1993.

Krepel VM, van Andel GJ, van Erp WFM: Percutaneous transluminal angioplasty of the femoropopliteal artery: initial and long-term results, *Radiology* 156:325-328, 1985.

Levin DC, Becker GJ, Dorros G, et al.: Training standards for physicians performing peripheral angioplasty and other percutaneous peripheral vascular interventions: a statement for health professionals from the Special Writing Group of the Councils on Cardiovascular Radiology, Cardio-thoracic and Vascular Surgery, and Clinical Cardiology, the American Heart Association, *Circulation* 86:1348-1350, 1992.

Nichols DA, Meyer FB, Piepgras DG, Smith PL: Endovascular treatment of intracranial aneurysms, *Mayo Clin Proc* 69:272-285, 1994.

Novick AC, Textor SC, Bodie B, Khauli RB: Revascularization to preserve renal function in patients with atherosclerotic renovascular disease, *Urol Clin N Am* 11:477-490, 1984.

Rose JS, editor: *Invasive radiology: risks and patient care,* Chicago, 1983, Year Book Medical Publishers, p 73.

Scoccianti M, Verbin CS, Kopchok GE, et al.: Intravascular ultrasound guidance for peripheral vascular interventions, *J Endovasc Surg* 1:71-80, 1994.

Sos TA: Angioplasty for the treatment of azotemia and renovascular hypertension in atherosclerotic renal artery disease, *Circulation* 83:I-162, 1991.

Sundt TM, Smith HC, Campbell JK, Vlietstra RE, Cucchiara RF, Stanson AW: Transluminal angioplasty for basilar artery stenosis, *Mayo Clin Proc* 55:673-680, 1980.

Tegtmeyer CJ, Kellum CD, Kron IL: Percutaneous transluminal angioplasty in the region of the aortic bifurcation, *Radiology* 157:661-665, 1985.

Udoff EJ, Barth KH, Harrington DP, et al.: Hemodynamic significance of iliac artery stenosis: pressure measurement during angiography, *Radiology* 132:289-293, 1979.

Van Andel GJ, van Erp WFM, Krepel VM, et al.: Percutaneous transluminal dilatation of the iliac artery: long term results, *Radiology* 156:321-323, 1985.

Van Breda A, Katzen BT: Femoral angioplasty, *Semin Intervent Radiol* 1:251-268, 1984.

Vetrovec GW, Landwehr DM, Edwards VL: Incidence of renal artery stenosis in hypertensive patients undergoing coronary angiography, *J Interven Cardiol* 2:69-76, 1989.

Wardlaw JM, Warlow CP: Thrombolysis in acute ischemic stroke: does it work? *Stroke* 23:1826-1839, 1992.

White CJ, Ramee SR, Collins TJ, et al.: Guiding catheter assisted renal artery angioplasty, *Cathet Cardiovasc Diagn* 23:10, 1991.

White CJ, Ramee SR: *Interventional cardiology. Clinical applications of new technologies*, New York, 1991, Raven Press, pp 1-55.

Working Group on Renovascular Hypertension of the National Heart, Lung and Blood Institute: Detection, evaluation and treatment of renovascular hypertension: final report, *Arch Intern Med* 147:820, 1987.

12

INOUE BALLOON MITRAL COMMISSUROTOMY AND AORTIC VALVULOPLASTY

Ted Feldman and John D. Carroll

MITRAL COMMISSUROTOMY
Background

Inoue described the single-balloon technique of mitral commissurotomy in 1984, having first performed the procedure
in 1982. Although a number of other techniques have been
described, the Inoue balloon technique and the double-
balloon technique have been the most commonly used. Today,
the Inoue technique is probably the most frequently used
technique internationally, and it is at present the only approved mitral dilatation balloon technique in the United
States.

Hemodynamic results have been well characterized by the
Inoue multicenter registry. On average there is >80% increase
in mitral valve area. Balloon inflation results in splitting of
the fused commissures with reductions in the transmitral
pressure gradient, the mean left atrial pressure, and the pulmonary artery pressure. The cardiac output and mitral valve
area increase (Table 12-1).

TABLE 12-1.   Hemodynamic results of balloon mitral valvotomy

	Pre	Post	p
Left atrium (mmHg)	24 ± 8	19 ± 12	<.001
Pulmonary artery (mmHg)	34 ± 14	29 ± 12	<.001
Mitral gradient (mmHg)	13 ± 6	6 ± 3	<.001
Cardiac output (L/min)	4.1 ± 1.1	4.4 ± 1.3	<.001
Mitral area (cm²)	1.0 ± 0.3	1.7 ± 0.6	<.001

The most important complication of the procedure is mitral regurgitation. Mitral valve replacement is needed during the initial hospitalization in 1% of patients. An additional 3% to 4% of patients have resultant 3+ or greater mitral regurgitation without need for immediate mitral valve replacement. Other complications are shown in Table 12-2.

The durability of results is excellent. Figure 12-1 shows the stability of the achieved valve area over a period of years. The 5-year actuarial freedom from death, mitral valve replacement, or repeat balloon commissurotomy for the Inoue registry population was 71%. More than 80% of patients were symptomatically improved.

TABLE 12-2.   Complications of PTMC

	Percent
Hospital MVR	1.0
Hospital death	1.4
TIA	0.6
Stroke	0
Cardiac perforation Pericardiocentesis	1.4
MI	0.3
DC shock for AF or VF	1.0
Vascular repair	0.6
Transfusion	0.3
Temporary pacer	0
MR 3+ or more (no MVR)	3.8
ASD > 1.5	3.1
Failure to cross MV	1.7

MVR, Mitral valve replacement; MI, myocardial infarction; AF, atrial fibrillation; VF, ventricular fibrillation; ASD, atrial septal defect; MV, mitral valve; MR, mitral regurgitation; TIA, transient ischemic attack.

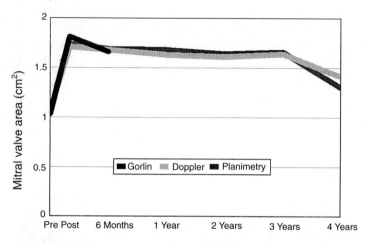

Fig. 12-1. Mitral valve area before PTMC, immediately after, and 4 years following PTMC. Gorlin calculated valve areas were obtained in 86 patients at repeat catheterization. Doppler and planimetry areas remained relatively constant for 3 years and then fell off slightly in the fourth year.

Technique

The Inoue balloon.   The Inoue device differs substantially from conventional balloons. It is constructed of two layers of latex with a nylon mesh in between. The latex is compliant, whereas the nylon mesh limits the maximum inflated diameter of the balloon and gives it its unique shape and three-stage inflation characteristics (Fig. 12-2). The front half of the balloon inflates, giving the appearance of a balloon flotation catheter. The proximal half of the balloon inflates next, creating a dumbbell shape. When it is positioned across the mitral valve, this facilitates positioning of the balloon device in the valve orifice. Last, the center portion of the balloon inflates, resulting in commissurotomy. The distensibility of the latex material allows each balloon to be inflated over a 4-mm range of diameter sizes (i.e., 26 to 30 mm for the largest available model). A single balloon can thus be used to effect sequential dilatation of the valve, by inflating it to serially larger diameters, without removing it from the patient. This procedure is thus analogous to coronary angio-

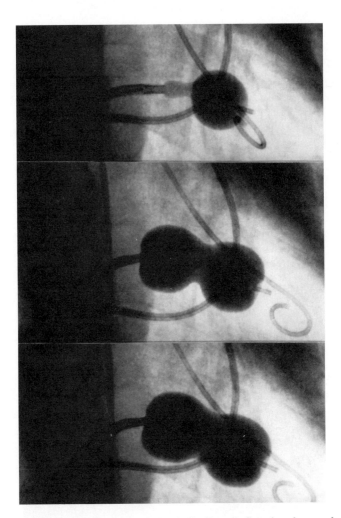

Fig. 12-2.   *Upper panel,* Front half of balloon inflated and passed across the mitral valve orifice. This is analogous to the manner in which a balloon flotation catheter is maneuvered from the right atrium to the right ventricle during right heart catheterization. The partially inflated balloon is pulled back until it engages the mitral valve. *Middle panel,* Front and back portions of balloon inflated, creating a "dogbone" shape, that self-positions the balloon in the mitral orifice. *Bottom panel,* Almost fully inflated balloon opening the commissures. Note that the inferior indentation in the balloon was not as pronounced as the superior, signifying incomplete commissural separation.

plasty, for which the result of a balloon inflation is evaluated and additional inflations are performed if necessary.

Patient evaluation. Evaluation by two-dimensional echocardiography and transesophageal echocardiography are essential before mitral valvotomy. Patients with thin, pliable mitral valve leaflets and minimally diseased subvalvular apparatus have the best long-term outcome from surgical commissurotomy (Fig. 12-3). This is no less true when using percu-

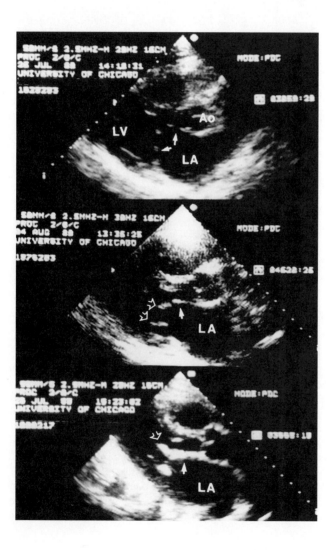

taneous methods to achieve commissurotomy. Although the immediate results of percutaneous transvenous mitral commissurotomy (PTMC) are acceptable in patients with significant valve deformity, the restenosis rate and need for late mitral valve replacement remains higher in these patients. The goals of therapy and long-term prospects for event-free survival must be appropriate for patients with significant valve deformity and echocardiographic scores greater than 10 to 12.

Transesophageal echocardiography before PTMC is useful for the detection of atrial thrombi. PTMC performed in patients before the widespread use of transesophageal echocardiography was not associated with frequent embolic events. Nonetheless, experience and common sense both argue that transesophageal echo screening virtually eliminates the chance of this devastating complication. Thrombi are a strong

Fig. 12-3.   *Upper panel,* Long-axis two-dimensional echocardiographic image from an ideal candidate for mitral commissurotomy. The solid arrows show the thin, domed leaflets. The mitral apparatus is not visible in the left ventricle, signifying its freedom from significant thickening. *Middle panel,* Typical valve replacement candidate. The solid arrow points at a thickened and calcified anterior mitral leaflet. The open arrows show the thickened submitral apparatus. These patients have echocardiographic scores between 8 and 12 and are reasonable candidates for PTMC, although they may have a less good long-term freedom from mitral valve replacement. *Bottom panel,* Elderly patient, not likely a candidate for surgical therapy of any kind. This patient was an 88-year-old woman. The solid arrow shows a densely calcified, thickened, and rigid anterior mitral leaflet. The open arrow points at the similarly thickened and calcified mitral apparatus. Balloon dilatation may be accomplished successfully in these patients but with acute results that are not as good as those in patients with less deformed valves. The long-term event-free outcome for these patients is poor. (From Feldman T, Carroll JD: Cardiac catheterization, balloon angioplasty, and percutaneous valvuloplasty, in Hall JB, Schmidt GA, Wood LDH, editors: *Principles of critical care,* New York, 1992, McGraw-Hill, pp 343-360.)

relative contraindication to the performance of both transseptal puncture and balloon mitral valvotomy. Atrial thrombi are found in 15% to 25% of patients with mitral stenosis being considered for PTMC, many of whom have been on long-term coumadin anticoagulation therapy, even when sinus rhythm is present. In many cases, when atrial thrombi are noted, it is possible to either institute or intensify anticoagulation therapy for 3 to 12 months and achieve resolution of thrombi. PTMC may then be undertaken without unnecessary risk. In carefully selected cases, small, densely organized thrombi in the atrial appendage may be present. These thrombi are not as likely to contain fresh clots or to be mobile. It is possible to do PTMC in these cases without complications, though this must be done with extreme care and recognition of the serious risk of stroke. Operator experience with the handling characteristics of the Inoue balloon steering stylet is essential in this setting. Some patients in atrial fibrillation without prior anticoagulation therapy are found not to have atrial thrombi upon transesophageal echo exam. In these cases, balloon dilatation may proceed without a prior course of anticoagulation.

Cardiac catheterization technique

1. The left femoral arterial and venous sheaths are placed. Because a pigtail catheter will be left in the ventricle for a relatively long period of time, we prefer to use 5 or 6 French arterial catheters.
2. A multilumen pulmonary artery balloon catheter with thermodilution cardiac output capability may be used for right heart catheterization. Left femoral access is preferred for these catheters, leaving the right side for balloon catheter insertion. Pulmonary artery catheters with oximetric monitoring greatly simplify the evaluation of venous saturations for detection of atrial shunting following the procedure. When significant right atrial dilatation is present, passage of the pulmonary artery catheter is facilitated by the use of an extra-stiff guidewire.
3. Left ventriculography and coronary arteriography are performed when indicated.
4. Right heart pressures and cardiac output are measured before the procedure.

5. Right femoral venous puncture is performed for placement of an 8F Mullins sheath. The pulmonary artery
   catheter does not interfere with the performance of the
   transseptal catheterization.
6. Following transseptal puncture, heparin, 100 μ/kg, is
   administered. When the transseptal catheterization has
   been completed successfully, the transmitral pressure
   gradient is measured using the Mullins sheath for left
   atrial and the pigtail for left ventricular pressures. If the
   Mullins sheath can be passed into the left ventricle with
   gentle counterclockwise rotation, a transaortic gradient
   is measured with the Mullins and pigtail. A Fick cardiac
   output in addition to the thermodilution output is usually obtained.

A simplified procedure with no arterial access and no pulmonary artery catheterization is not recommended. The safety
of the procedure and the evaluation of the results and possible
complications mandate continuous arterial pressure monitoring, a full right heart catheterization before and after the
procedure, and accurate cardiac output determination.

Selection of balloon size.   Balloon sizing has not been
rigorously defined by any study. Rather, a combination of
experience in the first decade of balloon mitral valvotomy,
common sense, and data from a few studies has established
several reasonable, simple approaches to balloon sizing. Maximum expected inflated balloon diameter may be selected
based on patient height (Table 12-3). This value provides a
guideline for balloon selection, and with the stepwise technique a first inflation is always performed at a diameter
smaller than the maximum possible for the selected balloon
(usually 4 mm less than the maximum). An alternative
method for selecting balloon size is to calculate the ratio of

TABLE 12-3.   Selection of balloon size for PTMC

Balloon diameter (range, mm)	Balloon dilating area (cm²)	Patient height, cm (in.)
26 to 30	7.07	>180 (70.9)
24 to 28	6.16	>160 (62.9)
22 to 26	5.13	<160

inflated balloon dilating area to the body surface area (effective balloon dilating area, EBDA):

EBDA = $[\pi * (\text{balloon diameter}/20)^2]/\text{body surface area (BSA) (m}^2)$

An effective balloon dilating area of 4.0 is the largest probable inflated balloon diameter necessary:

Largest probable balloon inflation diameter (EBDA 4.0)

$$= 20 * [\sqrt{(4 * \text{BSA})}/\pi]$$

Alternatively, a simple formula may be used for selecting maximal Inoue balloon size:

Maximum balloon diameter = [(height in cm/10) + 10]

This method results in somewhat different values for maximal balloon size in a given patient compared to the recommendations originally made by Inoue based on his empirical observations. The EBDA method is effective for balloon size selection using the double-balloon technique. Park and Kim employed this method in balloon size selection for PTMC with the Inoue balloon. They inflated the Inoue balloon to an EBDA of 4.0 using a single inflation without the stepwise technique and achieved results similar to those reported for the stepwise technique.

EBDA may not be equally useful in all patient populations. For overweight or obese patients in particular, a better estimate of largest expected balloon inflation diameter may be based on height alone.

For patients with pliable valves, the first balloon inflation can be made with a balloon 2 or 3 mm smaller than the reference size, and then increased in increments of 1 mm until either a maximal diminution of gradient has occurred or mitral regurgitation has begun to worsen significantly. For patients with more deformed valves, the first inflation can be performed at 4 mm less than the reference size, with increments of 1 mm in size while the balloon is on the shallow or low-pressure portion of the pressure–volume curve. Half-millimeter increments may be used over the last couple of millimeters of balloon diameter size when the balloon reaches the high-pressure portion of its pressure–volume curve.

Special considerations.   There are a number of special considerations in balloon size selection. Smaller balloons than

initially estimated may be us
age, subvalvular disease, or
marked constriction of the ball
cates that balloon pressure ma
situation, use of a smaller balloc
ter will result in greater inflatio

The stepwise technique. The
technique obviates the need for pi
imal inflated balloon diameter. Be ....y
be inflated over a range of sizes, ...c selection need
only be accurate enough to address this range. Although
patient and balloon characteristics may be evaluated in a
consistent manner, the inhomogeneity of the valve pathology
and the limitations of our ability to predict what balloon size
and pressure will produce commissural splitting make the
stepwise approach ultimately more practical than preprocedure predictions of expected balloon size.

Balloon preparation. Once a diagnosis of mitral stenosis
is confirmed after successful transseptal puncture, the balloon
catheter can be prepared. The balloon catheter comes packaged with all of the components necessary for the balloon
dilatation procedure. These include:

1. A rigid, 14F plastic dilator
2. A 0.025-in. spring-tip exchange guidewire
3. A balloon stretching tube
4. Calipers for measuring balloon diameter
5. A calibrated inflation syringe for the balloon
6. A stylet for manipulating the balloon across the mitral
   valve after it has been placed in the left atrium

The balloon catheter lumen is flushed with saline. Dilute
contrast (4 saline : 1 contrast) is injected through the blue vent
lumen to purge air from the inflate/deflate channel to the
balloon and the stopcock is closed on the vent lumen.

The precalibrated balloon inflation syringe is filled to the
calibration corresponding to the smallest inflated diameter
(for a nominal 28-mm balloon, this would be 24 mm in diameter).

After connecting the inflation syringe to the inflation port
and checking that all connections are secure, the balloon is
slowly inflated over a period of 10 to 20 sec so that the nylon
mesh may be slowly stretched without risking rupture.

is allowed to deflate passively in a bath of ... . Small bubbles will escape from within the ...r of the balloon. The balloon is then inflated rapidly, ...e inflated diameter is measured using calipers to verify ...t the precalibrated inflation syringe achieves the correct minimum inflated diameter. If the balloon does not inflate to the desired diameter, small amounts of contrast are added or subtracted to achieve proper calibration.

The syringe is then filled to the calibration corresponding to maximal nominal inflated size. The balloon may be tested to ensure that the maximum-size calibration is also correct.

The next step in balloon preparation is to stretch the balloon catheter along its long axis, causing it to become more slender. A metal tube (balloon stretching tube) is inserted into the center lumen of the balloon over the guidewire and advanced until it locks into the metal hub at the proximal end of the balloon. The hub and slenderizing tube are then advanced into the balloon catheter until they engage the plastic luer lock. This leaves the balloon in its elongated, slenderized form to ease not only percutaneous insertion but also delivery across the interatrial septum.

Balloon valvotomy. The major steps in the valvotomy procedure are illustrated schematically in Fig. 12-4. The 0.025-in. spring guidewire is advanced through the Mullins sheath into the left atrium with the full coiled distal portion out of the sheath and positioned in the roof of the atrium.

The Mullins sheath is withdrawn with the guidewire remaining in the left atrium. The 14F dilator is advanced through the skin and then to the atrial septum, where it may be passed through the septal puncture (Fig. 12-5).

The dilator is removed and the balloon catheter passed over the guidewire directly through the skin and across the atrial septum. Resistance at the skin is common but may be overcome most of the time by twisting the balloon catheter so that the angled tip finds its way through the subcutaneous tissues. Care must be taken not to unlock the metal luer lock connection. Lubricating the balloon with water before passing through the skin is sometimes helpful, as is a posteriorly directed insertion angle. A 14F sheath may be used if direct insertion is not feasible.

As the balloon is passed through the atrial septum, it must be allowed to resume its unstretched conformation to prevent

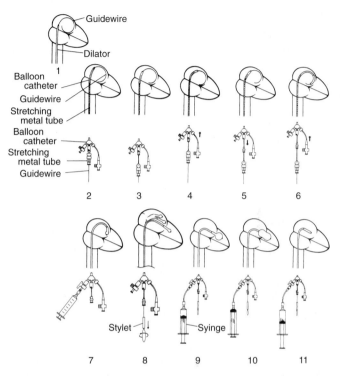

Fig. 12-4. Schematic illustration of the Inoue balloon mitral valvotomy procedure. (1) After a spring guidewire is introduced via a Mullins sheath into the left atrium, the interatrial septum is dilated using a rigid 14F plastic dilator. (2) The elongated balloon catheter is advanced over the wire through the interatrial septum. (3) The stretching metal tube is partially withdrawn, allowing the balloon to shorten and curl within the left atrium. (4) The balloon is advanced through the interatrial septum. (5) The stretching metal tube and balloon straightening device are withdrawn further. (6) The balloon is advanced beyond the mitral orifice. (7) The distal portion of the balloon is partially inflated with a contrast–saline mixture. (8) With counterclockwise rotation of the stylet, slight advancement of the catheter shaft, and withdrawal of the stylet, the balloon is directed through the mitral orifice and left ventricle. (9) The partially inflated balloon is withdrawn against the mitral orifice. (10) The balloon is fully and rapidly inflated and allowed to deflate. (11) After deflation, in most instances, the balloon passively returns to the left atrium from the left ventricle. (From Toray, Inc., Tokyo, Japan.)

the very stiff slenderizing tube from puncturing the roof of the left atrium. In some cases the blunt tip of the balloon will catch on the right atrial side of the septal puncture. Rotating the catheter slowly with gentle probing pressure will allow it to find its way through the septal puncture into the left atrium. After the tip of the balloon has passed across the atrial septum, the stretching metal tube is disengaged from the catheter metal hub and withdrawn as the balloon catheter is advanced. The tip of the balloon will then begin to track

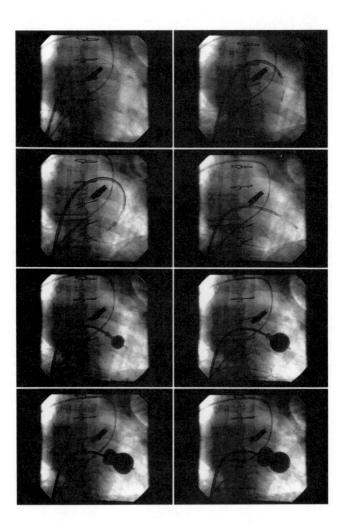

around the coiled spring guidewire. As the balloon reaches the roof of the left atrium, the plastic luer lock is disconnected, allowing the balloon to shorten as it enters the left atrium. The balloon catheter is then advanced over the spring-tipped guidewire. The balloon stretching tube and spring guidewire are removed from the patient, and cleaned and prepared for later use to remove the balloon.

The balloon catheter can then be flushed and connected to a pressure transducer. The transmitral pressure gradient can be remeasured through the balloon catheter to verify that the pressure waveform is similar to that obtained through the Mullin sheath. The waveform may appear slightly damped through the lumen of the Inoue balloon.

Before crossing the mitral valve with the balloon, it is useful to change the x-ray projection from A-P to 20° to 30° right anterior oblique.

Fig. 12-5.   The major steps in PTMC. *Upper left,* A 14F dilator is advanced over a spring-coiled guidewire. The guidewire has been introduced into the left atrium via a transseptal puncture. The 14F dilator dilates both the subcutaneous tissue at the groin catheter insertion site and the left atrial puncture. A prosthetic aortic valve marks the location of the aortic root. A pulmonary artery catheter traverses the right atrium, right ventricular outflow, and pulmonary artery. *Upper right,* The uninflated balloon catheter has been introduced over the course of the spring wire. The wire has been removed. The tip of the catheter overlays the mitral orifice. *Left second from top,* The tip of the balloon catheter is partially inflated so that it may be manipulated across the mitral valve using a steering stylet. This is analogous to crossing the tricuspid valve from the right atrium to the right ventricle using a flow-directed balloon tip catheter. *Second upper right,* The uninflated balloon is now in the left ventricular apex. *Left third from top,* The front portion of the balloon has been inflated and pulled back until it engages the mitral valve orifice. *Third from top right,* The balloon is inflated further. *Bottom left,* Additional inflation of the balloon causes the proximal portion to inflate leaving a waist in the middle. *Bottom right,* Full inflation of the balloon results in expansion of the center of the balloon, splitting the fused mitral commissures.

Passing the Inoue balloon from the left atrium to the left ventricle is analogous to passing a pulmonary artery balloon flotation catheter from the right atrium into the right ventricle. The steering stylet is introduced into the shaft of the balloon catheter. The distal portion of the balloon is inflated with a small amount of dilute contrast. The stylet, and if necessary the balloon catheter shaft, is rotated in a counterclockwise direction to bring the tip anterior toward the mitral orifice. Once again, care must be taken not to twist or rotate the metal luer lock. The stylet does most of the work, and ordinarily must be rotated 180°.

As the balloon passes across the mitral valve orifice, the stylet is withdrawn about 5 to 10 cm. The balloon catheter must be advanced gently and moved forward and backward to be sure that it is free of entanglements in the subvalvular apparatus.

The stylet may be bent to facilitate passage of the balloon across the mitral valve (Fig. 12-6).

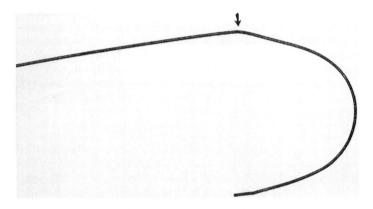

Fig. 12-6.   The arrow denotes an angulation placed in the curve of the steering stylet, used to direct the balloon catheter from the left atrium across the mitral valve into the left ventricle. When the septal puncture is high or the left atrium is very large, this angulation will facilitate crossing the mitral valve. (From Feldman T, Herrmann HC, Inoue K: Technique of percutaneous transvenous mitral commissurotomy using the Inoue balloon catheter, *Cathet Cardiovasc Diagn Suppl* 2:26-34, 1994.)

The distal half of the balloon is fully inflated and gently withdrawn until the mitral valve is engaged. The proximal half of the balloon is inflated, and when the position of the balloon appears correct, full inflation is achieved. The entire cycle of inflation and deflation takes 5 sec or less and it is unusual for patients to sense the inflation, as frequent ventricular ectopy does not usually occur and hypotension persists for no more than a few cardiac cycles.

As the balloon deflates, it usually falls back into the left atrium with no specific manipulation. If it does not, a gentle clockwise rotation of the balloon catheter will move the balloon catheter back in the left atrium. The stylet is withdrawn and the balloon shaft connected to a pressure transducer for reassessment of the transmitral gradient. A Doppler/echo examination is performed to evaluate any change in mitral regurgitation and to assess whether either fused commissure has been opened.

Stepwise balloon inflation.   If a transmitral gradient persists and no significant increase in mitral regurgitation has occurred, another balloon inflation is performed at an inflated diameter 1 mm greater than the preceding inflation (Fig. 12-7). This sequence is repeated until either an increase in mitral regurgitation or a sufficient decrease in the transmitral gradient occurs. Balloons can be overinflated by 1 to 2 mm diameter by using an additional 1 to 2 cc's inflation volume above the maximal calibrated balloon size. If sufficient reduction in gradient is not achieved after maximal or supermaximal inflation, a larger-size balloon can be utilized.

It is very useful to monitor the effect of each balloon inflation on the mitral valve by echocardiography in the catheterization laboratory. An in-lab Doppler exam will demonstrate whether mitral regurgitation has increased. More important, the short-axis two-dimensional examination will demonstrate the degree of commissural separation (Fig. 12-8). Note the degree of commissural fusion on the short-axis exam before balloon dilatation. Separation of one commissure while the other remains fused will facilitate the decision to proceed with further balloon inflations. If mitral regurgitation has not worsened, attempt to complete the commissurotomy. Conversely, if one commissure has opened completely and a significant amount of mitral regurgitation has developed, this will signify at least an adequate result.

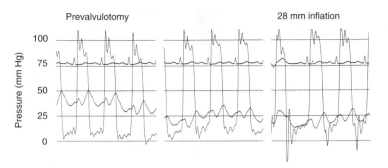

Fig. 12-7. Stepwise dilatations result in a progressive decline in left atrial pressure and transmitral pressure gradient. In the prevalvulotomy tracing, the mean left atrial pressure is well over 25 mmHg and the gradient is extreme. After a 27-mm-diameter balloon inflation, the transmitral gradient and left atrial pressure have declined significantly. On the right, after only one additional millimeter increment in inflated balloon diameter, there is dramatic improvement in the transmitral gradient. (From Feldman T, Herrmann HC, Inoue K: Technique of percutaneous transvenous mitral commissurotomy using the Inoue balloon catheter, *Cathet Cardiovasc Diagn Suppl* 2:26-34, 1994.)

A useful observation during balloon inflation is the "popping sign" denoting splitting of one or both commissures. During the final portion of the inflation one observes the inferior or superior margin of the mid-balloon suddenly popping out. This is a welcome sign that heralds a clear decrease in gradient due to the occurrence of a true commissurotomy. The transmitral pressure gradient is the simplest parameter to monitor between balloon inflations. The absolute level of left atrial pressure is extremely important as well. In general, if the left atrial pressure remains constant or decreases after successive balloon inflations, mitral regurgitation has not yet become limiting. When the mean left atrial pressure rises following a balloon inflation, even if a large V-wave has not occurred, mitral regurgitation may have worsened significantly. If in-lab echocardiography is not available, a repeat left ventriculogram should be done.

Decisions to proceed with further balloon inflations are among the most difficult to make. Use of all available informa-

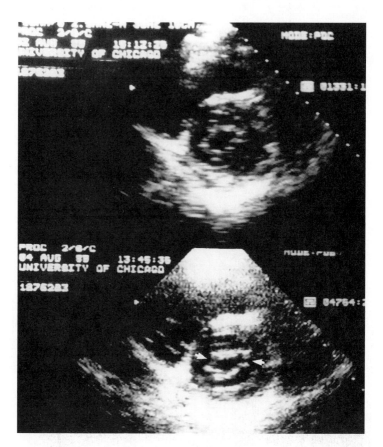

Fig. 12-8. Short-axis echocardiogram illustrating commissural splitting following balloon dilatation. *Upper panel,* Fishmouth orifice of the mitral valve. *Lower panel,* Bilateral commissural splitting, indicated by solid white arrows. (From Feldman T, Carroll JD: Cardiac catheterization, balloon angioplasty, and percutaneous valvuloplasty, in Hall JB, Schmidt GA, Wood LDH, editors: *Principles of critical care,* New York, 1992, McGraw-Hill, pp 343-360.)

tion, including two-dimensional and Doppler echocardiography, left atrial pressure level and waveform (Fig. 12-9), auscultation, and ventriculography, is important.

Technical considerations. If the interatrial septum is crossed in a relatively superior or anterior location, passing the balloon across the mitral valve may be difficult. In this

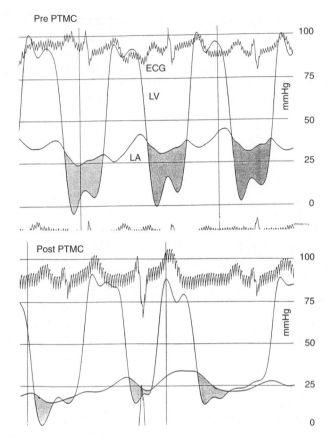

Fig. 12-9. Pre- and post-PBMC transmitral valve pressure gradients. In addition to evaluating the transmitral gradient, it is important to consider the magnitude of left atrial pressure and changes in left ventricular filling pressure. In this case, post-PBMC there is only a modest decline in left atrial pressure. Left ventricular filling pressure has risen significantly. In addition, the atrial fibrillation heart rate becomes irregular. These factors all can make evaluation of the success of a PTMC procedure difficult.

circumstance, clockwise rather than counterclockwise rotation of the stylet will "bounce" the balloon off the posterior atrial wall and allow it to cross into the left ventricle after making a loop (Fig. 12-10). This alternative approach is sometimes limited by the short length of the balloon catheter shaft.

In the event that the balloon is withdrawn toward the septal puncture during manipulations to cross the mitral valve, it is sometimes necessary to reinsert the coiled spring-tipped guidewire into the left atrium to be able to advance the balloon toward the mitral valve. This is especially true when the septum is markedly thickened and septal dilatation does not result in free movement of the balloon catheter shaft through the atrial septum.

Occasionally the catheter shaft may be seen to be pinched or bound by the atrial septum. Advancing the shaft of the catheter may cause it to buckle in the right atrium without causing the balloon to move forward in the left atrium toward the mitral valve. Redilatation of the interatrial septum with a 14F dilator, or even with a 6- or 8-mm peripheral arterial balloon, may sometimes be necessary.

Free movement of the balloon can be impaired by binding in the subcutaneous tissues at the groin puncture site. In very heavy patients the catheter may make a severe angle between the skin and the femoral vein. The use of a 14F sheath in these situations will greatly facilitate accomplishment of the procedure.

Post-PTMC evaluation and balloon withdrawal. Following dilatation, a left ventriculogram is repeated to evaluate mitral regurgitation. Cardiac output measurement is repeated while the balloon catheter remains across the interatrial septum. This is important because withdrawal of the balloon catheter will allow some shunt flow across the atrial septal puncture site and increase the cardiac output. This has been demonstrated to yield valve area results that are falsely elevated.

The balloon catheter must then be withdrawn across the atrial septum. This is accomplished by reintroducing the balloon stretching tube, which has been preloaded with the 0.025-in. spring-tipped guidewire. The guidewire is advanced and curled in the left atrium. The balloon stretching tube is then locked to the metal hub of the balloon catheter. These two metal units are then advanced together into the plastic luer lock to stretch the balloon. Special care must be taken not to stretch and stiffen the balloon through the roof of the

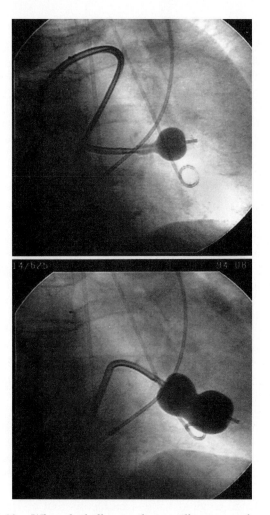

Fig. 12-10. When the balloon catheter will not cross the mitral valve using the conventional method, the catheter may be rotated clockwise and manipulated across the mitral valve using an alternative approach. The balloon is introduced into the left atrium in the usual manner and guided past the mitral orifice. With clockwise rotation of the stylet and catheter shaft, a loop is made directing the balloon off the posterior left atrial wall (*upper panel*). Withdrawal of the stylet and advancement of the catheter shaft direct the balloon catheter across the mitral valve into the left ventricle (*lower panel*).

left atrium. This is best accomplished by withdrawing the balloon backward onto the stretching metal tube and then withdrawing the plastic luer lock onto the assembled metal hub apparatus. The balloon catheter is thus pulled back across the atrial septum as it is stretched and elongated. The balloon and wire can then be withdrawn from the left atrium. The wire is best removed while the stretched balloon is part way across the septum to avoid any "slicing" action of the wire on the septal puncture, which could enlarge the septal defect. The balloon can be left in the inferior vena cava until it is ready to be withdrawn. Replace it with an 11 or 12 French sheath to facilitate patient movement and sheath removal. Finally, oximetry is repeated to evaluate left-to-right shunting across the atrial septal puncture site.

Atrial shunting.   Following double-balloon mitral valvotomy, some left-to-right shunting results in a spurious increase in cardiac output and artificially increased Gorlin mitral valve area calculation. Because the final cardiac output measurements after Inoue balloon PTMC are made while the 11.5F shaft of the Inoue catheter remains across the atrial septal puncture, the magnitude of spurious increase in Gorlin calculated mitral valve area is insignificant. Thus, use of a small balloon catheter to occlude the interatrial septum following balloon dilatation is not necessary for accurate post-PTMC valve area measurements.

Recognition and Management of Complications

The two most serious complications of PTMC are cardiac tamponade and acute mitral regurgitation. The recognition of pericardial tamponade requires a high degree of suspicion on an ongoing basis. It is very important to assess any chest, shoulder, or back pain of which a patient may complain during the procedure. Continuous attention to the pulsatile fluoroscopic cardiac borders is important. Make use of right heart pressures as well. Intraprocedure echocardiography is essential when the patient is hemodynamically unstable. It is not reasonable to perform PTMC without the ability to perform pericardiocentesis as well.

Acute mitral regurgitation is easily recognized by the left atrial pressure magnitude and waveform. It occurs in some cases with a single balloon inflation, or after even a $\frac{1}{2}$-mm-diameter increment in balloon inflation size. Confirmation of the diagnosis with ventriculography is important. Nitroprusside therapy is the mainstay of immediate management. One percent to 2% of patients undergoing PTMC will develop severe mitral regurgitation as a result of the procedure.

Postprocedure Care and Sheath Removal

A 5F arterial sheath and the large venous sheath do not require any special management. Sheaths may be removed when the activated clotting time falls below 180 sec. Younger patients with excellent hemodynamic results can be sent home on an outpatient basis at the end of the day of the procedure. For patients who require coumadin therapy, it is our usual practice to reinstitute coumadin therapy 1 or 2 days post-PTMC without a loading dose. In patients at special risk for thrombosis or a history of prior thrombotic episodes, heparin therapy following sheath removal and a transition to coumadin therapy may be necessary.

AORTIC VALVULOPLASTY
Background

Balloon aortic valvuloplasty showed great promise as an alternative to surgical aortic valve replacement when the procedure was initially described. Balloon dilatation of the aortic valve results in an immediate increase in the aortic valve area, with the expected fall in transvalve pressure gradient and a rise in cardiac output. Most patients show immediate clinical improvement. This is accomplished using a percutaneous procedure with substantially less morbidity than valve replacement surgery. Unfortunately, it was quickly discovered that the durability of these results is short-lived. Disappointment with the clinical results of this procedure over a 1- to 2-year follow-up period resulted in a pendulumlike movement away from the performance of balloon aortic valvuloplasty. However, a number of important clinical indications still exist for this procedure.

Indications

There are currently five clinical situations in which balloon aortic valvuloplasty is useful (see the accompanying box). First, patients who present with aortic stenosis and cardio-

Current Indications for Balloon Aortic Valvuloplasty

---

1. Cardiogenic shock/pre-op for aortic valve replacement (AVR)
2. Severe LV failure/bridge to AVR
3. Prior to major noncardiac surgery
4. To allow discharge of hospital-bound patients
5. Diagnostic test for low-gradient, low-output AS with poor LV function in consideration of surgery

---

genic shock may be stabilized for the short term. Balloon dilatation can be accomplished with diagnostic catheterization, and further decisions regarding therapy can be made after the patient has stabilized. Second, in patients with severe left ventricular dysfunction or shock in whom aortic valve replacement is planned, balloon dilatation may be performed to allow improvement in left ventricular performance before surgery. This can reduce a major co-morbid factor for valve replacement surgery, because left ventricular function is directly associated with surgical mortality. In addition, in these patients it is usual for the prerenal azotemia associated with their medical therapy to improve. Third, patients found to have aortic stenosis in the evaluation for major noncardiac surgery may undergo balloon dilatation. This is especially useful for patients with malignancies. Fourth, patients who are hospital bound with severe aortic stenosis, and who are not candidates for valve replacement surgery, may undergo balloon dilatation with a successful short-term improvement. This is useful for patients who are dependant on intravenous pressors in an ICU. Although valvuloplasty does not improve their long-term prognosis, it may allow them to be discharged from the hospital so that they may have some better quality of life.

Last are patients in whom balloon valvuloplasty may be performed as a diagnostic test. This is useful when the valve area is between 0.8 and 1.0 cm^2 with low cardiac output and low transvalve pressure gradient. In this group of patients the severity of valvular stenosis is especially difficult to ascertain. Poor ventricular function has made therapy in this group difficult. In the past, valve replacement could be performed, and if the patient showed improvement in ventricular function, then survival was good. Unfortunately, for those patients who do not show improvement in LV performance, perioperative mortality is high. Balloon dilatation may be performed and serial echocardiography used to monitor any changes in left ventricular function. If symptoms and left ventricular performance improve with opening of the aortic valve, valve replacement surgery can be undertaken with a high expectation of long-term success.

Prosthetic Aortic Valves

In-vitro evaluation of balloon dilatation for stenotic bioprosthetic valves has been very disappointing. Prosthetic tissue is often very friable, and frequently not severely calcified. The potential for leaflet perforation or avulsion is significant.

Results of Balloon Dilatation for Aortic Stenosis

Aortic valve area usually increases between 80% and 100%. The transvalve pressure gradient declines by more than 50%. Postdilatation valve areas range between 0.7 cm^2 and 1.1 cm^2. An increase in valve area from ≤ 0.5 cm^2 to >0.7 cm^2 will be associated with a dramatic clinical improvement. Predilatation valve areas >0.5 cm^2 may ultimately yield postdilatation valve areas of 1.0 cm^2 or more. It is notable that prosthetic aortic valves have an area between 0.9 and 1.2 cm^2, especially in the substantial subpopulation of aortic stenosis patients who are small women with small aortic annuli. Though substantially less than the normal 2.5- to 4-cm^2 valve area, these prostheses provide adequate hemodynamics even though prosthetic valve patient mismatch syndromes are still seen occasionally.

The greatest limitation of this procedure is the almost inevitable occurrence of restenosis following dilatation. The majority of patients have anatomic and symptomatic restenosis between 6 and 18 months after the procedure. Survival is not clearly improved by balloon aortic valvuloplasty. The mechanism of restenosis may be related to the mechanism of relief of aortic stenosis. A majority of these elderly patients have calcific trileaflet aortic stenosis with calcification and thickening of the valve cusps and no commissural fusion. The calcium deposits are nodular when viewed grossly. Histologically, the nodules are densely encased in fibrous tissue. This explains the striking lack of embolization during this procedure. After balloon dilatation, small fractures or cracks may be seen in the calcific nodules. This allows increased leaflet mobility due to the presence of many "hinge points" or fissures. The restenosis process involves regrowth of granulation tissue, fibrosis, and possibly true ossification of these fissures. This active process of restenosis follows a time course that is consistent with new scar formation.

Technique

In most cases, diagnostic coronary arteriography and ventriculography are performed immediately before balloon dilatation. It is unusual to encounter a new patient with aortic stenosis who has not had adequate echocardiographic evaluation before catheterization. Single-session diagnostic and therapeutic catheterization procedures may decrease morbidity in this very ill population.

Arterial access.   It is important to place the femoral puncture comparatively high (cranial) so that the large sheath necessary for valvuloplasty will not be inserted into a branch vessel. Before placing a sheath over the initial arterial wire, it is our practice to examine the course of the wire fluoroscopically. If the ilio-femoral system is extremely tortuous, we may pass a wire on the contralateral side and choose the straighter course for sheath placement and the eventual passage of the balloon. Lower abdominal angiography may be helpful. Specialized catheters can facilitate crossing the stenotic valve rapidly.

Heparin.   Heparinization is recommended at a dose of 5000 units for the average-size person. Supplemental doses will only be necessary for prolonged procedures. Early sheath removal is an important goal. Excessive anticoagulation is to be avoided.

Balloon catheter placement.   After the transvalve gradient and cardiac output determinations confirm the presence of severe aortic stenosis, the arterial sheath is exchanged for a 12.5F sheath. This exchange is performed over an extra-stiff 0.038-in. guidewire to minimize the chance of the large arterial dilator perforating the iliac vessels. The sheath is exchanged over a 360-cm extra-stiff wire that is left curled in the left ventricular apex. To maximize the safety of the tip of this wire in the left ventricle, a "ram's horn" curve is put on the end of the guidewire (Fig. 12-11). This is done by grasping the wire between the thumb and the edge of a curved hemostat and pulling along the wire rapidly in the same manner one uses to put a curl on gift-wrapping ribbon. After the sheath is exchanged, flushed, and connected to arterial pressure monitoring, a 20-mm-diameter by 5.5-cm-long aortic valvuloplasty catheter (Mansfield, Inc., Watertown, Mass.) is passed over the wire and across the aortic valve.

Balloon inflation.   The technique of balloon inflation in the aortic valve is especially important. The balloon is positioned midway across the valve. When ventricular function is poor, maintaining balloon position is very simple. A dynamic or vigorous left ventricle will typically eject the balloon during attempts to inflate it. Substantial forward pressure

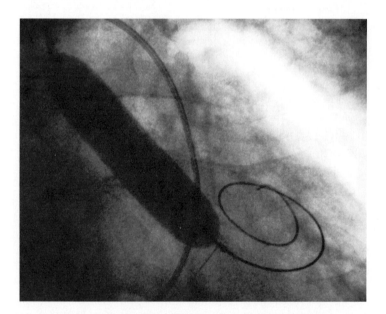

Fig. 12-11.   A 5.5-cm-long, 20-mm-diameter Mansfield aortic valvuloplasty catheter. The extra-support exchange guidewire has been looped into a ram's horn configuration by pulling it over the end of a hemostat as one would curl ribbon when wrapping a package.

may be necessary to maintain the position of the balloon in the valve in that case. Initially the balloon is inflated via a high-pressure stopcock using a 60-cc syringe partially filled with dilute saline contrast mixture. The diluted mix (7 parts of saline to 1 part contrast) minimizes the viscosity of the solution while at the same time maintaining fluoroscopic visibility. A 10-cc syringe filled with contrast mixture is placed on the side arm of the high-pressure stopcock used for inflating the balloon. After the 60-cc syringe has been used to inflate the balloon as much as possible, the operator flips the stopcock so that the smaller syringe can be used to inject additional saline contrast mixture under very high pressure. This "boost" in inflation is very important to achieve maximal balloon expansion. The balloon can be appreciated to fully expand or "plump" out along its sides when this is done. Adequate valve dilatation is usually not achieved unless this can be accomplished. Hypotension and ventricular tachycardia are usual during inflations (Fig. 12-12). Therefore, as soon as balloon deflation commences, the balloon can be pulled back in the aortic root while maintaining the guidewire in the left ventricle.

One balloon inflation is performed without boosting to determine how well the patient will tolerate inflations. A second inflation is performed to maximal balloon inflation (Fig. 12-13). If the balloon has not ruptured, a third inflation is performed with the intent of rupturing the balloon. It is thus very important to prepare the balloon very carefully and to be sure that no small air bubbles remain during test inflations outside the body. After maximal inflation or balloon rupture, the balloon is withdrawn over the guidewire and the balloon and sheath are removed together as a unit. The ruptured balloon material is often hard to get all the way back into the sheath. Pulling too hard will tear off the end of the balloon shaft. Frequently the balloon is pulled into the sheath until resistance is substantial and the sheath is close to being folded. The combined catheter and sheath are removed as a unit. A new sheath is then introduced over the wire, and then a diagnostic pigtail catheter is inserted over the wire into the left ventricle to evaluate the final valvuloplasty result.

Procedural end point. If the transvalve gradient has fallen by 50% or more, and if the cardiac output is at least

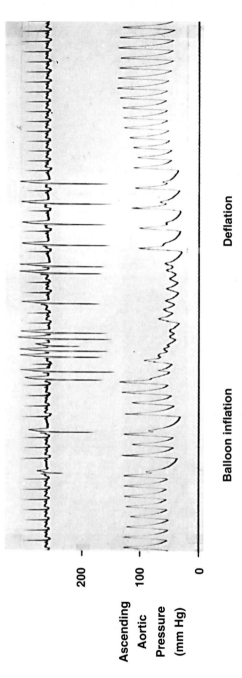

Aortic valvuloplasty

Ascending
Aortic
Pressure
(mm Hg)

200 —

100 —

0 —

Balloon inflation

Deflation

Fig. 12-12.   Hemodynamic tracing during balloon inflation in a patient undergoing aortic valvuloplasty. Ventricular tachycardia and hypotension are usual during balloon inflations. (From Feldman T, Carroll JD: Cardiac catheterization, balloon angioplasty, and percutaneous valvuloplasty, in Hall JB, Schmidt GA, Wood LDH, editors: *Principles of critical care,* New York, 1992, McGraw-Hill, pp 343-360.)

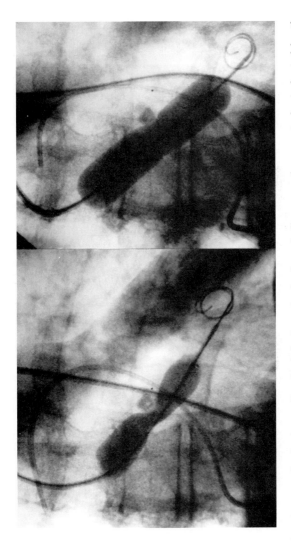

Fig. 12-13. Aortic valvuloplasty. On the left the valvuloplasty balloon can be seen to be indented by the calcified aortic valve leaflets. On the right the indentation has expanded as the calcific nodules in the rigid valve leaflets have been fractured. (From Feldman T, Carroll JD: Cardiac catheterization, balloon angioplasty, and percutaneous valvuloplasty, in Hall JB, Schmidt GA, Wood LDH, editors: *Principles of critical care*, New York, 1992, McGraw-Hill, pp 343-360.)

unchanged or has risen, successful valve dilatation has been accomplished (Fig. 12-14). In some cases, evaluation of valve resistance is helpful (Fig. 12-15). Resistance over 250 dynes-sec-cm^{-5} is consistent with persistent stenosis, while values below 200 dynes-sec-cm^{-5} signify relief of obstruction. Infrequently, it is necessary to size up to a 14F arterial sheath so that a 23-mm-diameter balloon can be used. A 23-mm balloon is commercially available, but it is only 3 cm in length. This is insufficient for aortic dilatation, so we keep special-order 4-cm-long $\times$ 23-mm-diameter balloons available for this purpose.

Sheath removal and postprocedure management. Heparin, 5000 units, is given during the procedure, and then none afterward. Antibiotic prophylaxis is not used for these procedures. The sheaths are removed as soon as the activated clotting time falls below 180 sec. After hemostasis has been achieved, a 10-lb sandbag is left on the groin for 6 hr, and then patients are allowed to sit up. A few hours later they are gradually ambulated. Most patients who are not in critical condition before the procedure are able to leave the hospital on the morning following balloon aortic valvuloplasty. It is

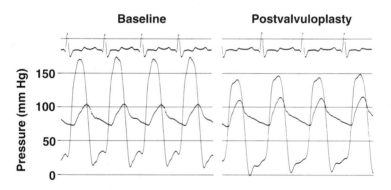

Fig. 12-14.   Pre- and postaortic valvuloplasty pressure tracings. Not only has there been a marked decline in the transaortic pressure gradient, aortic pressure has risen and left ventricular systolic pressure has fallen. The upstroke of the aortic pressure wave has become deeper. The left ventricular end-diastolic pressure has fallen. This 64-year-old man had an increase in valve area from 0.5 cm^2 to 1.0 cm^2.

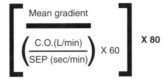

Fig. 12-15. Calculation of valve resistance (dynes/sec/cm^{-5}) may be very helpful in evaluating patients before and after aortic valvuloplasty. (From Kern MJ, Deligonul U, Donohue T, Caracciolo E, Feldman T: Hemodynamic data, in *The cardiac catheterization handbook,* St. Louis, 1994, Mosby, p 124.)

important to obtain a postprocedure echocardiogram prior to hospital discharge, so that serial comparisons can be made.

Complications

The major complications of aortic balloon valvuloplasty are ventricular perforation from the catheter or guidewires used in the left ventricle, and femoral arterial complications related to the large sheath size necessary. Cardiac tamponade from catheter perforation has been reported in about 1% of cases. Vascular surgery for femoral arterial complications is required in as many as 5% of patients. Significant hematomas occur in up to 10% of patients, and transfusion rates in some series are as high as 20%. Since the balloon catheter abrades the ventricular septum during balloon inflations, bundle branch block may occur that requires pacing in some cases, and rarely, permanent pacemaker implantation. Severe aortic regurgitation is infrequent. Leaflet avulsion may occur, usually with oversized balloons. Aortic valvuloplasty in the setting of regurgitation as the predominant valve lesion will not result in improvement. Rarely, a progressive low-output state has been reported after valvuloplasty, frequently ending in death. Each "therapeutic" balloon inflation causes a transient but substantial stress on the left ventricle. Outflow obstruction is acutely worsened, chamber dilatation occurs, ventricular pressure generation decreases, and coronary perfusion pressure drops. Several technical factors probably cause this disastrous syndrome. First, inadequate valve dilatation occurs, often from inability to position the balloon properly. Second, repeated inflations may be excessively prolonged. Third, ventricular tachycardia may contribute to left ventricular depression. And finally, a "rest" period between inflations of several minutes is needed. During this rest period one should observe a rebound in aortic pressure, resolution of any ischemic ECG changes, and resolution of any symptoms that occurred during the inflations.

Bicuspid aortic valves may resist dilatation more than degenerative tricuspid valves.

SUMMARY

Mitral stenosis can be treated successfully with PTMC with good long-term results and an acceptably low complication rate.

Aortic balloon valvuloplasty is reserved for selected patients at high risk of death from aortic stenosis or those who require a bridge to surgery or temporary relief for other medical treatment.

SUGGESTED READINGS

A report from the National Heart, Lung and Blood Institute: Balloon valvuloplasty registry: complications and mortality of percutaneous balloon mitral commissurotomy, *Circulation* 85:2014-2024, 1992.

Al Zaibag M, Al Kasab S, Ribeiro PA, Al-Fagih MR: Percutaneous double-balloon mitral valvotomy for rheumatic mitral valve stenosis, *Lancet* 757-761, April 5, 1986.

Babic U, Pejcic P, Djurisic Z, Vucinic M, Grujicic SM: Percutaneous transarterial balloon valvuloplasty for mitral valve stenosis, *Am J Cardiol* 57:1101-1104, 1986.

Bernard Y, Etievent J, Mourand JL, et al.: Long-term results of percutaneous aortic valvuloplasty compared with aortic valve replacement in patients more than 75 years old, *J Am Coll Cardiol* 20(4):796-801, Oct. 1992.

Carlson MD, Palacios I, Thomas JD, et al.: Cardiac conduction abnormalities during percutaneous balloon mitral or aortic valvotomy, *Circulation* 79(6):1197-1203, 1989.

Chen WJ, Chen MF, Liau CS, Wu CC, Lee YT: Safety of percutaneous transvenous balloon mitral commissurotomy in patients with mitral stenosis and thrombus in the left atrial appendage, *Am J Cardiol* 70:117-119, 1992.

Chow WH, Chow TC, Yip ASB, Cheung KL: Percutaneous balloon mitral valvotomy in patients with history of embolism, *Am J Cardiol* 71:1243-1244, 1993.

Cohen DJ, Kuntz RE, Gordon SPF, et al.: Predictors of long-term outcome after percutaneous balloon mitral valvuloplasty, *N Engl J Med* 327:1329-1335, 1992.

Cribier A, Remadi F, Koning R, Rath P, Stix G, Letac B: Emergency balloon valvuloplasty as initial treatment of patients with aortic stenosis and cardiogenic shock, *N Engl J Med* 326(9):646, 1992.

Feldman T: Hemodynamic results, clinical outcome, and complications of Inoue balloon mitral valvotomy, *Cathet Cardiovasc Diagn Suppl* 2:2-7, 1994.

Feldman T, Carroll JD, Herrmann HC, Holmes DR, Bashore TM, Isner JM: Effect of balloon size and stepwise inflation technique on the acute results of Inoue mitral commissurotomy, *Cathet Cardiovasc Diagn* 28:199-205, 1993.

Feldman T, Carroll JD, Herrman HC, et al.: N. American Inoue Investigation. Mitral regurgitation (not restenosis) is the most frequent indication for valve replacement after balloon mitral valvotomy, *J Am Coll Cardiol* 25:64A, 1995.

Feldman T, Glagov S, Carroll JD: Restenosis following successful balloon valvuloplasty: bone formation in aortic valve leaflets. *Cathet Cardiovasc Diagn* 29(1):1-7, 1993.

Feldman T, Herrmann HC, Carroll JD, et al.: N. American Inoue Investigation. Balloon valvotomy for non-ideal commissurotomy candidates, *J Am Coll Cardiol* 25:90A, 1995.

Feldman T, Herrmann HC, Inoue K: Technique of percutaneous transvenous mitral commissurotomy using the Inoue balloon catheter. *Cathet Cardiovasc Diagn Supp* 2:26-34, 1994.

Hung JS, Lin FC, Chiang CW: Successful percutaneous transvenous catheter balloon mitral commissurotomy after warfarin therapy and resolution of left atrial thrombus. *Am J Cardiol* 64:126-128, 1989.

Inoue K, Feldman T: Percutaneous transvenous mitral commissurotomy using the Inoue balloon catheter, *Cathet Cardiovasc Diagn* 28:119-125, 1993.

Isner JM: Acute catastrophic complications of balloon aortic valvuloplasty. The Mansfield Scientific Aortic Valvuloplasty Registry Investigators, *J Am Coll Cardiol* 17(6):1436-1444, 1991.

Lababidi Z, Wu JR, Walls JT: Percutaneous balloon aortic valvuloplasty: results in 23 patients, *Am J Cardiol* 53:194-197, 1984.

Lau KW, Hung JS: A simple balloon sizing method in Inoue balloon percutaneous transvenous mitral commissurotomy, *Cathet Cardiovasc Diagn* (in press).

Letac B, Crivier A, Koning R, Lefebvre E: Aortic stenosis in elderly patients aged 80 or older. Treatment by percutaneous balloon valvuloplasty in a series of 92 cases, *Circulation* 80(6):1514-1520, 1989.

Levin T, Feldman T, Carroll JD: Effect of atrial septal occlusion on mitral area after Inoue balloon valvotomy, *Cathet Cardiovasc Diagn* 29:88, 1993.

Lewin RF, Dorros G, King JF, Mathiak L: Percutaneous transluminal aortic valvuloplasty: acute outcome and follow-up of 125 patients, *J Am Coll Cardiol* 14(5):1210-1217, 1989.

Manga P, Singh S, Brandis S, Friedman B: Mitral valve area calculations immediately after percutaneous balloon mitral valvuloplasty: effect of atrial septal defect, *J Am Coll Cardiol* 21:1568-1573, 1993.

McKay CR, Kawanishi DT, Rahimtoola SH: Catheter balloon valvuloplasty of the mitral valve in adults using a double-balloon technique, *JAMA* 257:1753-1761, 1987.

McKay RG, Safian RD, Lock JE, et al.: Balloon dilatation of calcific aortic stenosis in elderly patients postmortem, intraoperative, and percutaneous valvuloplasty studies, *Circulation* 74:119-125, 1986.

Moreno PR, Jang IK, Newell JB, Block PC, Palacios IF: The role of percutaneous aortic balloon valvuloplasty in patients with cardiogenic shock and critical aortic stenosis, *J Am Coll Cardiol* 23(5):1071-1075, 1994.

Nishimura RA, Holmes DR Jr, Michela MA: Follow-up of patients with low output, low gradient hemodynamics after percutaneous balloon aortic valvuloplasty: the Mansfield Scientific Aortic Valvuloplasty Registry, *J Am Coll Cardiol* 17(3):828-833, 1991.

Otto CM, Mickel MC, Kennedy JW, et al.: Three year outcome after balloon aortic valvuloplasty. Insights into prognosis of valvular aortic stenosis, *Circulation* 89(2):642-650, 1994.

Percutaneous balloon aortic valvuloplasty. Acute and 30-day follow-up results in 674 patients from the NHLBI Balloon Valvuloplasty Registry, *Circulation* 84(6):2383-2397, 1991.

Petrossian GA, Tuzcu EM, Ziskind AA, Block PC, Palacios I: Atrial septal occlusion improves the accuracy of mitral valve area determination following percutaneous balloon mitral valvotomy, *Cathet Cardiovasc Diagn* 22:22-24, 1991.

Post JR, Feldman T, Isner J, Herrmann HC: Inoue balloon mitral valvotomy in patients with severe valvular and subvalvular deformity, *J Am Coll Cardiol* 25:1129-1136, 1995.

Safian RD, Berman AD, Diver DJ, et al.: Balloon aortic valvuloplasty in 170 consecutive patients, *N Engl J Med* 319(3):125-130, 1988.

Sherman W, Hershman R, Lazzam C, Cohen M, Ambrose J, Gorlin R: Balloon valvuloplasty in adult aortic stenosis: determinants of clinical outcome, *Ann Intern Med* 110(6):421-425, 1989.

The National Heart, Lung, and Blood Institute Balloon Valvuloplasty Registry Participants. Multicenter experience with balloon mitral commissurotomy: NHLBI balloon valvuloplasty registry report on immediate and 30-day follow-up results, *Circulation* 85:448-461, 1992.

Waller BF, McKay C, VanTassel J, Allen M: Catheter balloon valvuloplasty of stenotic porcine bioprosthetic valves: part II: mechanisms, complications, and recommendations for clinical use, *Clin Cardiol* 14(9):764-772, 1991.

13

PERICARDIOCENTESIS, BALLOON PERICARDIOTOMY, AND SPECIAL TECHNIQUES

Ted Feldman, John D. Carroll,
Andrew A. Ziskind, and
Morton J. Kern

PERICARDIOCENTESIS

Pericardiocentesis, required for management of acute pericardial effusions and cardiac tamponade, is a life-saving technique. A sufficient degree of operator skill must be employed to prevent further damage to the heart and pericardium. Unexplained hypotension during interventional procedures may be due to unobserved right ventricular (RV) perforation during pacing catheter placement or coronary perforation during angioplasty. Pericardiocentesis is an essential skill that should be acquired during the diagnostic training experience. A complete description of the technique is available in *The Cardiac Catheterization Handbook*. The technique is reviewed here in the context of coronary, valvular, and pericardial interventions.

Procedure

Pericardiocentesis often is preceded by echocardiographic confirmation of pericardial fluid. However, in interventional coronary cases in which tamponade is acute, echocardiography is not required and may be detrimental by delaying needed intervention. Although monitoring of pericardial pressure is not essential, evidence of cardiac tamponade and resolution of pericardial pressure restricting cardiac output are helpful. A long 16- or 18-gauge needle connected to a stopcock and tubing to a pressure transducer can be used. A standard 3.5-inch long, 18-gauge, thin-wall needle is usually sufficient.

Route to Pericardium

The preferred approach is the subxiphoid route, but other sites are acceptable depending on the location and volume of the effusion. The advantage of the subxiphoid approach is a decreased likelihood of coronary and internal thoracic artery laceration. In the acute setting, this approach is also easily identified and familiar to most operators.

Setup and Positioning

The patient is raised to a 30° to 45° head-up angle to permit pooling of pericardial fluid on the inferior surface of the heart. Local anesthesia is instilled through the pericardial needle as it is advanced initially perpendicularly to the skin and then at a sharp low angle (near parallel with horizontal plane) under the xiphoid toward the left shoulder. If the patient is obese, a larger needle and considerable force may be required to tip the syringe under the subxiphoid process toward the heart.

If access is available, a balloon-tipped catheter placed into the pulmonary artery via a femoral vein will assess equalization of diastolic right-sided pressures (and document the change with intervention). This catheter is withdrawn into the right atrium for pressure monitoring during pericardial puncture. Arterial pressure should be monitored closely.

Puncturing the Pericardium

Aspiration of the needle during passage through the skin may block the needle with subcutaneous tissue. Flush any tissue that may have accumulated before passing through the pericardium, a rigid fibrous membrane. A pericardial puncture feels similar to a lumbar puncture. Acute pericardial effusions during interventions are bloody, do not generally clot in the syringe, and have a lower hematocrit than intravascular blood.

Immediate confirmation that the needle tip has entered the pericardial space can be obtained by observing the pressure. Inadvertent right ventricular puncture can be recognized immediately. In cases of tamponade, pericardial pressure will resemble right atrial pressure. Hemodynamic monitoring is preferred over echo- or ECG-guided pericardiocentesis for its ease of application in the catheterization laboratory.

Once the needle is in the pericardial space, a 0.035-in. to 0.038-in. guidewire is inserted under fluoroscopic guidance high into the pericardial space and exchanged for a soft, multiple-side-hole plastic catheter (or sheath). Pericardial and right atrial pressures are measured. If there is a question as to the exact position of the needle or catheter, even after measuring the pressure, a small amount of radiographic contrast media may be injected. Contrast media pools in the dependent portion of the pericardial space, but will wash out of a vascular space rapidly if a cardiac chamber has been entered inadvertently.

Pericardial drainage catheters can be sutured in place and the output monitored while considerations for conservative or surgical management are made. RV and most coronary guidewire perforations can be managed conservatively, but reversal of heparin may cause PTCA vessel closure. Elective surgery for bypass may be a preferred option under these circumstances.

PERCUTANEOUS BALLOON PERICARDIOTOMY
Background

Treatment options for patients with cardiac tamponade include percutaneous catheterization or surgical drainage of the pericardial effusion. Reaccumulation of fluid with recurrence of cardiac tamponade has been reported in 15% to 50% of patients treated with catheter drainage. Creation of a "window" using operative techniques has been a traditional therapy in this setting. Recently, methods for creating such a window using balloon catheters have been described (Fig. 13-1). In-vitro studies have demonstrated that balloon dilatation creates a 1.5- to 2.0-cm hole in the pericardium.

Malignancy is the most frequent cause of pericardial effusion and tamponade. Cancer patients have a very short life

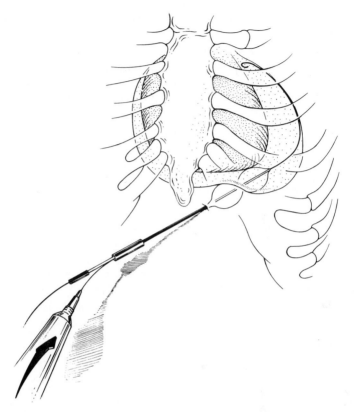

Fig. 13-1.   Schematic representation of percutaneous balloon pericardiotomy technique. (From Ziskin AA, Pearce AC, Lemmon CC, et al.: Percutaneous balloon pericardiotomy for the treatment of cardiac tamponade and large pericardial infusions: description of technique and report of the first 50 cases, *J Am Coll Cardiol* 21:1-5, 1993.)

expectancy and are often debilitated, making them poor candidates for surgical therapy. In addition, surgery may impair the quality of what remaining active life they have. Thus, the availability of a percutaneous method for pericardial drainage represents an important therapeutic option.

Patient Selection

Patients with large pericardial effusions who are felt to be at risk for tamponade are appropriate candidates for a balloon window. Contraindications include refractory coagulopathy, platelet dysfunction, thrombocytopenia with abnormal bleeding time, and clinical history suggestive of bacterial or fungal etiology of the effusion. Although malignancy is the major etiology in patients undergoing this procedure, some treated patients have had idiopathic, HIV-related, uremic, viral, hypothyroid, or posttraumatic effusions.

Patients with malignancy may be candidates for percutaneous balloon pericardiotomy (PBP) if they have undergone prior pericardiocentesis and have either persistent drainage (>100 ml/24 hr) or recurrent pericardial effusion after catheter removal. PBP may be offered as primary treatment at initial pericardiocentesis when the diagnosis of malignancy is clear.

Bleeding complications can occur in patients with coagulopathies or platelet disorders. Echocardiography should identify free pericardial fluid. Loculated effusions are best treated by surgery. Because left pleural effusions usually develop after PBP, patients with marginal pulmonary function should be evaluated carefully before undergoing the procedure.

Results

Results of percutaneous balloon pericardiotomy in 123 patients were reported from a national registry. Of these, 85% had malignancy as the underlying condition. Previous pericardiocentesis had been performed in 58%. Pericardial tamponade was the presenting problem in 72% of patients, whereas the remainder had large effusions. Balloon pericardiotomy was successful in 85%. Five (4%) patients were considered failures due to pericardial bleeding or persistent catheter drainage after the procedure. Recurrent pericardial effusion appeared in 10% of patients after a mean time of 54 days. Twelve of these 13 patients underwent surgical pericardial window, but 6 of these had recurrences. Thoracentesis or chest tube placement was required in 17% of patients with preexisting pleural effusions, and in 13% of patients without preexisting pleural effusions. Despite the short-term success of balloon window, the long-term survival for this group of patients was only 3 months.

Technique

Sedation. Liberal sedation is given, although caution should be used in patients in extremis from severe tamponade.

Antibiotics. For balloon pericardiotomy, prophylactic antibiotics are administered.

Pericardial puncture. Using a standard subxiphoid approach, special care must be taken not to make the needle insertion site too close to the inferior margin of the ribs. This will result in too sharp an angle for the wire and balloon catheter to turn from the skin to the pericardial space. Patients are placed on a 45° foam wedge. After local anesthesia to the skin, deeper anesthesia is given, because the passage of the balloon catheter causes significant discomfort. The pericardium is entered with an 18-gauge thin-wall needle. A 0.035-in. or 0.038-in. J-tip guidewire is advanced in the pericardial space and the needle is removed. The entry channel is dilated using an 8 or 9 French dilator. A straight pericardial drainage catheter with multiple side holes (Cook, Inc., Bloomington, Ind.) is placed in the pericardial space over the wire, and the wire is removed.

Hemodynamic measurements. Pericardial pressure is measured simultaneously with right atrial and right ventricular pressures (Fig. 13-2). Pericardial fluid is withdrawn for laboratory studies. Next, enough additional fluid to relieve hemodynamic evidence of pericardial tamponade is removed. It is important to leave at least 100 to 200 ml of fluid within the pericardium to provide a cushion of safety for balloon manipulation.

Balloon catheter insertion. If the patient has been elevated for the pericardial puncture, it is very important to remove the pillow or wedge before performing balloon pericardiotomy. If the patient is left sitting partially upright, an angulation is created between the lower margin of the ribs and the skin insertion site for the balloon. This makes passage of the balloon underneath the ribs very difficult. If the patient is placed supine before the balloon catheter is inserted, there is a much straighter path for the wire and the balloon to track over. A 0.038-in. extra-stiff J guidewire is then advanced into the pericardial space and placed in a generous-sized loop (Fig. 13-3). The pericardial catheter is removed and predilation performed with a 10F dilator, followed by a 20-mm-diameter × 3-cm-long Mansfield balloon catheter or a 26-mm Inoue balloon advanced over the guidewire to the pericardial membrane. Contrast can be injected into the pericardial space be-

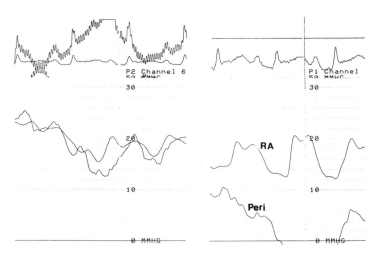

Fig. 13-2. On the left are simultaneous right atrial (RA) intra-pericardial (Peri) pressures from a patient with pericardial tamponade. On the right, following pericardiocentesis, the right atrial pressure remains above the zero line, while the pericardial pressure now shows respiratory variation with its nadir below zero.

fore passage of the balloon to make this position more identifiable.

Balloon inflation. Gentle inflation of the balloon may be helpful in locating the pericardial membrane (Figs. 13-4 and 13-5). When the location of the pericardium has been established by the appearance of a waist in the balloon, the balloon is inflated manually (Fig. 13-5). No more than two or three inflations are ordinarily required to be sure that a window has been created. Use of the Inoue balloon may facilitate positioning across the pericardium. If the pericardium is apposed to the chest wall, as indicated by failure of the proximal portion of the balloon to expand, a counter-traction technique can be used in which the catheter is firmly advanced while the skin is pulled in the opposite direction to isolate the pericardium for dilation (Fig. 13-6).

Balloon inflations are generally painful for the patient. After pericardiocentesis but before balloon pericardiotomy, we premedicate with intravenous analgesics. The balloon catheter is removed and the pericardial drainage catheter is

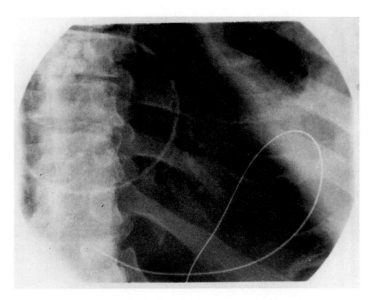

Fig. 13-3. Fluoroscopic image showing an extra-stiff guide-wire looped in the pericardium, outlining the pericardial space. Note that the silhouette defined by the wire is substantially wider than the border defined by the cardiac chambers.

replaced over the guidewire. X-ray contrast can be injected to demonstrate passage of pericardial fluid out of the pericardial space, into either the left chest or the abdomen. Any remaining fluid is drained from the pericardium. During the attempt at complete drainage it is very common for the patient to complain of typical pericardial pain. Forewarning the patient of this and giving adequate analgesics are important. The pericardial drain is connected to a collection bag.

The mechanism of PBP is tearing of the pericardium leading to a communication of the pericardial and pleural spaces. The use of a flexible fiber-optic pericardioscope introduced over a guidewire after PBP documents that a pericardial window communicates freely with the left pleural space (Fig. 13-7).

Postprocedure Management

Before the patient leaves the catheterization laboratory, a complete right heart catheterization is performed, including a

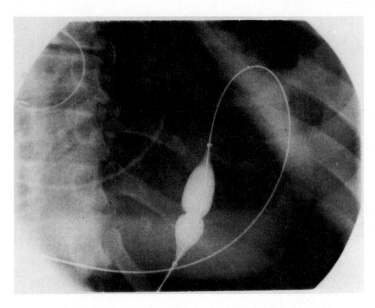

Fig. 13-4. Percutaneous balloon pericardiotomy: a 3-cm-long balloon is straddling the pericardial membrane. The membrane has indented the balloon.

cardiac output and recording of the final intrapericardial pressure. This has three substantial benefits. Postprocedure management of volume is clarified, the acute hemodynamic success of the procedure is proven, and residual hemodynamic abnormalities are evaluated. The incidence of effusive-constrictive pericardial syndrome is high in this patient population. A persistently elevated mean right atrial pressure of >10 mmHg with a 0 mmHg intrapericardial pressure suggests this syndrome. The pericardial catheter may be aspirated and flushed with 5 cc of heparinized saline every 6 hr to help maintain catheter patency. Antibiotics are administered while the drain is in place. When drainage decreases to less than 100 ml per day, the pericardial drain is removed. Usually this is within 24 to 48 hr, but occasionally substantial drainage may persist for a week and antiinflammatory medication may be useful. Echocardiography and chest x-rays are performed after the procedure to verify the results. Left pleural effusion may result from successful pericardial drainage and requires

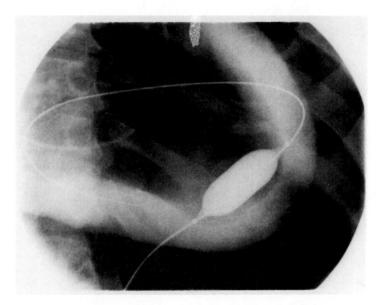

Fig. 13-5.   AP fluoroscopic images; 20 ml of radiographic contrast has been instilled into the pericardial space for illustration. A 0.038-in. guidewire has been advanced through the pigtail catheter and can be seen looping freely within the pericardial space. As the balloon is inflated manually, a waist is seen at the pericardial margin (Fig. 13-4). The waist disappears with full inflation of the balloon as the pericardial window is created.

thoracentesis or chest tube placement in some cases. Fever may occur after the procedure, and is often not attributable to any specific case.

Clinical Results

Multicenter registry data on 130 patients (Table 13-1) from 16 centers demonstrated that no recurrence of pericardial effusion on echocardiographic follow-up was present in 84% of patients at 5 ± 6 months. Five patients were failures due to bleeding and required surgery. Fever, a minor complication, occurred in 13%. No patient had bacteremia or positive pericardial cultures. Pleural effusions that required thoracentesis or chest tubes occurred in 17 patients, 12 with preexisting pleural effusions.

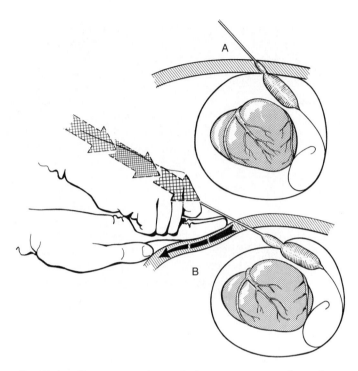

Fig. 13-6. Counter-traction technique to separate the epicardium from the adjacent chest wall (transverse view from below). **A,** Initial trial inflation of the balloon demonstrates trapping of the proximal portion of the balloon within the chest wall structures. **B,** Simultaneous traction on the skin and pushing of the balloon catheter results in displacement of the pericardium away from the chest wall, allowing proper inflation to occur. (From Ziskind AA, et al.: Percutaneous balloon pericardiotomy for patients with pericardial effusion and tamponade, in Topol EJ, editor: *Textbook of interventional cardiology,* Philadelphia, 1994, W.B. Saunders, p 1315.)

Ninety of 110 patients with malignancy died, compared to two of 20 patients with nonmalignant pericardial effusions. Mean survival for malignant pleural effusion patients was 3.6 ± 3.8 months. No procedure-related variables were found to influence survival or recurrence. There was no difference in recurrence rate when PBP was performed primarily or after failed pericardiocentesis.

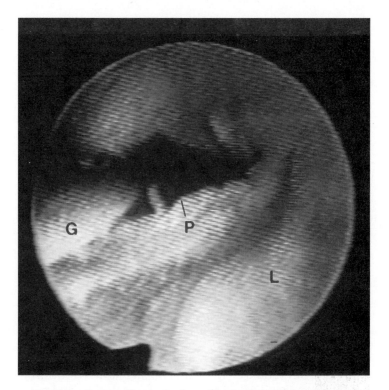

Fig. 13-7. Pericardioscopic view of the balloon pericardiotomy site. The fiber-optic scope has been withdrawn over a guidewire to visualize the external pericardial surface and demonstrate the free communication between pleural and pericardial spaces. G, Guidewire; P, pericardial window created by balloon dilation; L, lung in left pleural space immediately outside the pericardium. (From Ziskind AA, et al.: Percutaneous balloon pericardiotomy for patients with pericardial effusion and tamponade, in Topol EJ, editor: *Textbook of interventional cardiology*, Philadelphia, 1994, W.B. Saunders, p 1317.)

SPECIAL TECHNIQUES
Retained PTCA Equipment Components

Rarely, fragments of interventional equipment may be broken and remain in the coronary artery. This has occurred previously with guidewire tips from fixed-wire balloon systems, distal fragments of other guidewires, retained intravascular fragments associated with coronary artery occlusion, distal

TABLE 13-1. Clinical characteristics of 130 patients

Age (years, mean ± SD)	58 ± 13 (range 25 to 87)
Male/female	68/62
Tamponade present	90 (69%)
Prior pericardiocentesis	75 (58%)
Clinical history	
Known malignancy	110 (85%)
Lung	55
Breast	21
Other malignancies	34
Nonmalignant	20 (15%)
Idiopathic	5
HIV Disease	4
Postoperative/trauma	4
Uremia	2
Renal transplant	1
Hypothyroidism	1
Congestive heart failure	1
Viral	1
Autoimmune	1

embolization of clot, vessel perforation, infection, and ischemic complications. Removal of intravascular fragments and foreign bodies should be done immediately to avoid incorporation of this material after several days, during which the objects become coated and adhered within the vessel. There are several techniques that involve removal of retained intravascular foreign bodies. The most common is a loop made with a guidewire placed through a probing catheter. Baskets, forceps, and other snares have been available, but are, in general, too large to be placed within coronary arteries. Retrieval of foreign bodies from within the heart has been well described in *The Cardiac Catheterization Handbook* and will not be repeated in this section.

Special guidewire retrieval techniques. Multiple-catheter systems have been designed to retrieve foreign bodies, which are usually fragments of previous catheters or guidewires. Most catheter fragments result from injudicious insertion or removal of catheters inserted from the subclavian, jugular, or rarely, inferior vena caval approaches. Most recently, angioplasty guidewire fracture required refined removal techniques for coronary arteries. A catheter-housed wire loop or snare is commercially available. A loop passing through a very small intracoronary guiding catheter can be applied to retrieve intracoronary guidewire fragments from angioplasty systems. The snare and loop techniques have been used successfully in both venous and arterial applications. Extra care always must be employed with the snare, because its rigid tip may damage surrounding structures from which the catheter fragment is to be retrieved. In addition, the catheter fragment or guidewire material that is being retrieved also may scratch or tear the cardiac chamber unless it is captured at a distal end with the free sharp edge of the fragment contained so that it will not produce injury. In some cases it is possible to pass two intact coronary guidewires beyond a wire fragment and twist them together to ensnare and remove the fragment.

Shortening Guiding Catheters

Stratienko and Teirstein from Scripts Clinic, La Jolla, California, describe a technique for shortening angioplasty guide catheter length when therapeutic catheters fail to reach the target lesion. Most standard guide catheters are 100 cm long. The Y connector adds 6 to 10 cm in overall length. Because conventional angioplasty balloon catheters are 135 cm or less, the distal portion of the catheter extends <25 cm from the tip. In some cases, the limited balloon catheter length will prevent achieving successful dilatation in some individuals. The technique for shortening the guide catheter ex vivo or in vivo while maintaining both guide catheter and guidewire position is described next.

To shorten an in-dwelling guide catheter, a clamp is placed onto the guide catheter distal to the hub by a distance equal to the desired length of catheter reduction. The clamp prevents unnecessary blood loss during the shortening procedure. The guide catheter is cut with a scalpel proximal to the clamp, taking care not to damage the in-dwelling coronary guidewire. The guide catheter hub and hemostatic valve are removed. Next, a standard sheath one French smaller than the guide catheter is cut to approximately 2 cm of remaining sheath length from the hub. The newly shortened sheath is flared with a vessel dilator one French size larger than the nominal sheath size. This is accomplished by inserting the tapered end of the dilator retrograde into the sheath tip. The shortened and flared sheath is threaded over the in-dwelling guidewire, making sure that the stiff end of the guidewire does not perforate the diaphragm of the short sheath. A dilator placed through the sheath may facilitate the passage of the guidewire while threading it onto the guide catheter. The flared end of the sheath stub is advanced over the guide catheter with firm friction and the hemostatic clamp is removed. The side port of the sheath is connected to the manifold. The newly assembled system is carefully aspirated through the manifold to ensure that no air is trapped within it. The balloon catheter is then advanced over the guidewire through the diaphragm of the short sheath newly secured onto the in-dwelling guide catheter. The balloon catheter may now be advanced to the target lesion. Pressure-monitoring contrast injections are performed through the side port of the sheath stub.

SUGGESTED READINGS

Chow LT, Chow WH: Mechanism of pericardial window creation by balloon pericardiotomy, *Am J Cardiol* 72(17):1321-1322, 1993.

Chow WH, Chow TC, Cheung KL: Nonsurgical creation of a pericardial window using the Inoue balloon catheter, *Am Heart J* 124(4):1100-1102, 1992.

Kopecky SL, Callahan JA, Tajik AJ, Seward JB: Percutaneous pericardial catheter drainage: report of 42 consecutive cases, *Am J Cardiol* 58:633-635, 1986.

Markiewicz W, Borovik R, Ecker S: Cardiac tamponade in medical patients: treatment and prognosis in the echocardiographic era, *Am Heart J* 111:1138-1142, 1986.

Patel AK, Koosolcharoen PK, Nallasivan M, Kroncke GM, Thomsen JH: Catheter drainage of the pericardium: practical method to maintain long term patency, *Chest* 92:1018-1021, 1987.

Stratienko AA, Ginsberg R, Schatz RA, Teirstein PS: Technique for shortening angioplasty guide catheter length when therapeutic catheter fails to reach target stenosis, *Cathet Cardiovasc Diagn* 30:331-333, 1993.

Ziskind AA, Lemmon CC, Rodriguez S, et al.: Final report of the percutaneous balloon pericardiotomy registry for the treatment of effusive pericardial disease, *Circulation* 90(I):121, 1994.

Ziskind AA, Pearce AC, Lemmon CC, et al.: Percutaneous balloon pericardiotomy for the treatment of cardiac tamponade and large pericardial effusions: description of technique and report of the first 50 cases, *J Am Coll Cardiol* 21:1-5, 1993.

14

LASER CORONARY ANGIOPLASTY

Herbert J. Geschwind

BACKGROUND

Laser stands for "light amplification of stimulated emission of radiation." The light is emitted at the same time and in the same direction. For this reason it is called "coherent" light. Lasers emit radiation at a very high level of energy, which is able to destroy any kind of tissue regardless of its density. The coherent light beam is coupled to optical fibers as it exits from the laser cavity. The energy is passed through the silica fibers without any loss of efficiency. The radiation is produced in the laser cavity by exciting electrons that are moved from the ground state to the excited state. As the electrons return to the ground state, photons are emitted that are reflected in a semitransparent mirror and exit from the cavity through a transparent mirror. Laser energy may be emitted from a gas, liquid, or solid-state source. Solid-state lasers are more reliable, easier and cheaper to maintain than gas lasers, but less clinically applicable. The most commonly used laser sources are made of gases, mainly the xenon chloride excited dimer laser, which emits at a wavelength of 308 nm in the ultraviolet spectrum. A less commonly used laser is emitted from a garnet of yttrium and aluminum doped with holmium (Ho-YAG) at 2100 nm in the midinfrared spectrum. All lasers utilized for coronary angioplasty are delivered in the pulsed mode because delivery in this way provides more energy and less thermal effects than the continuous-wave mode.

Laser angioplasty was used clinically for peripheral angioplasty first in 1983 and 1984 by Ginsburg* and Geschwindt using an argon continuous-wave mode and an Nd-YAG laser coupled to a single 0.400-mm optical fiber. The thermal effects have been studied extensively by Abela, who advocated the use of laser for angioplasty in the early 1980s. In clinical practice, laser angioplasty was used first in peripheral arteries for recanalization of totally occluded vessels, mainly the superficial femoral artery. One of the first devices to be used was the "hot tip" laser, consisting of a rugby balloon-shaped metal tip that delivered thermal energy from an argon laser to vaporize the obstructing material within the vessel lumen. Although some clinical successes were obtained in diseased peripheral vessels, major complications occurred in the coronary arteries. For this reason the system is no longer used.

Catheter design improved over time. In order to replace the sharp-edged, bare optical-fiber tip by an atraumatic tip and to increase the diameter of the channel created by the laser catheter, a round, smooth, sapphire tip was used in leg arteries. This system delivered a continuous-wave infrared Nd-YAG laser. The system had a low ablating effect due to the direct emission of light through the sapphire and mostly a heating effect, similar to that obtained by the "hot tip." Because of the thermal effect and the relative catheter stiffness, this device was also inappropriate for coronary arteries. Access to coronary arteries was not obtained until the late 1980s, using an excimer pulsed laser coupled onto a multifiber catheter that was mechanically guided by an angioplasty guidewire.

MECHANISM

The delivery of high-energy pulses was shown to be associated with the formation of fast-expanding and -collapsing gas bubbles, which develop high-pressure photoacoustic shock

* Ginsburg R, Kim DS, Guthaner D, Tots J, Mitchell RES: Salvage of an ischemic limb by laser angioplasty: description of a new technique, *Clin Cardiol* 7:54-58, 1984.
† Geschwind H, Boussignac G, Teisseire B, Vieilledent C: Percutaneous transluminal laser angioplasty in man, *Lancet* II:844, 1984.

waves (Fig. 14-1). The latter are thought to be involved in the process of vessel wall damage, splitting the media and flattening the internal elastic lamina. Both mechanisms are associated with the clinical occurrence of dissections, perforation, aneurysm formation, vasospasm, acute closure, and possibly restenosis. Bubble size is significantly reduced by saline infusion and scanned laser beam delivery. The photoacoustic effects were postulated to contribute to tissue softening by splitting and redistributing hard calcified material within the arterial wall, increasing vessel compliance for improved dilatation results. Angioscopy has shown a smooth-edged channel created by laser irradiation without thermal effects and less intimal hemorrhage than after balloon dilatation. Intracoronary ultrasound demonstrated that little obstructing

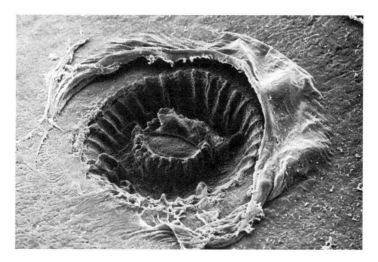

Fig. 14-1. Scanning electron photomicrograph of a crater created by excimer laser irradiation of a human postmortem aortic wall sample through a multifiber catheter. The three major effects of laser irradiation are displayed: a central crater; a pattern of remaining tissue between laser fibers ("dead space") and the center of the crater, corresponding to the nonirradiated area of the central lumen for the guidewire; and a surrounding zone of tissue elevation, tearing, and splitting due to the collateral damage effects of pulsed laser delivery by photoacoustic shock waves.

calcified tissue was ablated, although the vessel compliance was increased.

EQUIPMENT
Laser Emitter

Excimer lasers, emitting at 308 nm with a pulse length of 135 to 250 nm at a repetition rate of 25 to 40 Hz and an energy density of 40 to 60 mJ/mm^2, are the most commonly used. The laser device is large, with a weight of approximately 300 kg and dimensions of 110 × 110 cm and a width of 65 cm. The laser is triggered by a fast electrical discharge in a mixture of rare gases and halogens, which react to form an XeCl compound. Most devices deliver the energy in sequences of 5 sec separated by an automatic minimal resting interval of 15 sec. The system should be serviced at least two or three times a year for optical adjustment and gas filling.

Laser Catheter

The laser catheter is 135 cm long and varying diameters of 1.2 to 2.5 mm. The most commonly used diameters are 1.4, 1.7, and 2.0 mm. The catheters are made of a varying number of optical fibers measuring 50 to 100 μm in diameter, arranged concentrically around a central lumen for the passage of a 0.014- to 0.018-in. guidewire. The most densely packed catheters are made of 350 optical fibers. The advantages of multifiber-wire-guided catheters include: (1) high flexibility, (2) safe guidance and positioning derived from that commonly used for balloon dilatation; (3) coaxial positioning, which is likely to avoid laser radiation of the vessel wall and subsequent perforation; and (4) wider channels than those obtained with a single fiber. Recent devices have an asymmetrical configuration to increase the channel size by mechanically torquing the catheter over the guidewire. A monorail delivery system facilitates the procedure.

TECHNIQUE

The percutaneous approach is similar to that commonly used for balloon dilatation. Preangioplasty medications and intravenous heparin are administered exactly as for routine balloon angioplasty. Because of the relatively large size of the catheters, an 8 or 9 French guiding catheter precludes the common use of 6 French systems and the brachial or radial approach. Selection of the appropriate catheter size depends on the catheter/vessel diameter ratio. Optimal debulking is obtained with a catheter/vessel ratio close to 1, which is associated with a higher risk of complications. Small catheter diameters are safer but less efficient. A reasonable compromise consists of a 0.8 catheter/vessel ratio, which is able to debulk effectively without an excessively high risk of vessel wall damage.

After coronary angiography and positioning of the guiding catheter in the coronary ostium, the guidewire is passed into the diseased artery, penetrates the stenosis, and is positioned distal to the lesion. The laser catheter is gently advanced over the guidewire and positioned at the entrance of the stenosis. Repeat injections of contrast medium establish the precise position of the laser catheter tip. The distal tip should be kept in a coaxial position by using various angiographic projections. Before activating the laser, a saline flush should be delivered from the distal tip of the guiding catheter to wash out contrast and blood from the laser-radiated field. The laser is then activated and advanced gently at a slow pace to avoid any deleterious effect on the arterial wall and any "dottering" effect. Sufficient time should be provided to permit laser radiation to produce tissue ablation. The tissue ablation rate is approximately 5 to 10 μm per pulse. The position of the catheter tip should be viewed angiographically after each sequence of 5 sec or less. Multiple passes have been recommended to improve the results, although this method is associated with a higher risk of complications. After debulking the lesion, repeat angiography in at least two views should be performed to assess the angiographic result. Angiography is best obtained after pullback of the catheter, which may not allow contrast material to penetrate the residual stenosis.

If the result is considered satisfactory with a residual stenosis <30% diameter, the procedure may be considered a successful "stand alone," and the patient may be discharged from the catheterization laboratory. When the residual stenosis is >30%, an adjunctive balloon angioplasty should be performed to achieve the optimal angiographic result. After the procedure, heparin, vasodilators, and sheath removal should be performed per the laboratory angioplasty routine.

INDICATIONS

Coronary laser angioplasty is indicated for lesions that cannot be treated successfully with balloon dilatation, such as long diffuse lesions (>10 to 20 mm), moderately calcified, aorto-ostial, saphenous vein graft lesions, total occlusions that can be crossed with a guidewire, suboptimal results following balloon dilatation, stenoses that cannot be crossed with a balloon catheter, and restenoses.

Recently developed devices such as the laser guidewire consisting of a 0.018-in. guidewire with 12 optical fibers of 45 μm each have been able to cross total occlusions. Lasers such as the Ho-YAG or dye lasers have been shown to destroy acute thrombi in myocardial infarction and can be used in patients in whom thrombolysis is contraindicated.

CLINICAL RESULTS

Laser success is defined as a reduction by >20% of the narrowing of the vessel diameter. Procedure success is defined as a reduction to <50% of the residual stenosis in the absence of a major in-hospital complication such as myocardial infarction, death, or emergency coronary artery bypass graft surgery (CABG), whether the procedure is performed by laser alone or laser followed by an adjunctive balloon dilatation. The laser success is 82% to 85% and the procedural success is 86% to 94%. Stand alone laser angioplasty without the need for adjunctive balloon dilatation can be performed in 15% to 20% of patients. Results from several registries show that the mean lesion percent stenosis of 80% to 87% was reduced to 43% to 50% following laser angioplasty and to a final residual stenosis of 21% to 30% following adjunctive balloon dilatation. Procedural success is slightly lower in complex lesions: 86% in type C as compared to 88%, 95%, and 92% for types B2, B1, and A, respectively. Failures occur in 10% to 12% of patients and are related to treatment of long segmental lesions, calcified or thrombotic lesions, and total occlusions, or to the inability to position the catheter tip at the proximal segment of the stenosis due to severe prestenotic tortuosity.

COMPLICATIONS

Minor complications include vasospasm (13%), dissection (20%, 4% of which are flow-limiting), reclosure (8%), and perforation (2%). Major complications are myocardial infarction (2%), need for emergency CABG (2%), and death (1.5%). Arterial dissections are related to the use of a large catheter size, high energy per pulse, long lesions, or the presence of a side branch. The incidence of perforations is higher in women, in totally occluded vessels, and in the presence of a side branch. Fatal complications are correlated with multivessel-diseased patients with acute myocardial infarction, and patients >70 years old. The learning curve plays also an important role in the safety of the procedure. Rare complications include transient arrhythmia (<1%) and aneurysm formation (<1%). The complication rate may be reduced by saline perfusion during laser irradiation and by multiplexing laser delivery, which consists of a sequential distribution of the laser beam at the active radiation area of the multifiber catheter tip. The restenosis rate for laser-assisted balloon angioplasty is not lower than that observed following balloon dilatation alone. Comparison between atherectomy achieved with rotablation or laser and balloon dilatation showed a slightly higher angiographic restenosis rate for the former than for the latter method (55% to 62% versus 52%).

SUMMARY

Laser angioplasty is an atherectomy technique using flexible catheters designed to debulk coronary arteries or penetrate total occlusions for subsequent balloon dilatation. The concept of tissue ablation rather than compression has not been shown to improve the immediate and late results of coronary angioplasty. However, the procedure may facilitate dilatation in selected cases. Homogeneous laser light distribution through specialized windows to improve clinical results with the assistance of stent implantation is currently under investigation.

SUGGESTED READINGS

Abela GS, Conti CR, Geiser EA, Normann S: The effect of laser irradiation on atheromatous plaque: a preliminary report, *Am J Cardiol* 49:1008, 1982.

Baumbach A, Bittl JA, Fleck E, et al.: Acute complications of excimer laser coronary angioplasty: a detailed analysis of multicenter results, *J Am Coll Cardiol* 23:1305-1313, 1994.

Cumberland DC, Taylor DI, Welsh CL, et al.: Percutaneous laser thermal angioplasty: initial clinical results with a laser probe in total peripheral artery occlusions, *Lancet* 1:1457-1459, 1986.

Geschwind HJ, Boussignac G, Dubois-Rande JL, Zelinsky R, Jea Tahk S: Laser angioplasty in peripheral arterial disease, *Laser Med Surg* 6:307, 1991.

Geschwind HJ, Nakamura F, Kvasnicka J, et al.: Excimer and holmium yttrium aluminum garnet laser coronary angioplasty, *Am Heart J* 125:510-522, 1993.

Grundfest WS, Litvack F, Forrester JS, et al.: Laser ablation of human atherosclerotic plaque without adjacent tissue injury, *J Am Coll Cardiol* 5:929-933, 1985.

Isner JM, Donaldson RF, Deckelbaum KI, et al.: The excimer laser: gross, light microscopic and ultrastructural analysis of potential advantages for use in laser therapy in cardiovascular disease, *J Am Coll Cardiol* 6:1102-1109, 1985.

Isner JM, Rosenfield K, Losordo DW, et al.: Combination balloon-ultrasound imaging catheter for percutaneous transluminal angioplasty, *Circulation* 84:739-754, 1991.

Lammer J, Karnel F: Percutaneous transluminal laser angioplasty with contact probes. *Radiology* 168:733-737, 1988.

Larrazet FS, Dupouy PJ, Dubois-Rande JL, Hirosaka A, Kvasnicka J, Geschwind HJ: Angioplasty after laser and balloon coronary angioplasty, *Am Heart J* 23:1321-1326, 1994.

Litvack F, Eigler N, Margolis J, et al.: Percutaneous excimer laser coronary angioplasty: results in the first consecutive 3000 patients, *J Am Coll Cardiol* 23:323-329, 1994.

Tcheng JE, Phillips HR, Wells LD, et al.: A new technique for reducing pressure pulse phenomena during coronary excimer laser angioplasty, *J Am Coll Cardiol* 21:386A, 1993.

Topaz O, Rozenbaum EA, Battista S, Peterson C, Wysham DG: Laser facilitated angioplasty and thrombolysis in acute myocardial infarction complicated by prolonged or recurrent chest pain, *Cathet Cardiovasc Diagn* 28:7-16, 1993.

Total Investigators: Recanalization of chronic total coronary occlusions using a laser guidewire. The European multicentre surveillance study, *Eur Heart J* 16:488, 1995.

van Leeuwen TG, Meertens JH, Velema E, et al.: Intraluminal vapor bubble induced by excimer laser pulse causes microsecond arterial dilation and invagination leading to extensive wall damage in the rabbit, *Circulation* 87:1258-1263, 1993.

1

COMMON MEDICATIONS DURING CORONARY ANGIOPLASTY

TABLE I-I. Common medications during coronary angioplasty

Drug	Dose	Uses	Side effects	Comments
Analgesics				
Meperidine (Demerol)	IV, 5 to 25 mg × 5 to 25 min.	Analgesic	Urinary retention Rarely—allergic reaction	
Morphine	IV, 2 to 4 mg × 1 to 4 min.	Analgesic	Urinary retention Rarely—allergic reaction	Naloxone (Narcan), a pure opiate antagonist, reverses respiratory depression and hypotension (IV, 0.4 to 2 mg × push, repeat 2 to 3 min).
Diazepam (Valium)	IV, 2 to 5 mg slow push; rate not to exceed 5 mg/min.	Anxiolytic/muscle relaxant	Drowsiness, respiratory depression, disorientation, incoordination, paradoxical hypertension	Dose reduction advised in aged and in patients with hepatic insufficiency.
Diphenhydramine (Benadryl)	IV, 25 to 50 mg push.	Sedative (see antiallergy)	Drowsiness, dryness of mouth, urinary retention	
Antiallergic drugs				
Cimetidine	IV, 300 mg in 20-ml D5W or NS given over 2 to 5 min.			

| Epinephrine | 0.5 to 1 mg IV push. | For anaphylaxis *only* | Anxiety, tremor, headache, ↑ BP, arrhythmias | |
| Hydrocortisone sodium phosphate/ succinate | 100 mg IV push. | | | |

Antianginals

| Nitroglycerin | IV: Initially 5 μg/min, titrate to clinical situation.
IC: 100 to 200 μg; higher doses may be required; repeat as necessary.
SL: 0.4 mg. | Antihypertensive, Antiischemic/CHF
CHF
Coronary artery spasm | Hypotension, tachycardia, nausea, headache, dizziness | Heparin effects may be decreased by concurrent administration of IV nitroglycerin. |

Antiarrhythmics/antianginal (beta blockers)

| Esmolol | IV: Loading dose 0.5 mg/kg/min for 1 min, then maintenance dose of 2 mg/min; average dose 100 μg/kg/min. | SVT/antiischemic | Hypotension, dizziness, agitation, nausea | Titrate esmolol carefully in patients receiving morphine since morphine can ↑ esmolol concentration by about 50%; bronchospastic disease is relative contraindication. |

Continued on pages 506–507.

TABLE I-I. Common medications during coronary angioplasty—cont'd

Drug	Dose	Uses	Side effects	Comments
Antiarrhythmics/antianginal (calcium blockers)				
Diltiazem	1. Initial dose 0.25 mg/kg (TBW) as a bolus over 2 min (average dose 20 mg); if response is not adequate, a second dose of 0.35 mg/kg over 2 min (average dose 25 mg) may be administered after 15 min. 2. Continuous infusion in patients with A fib/A flutter immediately following bolus, administration of 0.25 mg/kg or 0.35 mg/kg; recommended initial infusion rate of cardizem is 5 to 10 mg/hr with increments of 5 mg/hr up to a maximum rate of 15 mg/hr; infusion may be maintained up to 24 hr.	1. Atrial fibrillation or atrial flutter 2. PSVT	Hypotension, flushing, burning at injection site, pruritus, dizziness	IV diltiazem and IV beta blockers should not be administered together or within hours of each other. Patients with impaired renal or hepatic function may be prone to side effects.

Verapamil	PSVT	IV: Initial dose 5 to 10 mg over 2 to 3 min. Repeat dose → 10 mg (0.15 mg/kg) 15 to 30 min after the first dose if the initial response is not adequate.	Hypotension, bradycardia, severe tachycardia, dizziness, headache, nausea	1. See diltiazem. 2. Avoid in suspected digitalis toxic patients.
		IC: 100 to 400 µg bolus.	Coronary spasm "No reflow"	Little hard data on benefit.
			Few systemic effects	

Miscellaneous antiarrhythmics

| Adenosine | PSVT | IV: Initially 6 mg as a *rapid* bolus (over 1 to 2 sec) to be given directly into a vein or proximal IV line followed by a *rapid* saline flush. A second and third dose (12 mg each) may be given as necessary every 1 to 2 min. | Facial flushing, headache, fatigue, light-headedness, nausea | Dipyridamole may potentiate the action of adenosine. Methylxantines (e.g., caffeine, theophylline) may antagonize the actions of adenosine. |

Continued on pages 508–509.

TABLE I-I. Common medications during coronary angioplasty—cont'd

Drug	Dose	Uses	Side effects	Comments
Bretylium	*For V-fib/V-tach* Administer undiluted, 5 mg/kg by rapid IV injection. If V-fib persists, increase dosage to 10 mg/kg every 15 min up to a total of 30 mg/kg. *Maintenance* 1 to 2 mg/min. Dilute 1 g bretylium in 250 ml D5W (or NS).	1. In the treatment of life-threatening ventricular arrhythmias that have failed to respond to lidocaine 2. Prophylaxis and therapy of ventricular fibrillation	Hypotension, bradycardia, PVCs, angina, nausea, vomiting, dizziness, syncope	Transient hypertension and increased frequency of arrhythmias may occur due to initial release of norepinephrine. Avoid use in patients with fixed cardiac output (i.e., severe aortic stenosis or severe pulmonary hypertension).
Lidocaine	IV: 50 to 100-mg IV bolus (1 mg/kg) given at a rate of 25 to 50 mg/min. Subsequent boluses may be necessary, not to exceed 200 to 300 mg/kg/hr. *Maintenance infusion* 1 to 4 mg/min. *Dilution* 2 g/500 ml D5W (or NS) (see infusion rate chart).	1. Acute ventricular arrhythmias 2. PVCs associated with MI	Light-headed, drowsiness, dizziness, confusion, double vision, vomiting, convulsions, hypotension, bradycardia	Do not use in patients who are hypersensitive to local anesthetics of the amide type (e.g., bupivicaine, dibucaine, efidocaine, mepivacaine, prilocaine). Caution advised in patients with liver and renal disease.

Drug	Indications	Dosage	Side Effects	Comments
Procainamide	PVCs, ventricular tachycardia, atrial fibrillation, SVT	IV: A loading dose of 500 to 600 mg over 30 min to a maximum of 1 g. Not to exceed rate of 50 mg/min. To maintain therapeutic plasma concentration, a continuous IV infusion of 1 to 5 mg/min may be administered. *Dilution:* 1 g procainamide in 250 ml D5W (or NS).	Hypotension, arrhythmias, bradycardia, AV block, ventricular arrhythmias, nausea, urticaria, rash, agranulocytosis, thrombocytopenia, lupus, erythematosus-like syndrome, dizziness, weakness	Caution advised in patients with myasthenia gravis, monitor blood levels, especially in patients with hepatic/renal disease.
Anticholinergic				
Atropine	Sinus bradycardia, high-grade AV block	IV: 0.5 to 1 mg every 5 min up to 2 mg.	Tachycardia, dry mouth, blurred vision, urinary hesitancy and retention, headache	
Antihypertensives				
Nifedipine	Antihypertensive Coronary artery spasm	SL: 10 to 20 mg, repeat as necessary.		

Continued on pages 510–511.

509

TABLE I-I. Common medications during coronary angioplasty—cont'd

Drug	Dose	Uses	Side effects	Comments
Nitroprusside	IV → 0.3 to 10 μg/kg/ min. *Dilution:* 50 mg nitroprusside in 250 ml D5W only. Protect from light. (See infusion rate chart.)	Hypertensive crisis	Hypotension, abdominal pain, apprehension, diaphoresis, dizziness, headache, bradycardia, tachycardia, methemoglobinemia, thiocyanate toxicity	Monitor cyanide and thiocyanate levels. Cyanide antidote kit (sodium nitrite, sodium thiosulfate, amylnitrite inhalant, and so on) should be available if needed.
Antithrombotics Heparin	IV: Intraprocedural dose individualized to maintain activated clotting time (ACT) >300 sec. Usual dose 10,000 to 15,000 units as bolus in those not previously anticoagulated. Following the procedure, rate adjusted to maintain ACT between 160 and 190 sec.	Antithrombotic	Hemorrhage, thrombocytopenia	Concomitant use of heparin, thrombolytics, and antiplatelet agents increase the risk of hemorrhage. IV nitroglycerin may antagonize heparin efficacy.

Protamine	*Dilution:* 15,000 units of heparin in 250 ml D5W (or NS). IV (not necessary to dilute): 1 mg of protamine neutralizes approximately 100 U heparin. Administer protamine within 30 to 60 min of last heparin bolus. 20 to 50 mg over 1 to 3 min. Do not exceed 50 mg in any 10-min period.	Treatment of heparin overdosage, heparin reversal	Hypotension, nausea, vomiting, lassitude	Too rapid administration of protamine sulfate can cause severe hypotension and anaphylactoid reactions.
Inotropes and vasopressors				
Dobutamine	IV → 2.0 to 20 µg/kg/min. *Dilution:* 500 mg of dobutamine in 250 ml of D5W (or NS). (See infusion rate chart).	Inotropic agent	Tachycardia. ↑ BP and ectopic activity	

Continued on pages 512–513.

TABLE I-I. Common medications during coronary angioplasty—cont'd

Drug	Dose	Uses	Side effects	Comments
Dopamine	IV → 2 to 20 µg/kg/min. Up to 50 µg/kg/min has been used. *Dilution:* 400 mg of dopamine in 250 ml D5W (or NS). (See infusion rate chart).	Inotropic agent/vasopressors	Tachycardia, angina, ectopic heart beats, dyspnea, headache, hypotension, vasoconstriction	The injection site should be carefully monitored. If extravasation occurs, 10 to 15 ml of NS injection containing 5 to 10 mg of phentolamine should be infiltrated liberally throughout the affected area. Administration of IV phenytoin to patients receiving dopamine has resulted in hypotension, bradycardia. Use phenytoin with extreme caution, if at all, in patients receiving dopamine.
Epinephrine	IV: 1 to 4 µg/min. *Dilution:* → 1 mg epinephrine in 250 ml D5W (or NS).	Inotropic agent (see antiallergy)	Anxiety, tremor, fear, headache, ↑ BP, arrhythmias, cerebral hemorrhage, nausea, vomiting	Beta blockers may block the beta-adrenergic effect of epinephrine, causing hypertension.
Metaraminol (Aramine)	IV: 0.5 to 5 mg as a single dose. IV infusion: 15 to 100 mg of metaraminol in 500 ml of D5W (or NS). Titrate to maintain desired blood pressure.	Vasopressor	Apprehension, restlessness, tremor, headache, dizziness, vasoconstriction, hypotension, tachycardia	(As above.)

Continued on pages 514–515.

Drug	Classification	Dose/Administration	Side Effects
Norepinephrine (Levophed)	Vasopressor	IV: Initial 8 to 12 μg/min. Average dose: 2 to 4 μg/min. *Dilution:* 4 mg (4 ml) of norepinephrine in 250 ml D5W (do not mix with normal saline alone). (See infusion rate chart).	(As above.)
Phenylephrine	Vasopressor	*Mild to moderate hypotension* IV → 0.1 to 0.5 mg over 2 to 3 min. 0.2 is usual dose. May repeat every 10 to 15 min. *Severe hypotension or shock* Following IV bolus initiate IV infusion at a dose of 0.2 to 0.18 mg/min until blood pressure is stabilized. Then average dose: 0.04 to 0.06 mg/min. *Dilution:* Mix 10 mg phenylephrine in 250 ml D5W (or NS). (See infusion rate chart.)	Anxiety, restlessness, weakness, dizziness, tremor, respiratory distress, vasoconstriction, decreased renal perfusion, bradycardia, decreased cardiac output

513

TABLE I-I. Common medications during coronary angioplasty—cont'd

Drug	Dose	Uses	Side effects	Comments
Thrombolytics Alteplase, Recombinant (t-PA, activase)	For lysis of coronary artery thrombi associated with AMI: 100 mg over a 3-hr period, given as an initial 60 mg over the first hour (of which 6 to 10 mg is given as a bolus over the first 1 to 2 min) followed by 20 mg/hr for the next 2 hr.	Thrombolytic agent	Bleeding, nausea, vomiting	Bleeding precautions should be used when thrombolytics used with agents such as heparin, warfarin, aspirin, and dipyridamole. *Contraindications:* see streptokinase.
	Anistreplase (APSAC, Eminase) IV: 30 units over 2 to 5 min.		Thrombolytic agent bleeding.	*Contraindications:* see streptokinase.
Streptokinase	IV → 1.5 million IU in NS infused over 60 min. IC → 10,000 to 30,000 IU in 3 to 20 ml of D5W or NS over 15 sec to 2 min followed	Thrombolytic agent	Allergic reactions (2% to 5%), bleeding, fever, hypotension (5% to 10%) associated with higher concentration and infusion rates	Patients who recently have had a streptococcal infection or streptokinase treatment may possess elevated levels of streptokinase antibodies.

by a maintenance infusion of 2000 to 4000 IU/min. The maximum recommended dose is 150,000 to 500,000 IU. (average rate of 2000 to 5000 IU/min).

Such patients have an increased likelihood of resistance to streptokinase therapy, and the drug may not be effective if administered between 5 days and 6 months after prior streptokinase therapy or streptococcal infection (e.g., pharyngitis, acute rheumatic fever). Rigors may respond to acetaminophen/meperidine.

Contraindications:
1. Active internal bleeding
2. Recent (within 2 months) cerebrovascular accident
3. Intracranial or intraspinal surgery
4. Intracranial neoplasm
5. Severe uncontrolled hypertension

Continued on page 516.

515

TABLE I-I. Common medications during coronary angioplasty—cont'd

Drug	Dose	Uses	Side effects	Comments
Urokinase	Commonly employed dose is 250,000 to 500,000 IU over 15 to 30 min (range 125,000 to 1.5 million units over 5 min to 2 hr). Concentration varies between 2000 and 10,000 U/ml IV → for lysis of coronary artery thrombi in patients with AMI, a dosage of 2 to 3 million units has been administered over 45 to 90 min, with half or all of the dose given as an initial rapid IV injection (e.g., over 5 min) and the remainder, if any, as a continuous infusion. Usual dose is 1.5 million units as a bolus followed by 1.5 million units over 60 min.	Thrombolytic agent	Bleeding	*Contraindications:* see streptokinase.

II

TECHNIQUES OF ARRHYTHMIA MANAGEMENT

VENTRICULAR TACHYCARDIA/FIBRILLATION

1. Three consecutive unsynchronized defibrillations in rapid sequence are recommended for adults. The first defibrillation is done at 200 J, the second at 200 to 300 J, and the third at 360 J. For children 2.5 to 50 J (2 J/kg) is used.
2. If defibrillation is unsuccessful, begin CPR, give 1 mg epinephine, intubate if possible, and ventilate the patient manually. If intubation is not possible, a mouthpiece should be inserted and the patient ventilated by a facemask. Epinephrine administration should be repeated at least every 5 min until a pulse is established. The success of treatment at this point depends, in large part, on the adequacy of the CPR. CPR should not be stopped for more than 5 sec except to defibrillate or intubate. Treatment of underlying abnormalities (e.g., hypokalemia, hypomagnesemia, ischemia, infarction, airway obstruction, or hypoxemia) that may be causing the arrhythmia is critical.
3. Defibrillate again at 360 J.
4. If unsuccessful, administer lidocaine (1 mg/kg bolus) and defibrillate again at 360 J.
5. If unsuccessful, administer bretylium (5 mg/kg bolus) and defibrillate at 360 J. Additional doses of lidocaine may be preferred.
6. At this time, the use of bicarbonate should be considered, particularly if there has been a delay in ventilating the patient.

7. Finish loading with either lidocaine or bretylium. Defibrillate at 360 J after each dose of antiarrhythmic agent.
8. If ventricular fibrillation is refractory to the above measures, one may consider Pronestyl, propranolol, or emergency cardiopulmonary bypass.
9. If ventricular fibrillation recurs during the arrest sequence, defibrillation should be reinitiated at the energy level that had previously resulted in successful defibrillation.

SUPRAVENTRICULAR ARRHYTHMIAS

1. In patients who are unstable (e.g., as a result of hypotension, chest pain, congestive heart failure, acute ischemia, or infarction), perform immediate synchronized cardioversion. Sedate with a rapidly acting IV agent (e.g., diazepam) in conscious, nonhypotensive patients as long as it does not delay the procedure. The recommended energy for the initial discharge is 75 to 100 J. If PSVT or atrial fibrillation immediately recurs, repeated electrical cardioversion is not indicated. If initial conversion is unsuccessful, repeat with increasing energy levels (e.g., 200 J, 360 J). If these maneuvers fail, treat with IV Pronestyl and repeated cardioversion. Relative contraindications to cardioversion include overt digitalis toxicity (severe bradycardia or asystole may occur after cardioversion). In stable patients with atrial fibrillation, the ventricular response can be controlled with digitalis, verapamil, or beta blockers. The rhythm can be converted later with procainamide or elective cardioversion.
2. In stable patients, PSVT initially should be treated with vagal maneuvers (Valsalva maneuver is the most successful, or, in the absence of known carotid disease or carotid bruit, carotid sinus massage). If vagal maneuvers are unsuccessful, verapamil (5 mg IV) or adenosine (5 to 12 mg IV bolus) are often successful. Patients who fail to respond to verapamil or adenosine can be treated with any of the following: overdrive pacing, Pronestyl, elective cardioversion, digitalis, or beta blockers.
   Verapamil is an available intravenous or oral calcium channel blocker with electrophysiologic effects on the AV node and, to a lesser extent, the SA node. It also has negative inotropic properties and is used to treat narrow QRS-complex

paroxysmal supraventricular tachycardia in stable patients. Verapamil is also useful for rate control in patients with atrial fibrillation and a rapid ventricular response. Initially, a 5-mg dose should be given IV over 1 min and additional doses of 2.5 to 5 mg given at 5- to 10-min intervals up to a maximal dose of 20 mg if PSVT persists without an adverse response to the initial dose. Contraindications to verapamil include history or presence of bradycardia, hypotension, decompensated congestive heart failure, or concomitant use of an IV beta blocker. The adverse reactions to verapamil include severe bradycardia, hypotension, congestive heart failure, and facilitated accessory conduction in patients with Wolff-Parkinson-White syndrome. Hypotension frequently can be reversed by the IV administration of 0.5 to 1.0 g of calcium chloride.

Adenosine is a naturally occurring agent that increases AV nodal blockade, as well as coronary blood flow. It is 90% to 100% effective in terminating reentrant supraventricular or AV nodal tachycardia in 5- to 12-mg IV bolus doses. It has a 30-sec onset of action and a 60-sec offset of action. Transient flushing is the only major side effect.

Digitalis is useful for controlling a rapid ventricular response in patients with atrial fibrillation, atrial flutter, or PSVT. The toxic/therapeutic ratio is narrow and the onset of action is slower than with verapamil (i.e., digitalis is not useful for acute situations).

Beta blockers (including esmolol and propranolol) can be used to control recurring episodes of PSVT. Beta blockers may be hazardous when cardiac dysfunction is present. The dosage for propranolol is 1 mg every 5 min intravenously up to a total of 0.1 mg/kg. Short-acting beta blockers (esmolol) are administered in 1- to 5-mg boluses and have 5- to 10-min half-lives.

CORONARY ANGIOGRAPHIC PROJECTIONS AND NOMENCLATURE

A-P PROJECTION

The A-P projection allows a good visualization of the left main coronary artery:

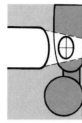

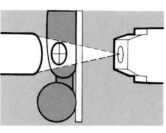

1. Left main coronary
2. Proximal part of LAD
3. Middle part of LAD
4. Distal part of LAD
5. Proximal circumflex artery
6. Distal circumflex artery
7. Left obtuse marginal artery
8. First diagonal artery
9. First septal perforating artery
10. Septal arteries
11. Auricular branch of the circumflex artery
12. Obtuse marginal artery number 2.

Fig. III-I. Left coronary artery. AP, Anteroposterior; LAD, left anterior descending artery; LAO, left anterior oblique; RAO, right anterior oblique. (From Bertrand ME, editor: *Coronary arteriography*, Lille, France, 1979, French Society of Cardiology.)

RIGHT ANTERIOR OBLIQUE PROJECTION AT 30° (R.A.O. 30°)

The R.A.O. projection at 30° permits the entire circumflex system to be studied, as well as the first centimeters of the anterior interventricular artery.

1. Left main coronary
2. Proximal part of LAD
3. Middle part of LAD
4. Distal part of LAD
5. Proximal circumflex artery
6. Distal circumflex artery
7. Obtuse marginal artery
8. First diagonal artery
9. Second diagonal artery
10. First septal perforating artery
11. Septal arteries
12. Auricular branch of the circumflex artery

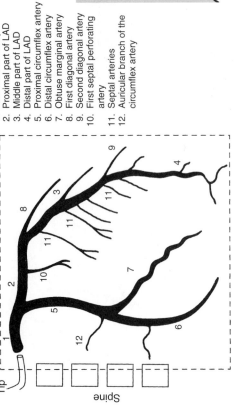

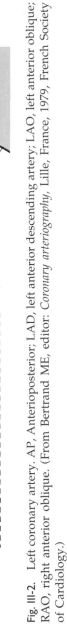

Fig. III-2. Left coronary artery. AP, Anterioposterior; LAD, left anterior descending artery; LAO, left anterior oblique; RAO, right anterior oblique. (From Bertrand ME, editor: *Coronary arteriography*, Lille, France, 1979, French Society of Cardiology.)

LEFT ANTERIOR OBLIQUE PROJECTION AT 55/60° (L.A.O. 55/60°)

The LAO projection at 55/60° mainly studies the diagonal arteries and the middle and distal parts of the LAD. On the other hand, the circumflex system is not well defined.

1. Left main coronary
2. Proximal part of LAD
3. Middle part of LAD
4. Distal part of LAD
5. Proximal circumflex artery
6. Distal circumflex artery
7. Left obtuse marginal artery
8. First diagonal artery
9. Second diagonal artery
10. First septal perforating artery
11 and 12. Septal arteries

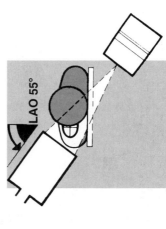

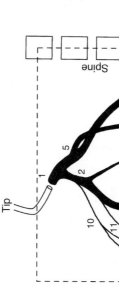

Tip

Spine

Fig. III-3. Left coronary artery. AP, Anterioposterior; LAD, left anterior descending artery; LAO, left anterior oblique; RAO, right anterior oblique. (From Bertrand ME, editor: *Coronary arteriography*, Lille, France, 1979, French Society of Cardiology.)

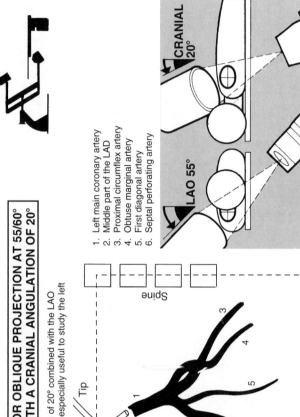

LEFT ANTERIOR OBLIQUE PROJECTION AT 55/60° COMBINED WITH A CRANIAL ANGULATION OF 20°

The cranial angulation of 20° combined with the LAO projection at 55/60° is especially useful to study the left main coronary artery.

1. Left main coronary artery
2. Middle part of the LAD
3. Proximal circumflex artery
4. Obtuse marginal artery
5. First diagonal artery
6. Septal perforating artery

Fig. III-4. Left coronary artery. AP, Anteriorposterior; LAD, left anterior descending artery; LAO, left anterior oblique; RAO, right anterior oblique. (From Bertrand ME, editor: *Coronary arteriography*, Lille, France, 1979, French Society of Cardiology.)

LEFT LATERAL PROJECTION

The left lateral projection, allows the study of the different segments of the anterior interventricular artery, the first diagonal artery, and the left marginal artery.

1. Left main coronary artery
2. Proximal part of LAD
3. Middle part of LAD
4. Distal part of LAD
5. Proximal circumflex artery
6. Distal circumflex artery
7. Obtuse marginal artery
8. First diagonal artery
9. Second diagonal artery
10. Septal arteries
11. Obtuse marginal artery number 2.

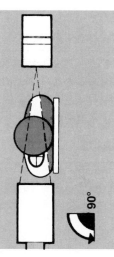

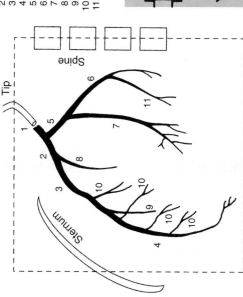

Fig. III-5. Left coronary artery. AP, Anterioposterior; LAD, left anterior descending artery; LAO, left anterior oblique; RAO, right anterior oblique. (From Bertrand ME, editor: *Coronary arteriography*, Lille, France, 1979, French Society of Cardiology.)

525

LEFT ANTERIOR OBLIQUE PROJECTION AT 45° COMBINED WITH A CAUDAL ANGULATION OF 15°

This projection allows the whole study of the RCA and, especially, clearly defines the region of the crux of the heart.

1. First (horizontal) segment of the right coronary artery
2. Second (vertical) segment of the right coronary artery
3. Third (horizontal) segment of the right coronary artery
4. Posterior interventricular

5. Retroventricular artery
6. Conus branch
7. Artery of the sinus node
8. Right ventricular artery
9. Right marginal artery
10. Artery of the A-V node
11. Diaphragmatic artery

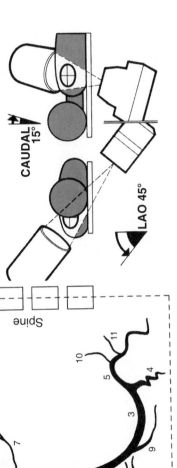

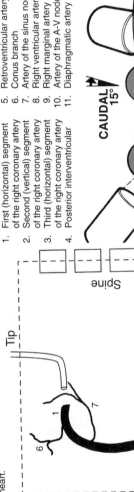

Fig. III-6. Right coronary artery. AP, Anterioposterior; LAD, left anterior descending artery; LAO, left anterior oblique; RAO, right anterior oblique. (From Bertrand ME, editor: *Coronary arteriography*, Lille, France, 1979, French Society of Cardiology.)

RIGHT ANTERIOR OBLIQUE PROJECTION AT 45°

The RAO projection at 45° permits the survey of the second (vertical) segment of the right coronary artery, the posterior interventricular artery, and the collateral branches (right ventricular and right marginal arteries). On the other hand, the first segment and the third segment, as well as the retroventricular artery, are not clearly defined. This projection also allows the visualization of the retrograde reopacification of the distal part of LAD proximally occluded.

1. First (horizontal) segment of the right coronary artery
2. Second (vertical) segment of the right coronary artery
3. Third (horizontal) segment of the right coronary artery
4. Posterior descending artery
5. Retroventricular artery
6. Conus branch
7. Artery of the sinus node
8. Right ventricular artery
9. Right marginal artery
10. Artery of the A-V node
11. Inferior septal arteries

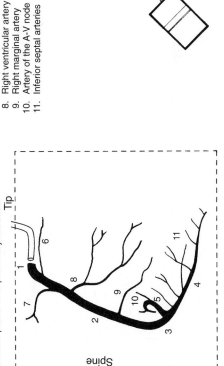

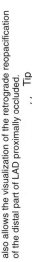

Fig. III-7. Right coronary artery. AP, Anterioposterior; LAD, left anterior descending artery; LAO, left anterior oblique; RAO, right anterior oblique. (From Bertrand ME, editor: *Coronary arteriography*, Lille, France, 1979, French Society of Cardiology.)

RIGHT ANTERIOR OBLIQUE PROJECTION AT 120° COMBINED WITH A CRANIAL ANGULATION OF 10°

This projection is very useful for studying the third horizontal segment, the crux of the heart and the retro-ventricular artery and its branches.

1. First (horizontal) segment of the right coronary artery
2. Second (vertical) segment of the right coronary artery
3. Third (horizontal) segment of the right coronary artery
4. Posterior interventricular artery
5. Retroventricular artery
6. Diaphragmatic artery

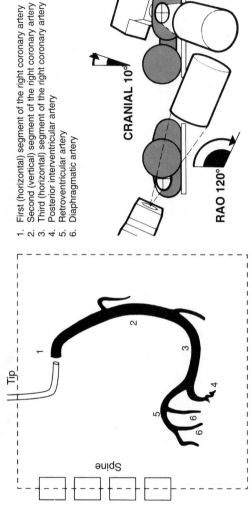

Fig. III-8.   Right coronary artery. AP, Anterioposterior; LAD, left anterior descending artery; LAO, left anterior oblique; RAO, right anterior oblique. (From Bertrand ME, editor: *Coronary arteriography,* Lille, France, 1979, French Society of Cardiology.)

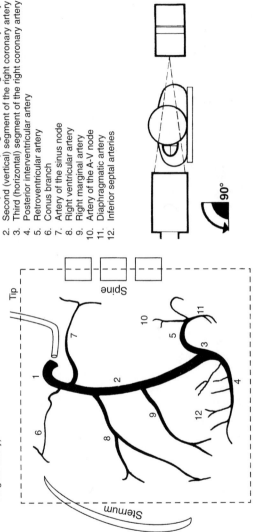

LEFT LATERAL PROJECTION

This projection permits the study of the second (vertical) segment of the right coronary artery and the collateral branches (conus branch, right ventricular artery, right marginal artery).

1. First (horizontal) segment of the right coronary artery
2. Second (vertical) segment of the right coronary artery
3. Third (horizontal) segment of the right coronary artery
4. Posterior interventricular artery
5. Retroventricular artery
6. Conus branch
7. Artery of the sinus node
8. Right ventricular artery
9. Right marginal artery
10. Artery of the A-V node
11. Diaphragmatic artery
12. Inferior septal arteries

Fig. III-9. Right coronary artery. AP, Anterioposterior; LAD, left anterior descending artery; LAO, left anterior oblique; RAO, right anterior oblique. (From Bertrand ME, editor: *Coronary arteriography,* Lille, France, 1979, French Society of Cardiology.)

INTERVENTIONAL
DEVICE
SPECIFICATIONS

Because of the proliferation of coronary angiography procedures, balloon and guiding catheters and guidewires are
available in a wide variety of configurations for general and
specific applications. The following tables in this section provide different specifications and a partial list of available
PTCA and other interventional device equipment in 1995.

TABLE IV-I. PTCA balloon catheter specifications

| System | Type | Shaft | | Balloon size (mm) | | | | | | Max guidewire size accepted (gw) (in.) | Balloon material | Nominal (atm) | RBP (atm) |
		Prox	Dis	1.5	2.0	2.5	3.0	3.5	4.0				
Over-the-Wire													
Cordis													
Sleek	OTW	3.2F	2.5F	.025	.027	.028	.030	.031	—	.014	DURALYN	8	10
Sleuth	OTW	3.5F	3.0F	—	.031	.031	.032	.033	.035	.018	DURALYN	8	8
Olympix	OTW	3.5F	3.0F	—	.030	.031	.031	.033	.035	.018	DURALYN	8	10
Olympix Long	OTW	3.5F	3.0F	—	.030	.031	.031	.033	.035	.018	DURALYN	8	10
ACS													
ACX II	OTW	3.3F	3.3F	.029	.031	.032	.034	.035	.037	.014	PE600	6	6
Omega	OTW	2.9F	2.9F	.022	.023	.025	.028	.030	.034	.010	VERBATIM	6	6
Pinkerton .018	OTW	3.6F	3.6F	—	.035	.037	.039	.040	.042	.018	PE600	6	6
Prism	OTW	3.3F	3.3F	.029	.031	.032	.034	.035	.037	.014	VERBATIM	6	6
RX .014	RX	3.3F	3.3F	—	.032	.034	.037	.039	—	.014	PE600	6	6
RX .018	RX	3.7F	3.7F	—	.035	.038	.040	.042	.046	.018	PE600	6	6

Continued on pages 532-533.

TABLE IV-I. PTCA balloon catheter specifications—cont'd

| System | Type | Shaft | | Balloon size (mm) | | | | | | Max guidewire size accepted (gw) (in.) | Balloon material | Nominal (atm) | RBP (atm) |
		Prox	Dis	1.5	2.0	2.5	3.0	3.5	4.0				
RX Alpha .014	RX	2.3F	3.3F	.029	.030	.031	.033	.034	.035	.014	PE600	6	8
RX Perfusion	RX	3.7F	4.2F	—	.053	.054	.055	.056	.059	.018	PE600	6	6
RX Streak	RX	2.3F	3.3F	.029	.030	.031	.033	.034	.035	.014	VERBATIM	6	8
RX Flowtrack 40	RX	2.3F	3.5F	—	.048	.049	.050	.051	.052	.018	PE600		6
Stack	OTW	3.9F	4.5F	—	.056	.057	.058	.060	.062	.018	PE600	6	6
Stack 40-S	OTW	3.9F	4.5F	—	—	.052	.053	.054	.055	.018	PE600	6	8
Ten	OTW	2.8F	2.8F	.024	.026	.027	.028	.030	.033	.010	PE600	6	6
Baxter													
Slinky	OTW	3.2F	3.0F	—	.028	.031	.032	.036	—	.014	POC	6	6-9
Reach	OTW	3.2F	2.9F	.028	.030	.032	.035	.037	.039	.014	POC	6	6-8
Mansfield													
Nitech	OTW	2.9F	2.9F	—	.029	.033	.035	.039	—	.014	HDPE	6	10
Slider .014	OTW	3.4F	3.4F	—	.035	.036	.040	.044	.045	.014	HDPE	6	10
Slider .018	OTW	3.4F	3.4F	—	.037	.038	.042	.044	.048	.018	HDPE	6	10
Slider ST	OTW	2.7F	2.7F	—	.029	.033	.035	.039	—	.014	HDPE	6	10

Continued on page 534.

Manufacturer	Device	Type										Material		
	Synergy	RX/OTW	2.9F	2.9F	—	.029	.033	.035	.039	.040	.014	HDPE	6	10
	Synergy	RX/OTW	2.9F	2.9F	—	.032	.035	.039	.041	.044	.018	HDPE	6	10
Medtronic	14K	OTW	2.9F	2.9F	.026	.030	.033	.036	.041	—	.014	PE	6	8
	18K	OTW	3.5F	3.5F	—	.032	.036	.038	.040	—	.018	PE	5	6
Schneider	Piccolino	RX	3.0F	3.2F	.025	.027	.029	.031	.034	.036	.014	PET	10	16
	Piccolino Forte	RX	3.0F	3.2F	.025	.027	.028	.031	.034	.036	.014	PET	10	16
	Speedy	RX	3.0F	3.3F	.030	.031	.032	.034	.036	.039	.016	PET	5	10
	Microsoftrac XLP	OTW	3.5F	3.0F	.025	.027	.029	.031	.034	.035	.014	PET	4	16
	Magnum-Meier	OTW	4.5F	4.5F	—	.039	.041	.043	.044	.047	.021	PET	N/A	16
	Mongoose	RX	3.2F	3.1F	.027	.029	.029	.032	.034	.038	.014	PET	N/A	16
SciMed	Cobra 10	OTW	2.8F	2.5F	.027	.029	.031	.033	.034	—	.010	POC	6	9
	Cobra 14	OTW	3.0F	2.7F	.030	.031	.033	.037	.039	.042	.014	POC	6	9
	Express	RX	1.8F	2.7F	.028	.029	.031	.035	.039	.040	.014	POC	6	9
	Mirage	OTW	3.6F	2.9F	.032	.034	.035	.038	.040	.044	.018	POC	6	9
	NC Shadow	OTW	3.6F	2.7F	—	.031	.032	.036	.040	.043	.014	TRIAD	6	16
	SC Shadow	OTW	3.6F	2.7F	.030	.031	.033	.037	.039	.042	.014	POC-8	8	9

TABLE IV-I. PTCA balloon catheter specifications—cont'd

System		Type	Shaft		Balloon size (mm)						Max guidewire size accepted (gw) (in.)	Balloon material	Nominal (atm)	RBP (atm)
			Prox	Dis	1.5	2.0	2.5	3.0	3.5	4.0				
	Shadow	OTW	3.6F	2.7F	.030	.031	.033	.037	.039	.042	.014	POC	6	9
	Skinny .014	OTW	3.5F	3.0F	.028	.031	.033	.037	.040	.042	.014	POC	8	9
	Skinny .018	OTW	3.5F	3.0F	.031	.034	.037	.039	.040	.044	.018	POC	8	9
USCI	Force	OTW	3.5F	3.5F	—	.031	.033	.034	.036	.036	.018	PET	5	12
	Solo	OTW	3.0F	3.0F	.028	.030	.030	.032	.034	.035	.014	PET	5	12
	Sprint	OTW	3.5F	3.5F	—	.031	.033	.035	.037	.039	.018	PET	5	12
Fixed-Wire														
Cordis	Orion	FW	2.4F	1.8F	—	.024	.028	.030	.032	—	FW	DURALYN	8	12
	Lightning	FW	2.4F	1.8F	—	.024	.027	.030	.032	—	FW	DURALYN	8	12
ACS	Slalom	FW	2.5F	2.0F	—	.023	.025	.029	.033	—	FW	PE600	6	8
SciMed	Ace	FW	1.8F	1.8F	.020	.022	.030	.032	.036	—	FW	POC	7	8
USCI	Probe III	FW	1.7F	1.7F	—	.019	.021	.026	—	—	FW	PET	5	10.6

Shaft/RBP specifications are for 3.0-mm catheters.
Courtesy of Cordis Corporation, Miami, FL.

TABLE IV-2.   PTCA guiding catheters

Company	Product name	French size	I.D.	Construction Top coat	Construction Braid type	Construction Lumen surface	Radiopaque tip marker	Metal curve support
ACS	Powerguide	7	.070″	Polyurethane	Kevlar	FEP	Yes	Yes
	Powerguide	8	.080″	Polyurethane	Kevlar	FEP	Yes	Yes
Baxter	Marathon	7	.070″	Pebax	Stainless steel	Silicone	No	No
	Marathon	8	.078″	Pebax	Stainless steel	Silicone	No	No
	Marathon Gold	8	.082″	Pebax	Stainless steel	Silicone	No	No
Cordis	Petite Brite Tip	6	.062″	Nylon blends	Stainless steel	PTFE	Yes	Yes
	Brite Tip	7	.072″	Nylon blends	Stainless steel	PTFE	Yes	Yes
	Brite Tip Large Lumen	8	.078″	Polyurethane	Stainless steel	PTFE	Yes	No
	New XL Brite Tip	8	.084″	Nylon blends	Stainless steel	PTFE	Yes	Yes
	Vista Brite Tip	9	.098″	Nylon blends	Stainless steel	PTFE	Yes	Yes
	Vista Brite Tip	10	.110″	Nylon blends	Stainless steel	PTFE	Yes	Yes
DVI	DVI	9.5	.104″	Polyurethane	Stainless steel	PTFE	Yes	No
	DVI	10	.104″	Polyurethane	Stainless steel	PTFE	Yes	Yes
	DVI	11	.111″	Polyurethane	Stainless steel	PTFE	Yes	Yes
Mansfield	Proformer	8	.081″	Polyur./Teflon	Stainless steel	Polyur./Teflon	No	Yes

Continued on page 536.

TABLE IV-2. PTCA guiding catheters—cont'd

Company	Product name	French size	I.D.	Construction Top coat	Construction Braid type	Construction Lumen surface	Radiopaque tip marker	Metal curve support
Medtronic	Sherpa	6	.057"	Polyurethane	Stainless steel	FEP	No	No
	Sherpa	7	.070"	Polyurethane	Stainless steel	FEP	No	No
	Sherpa Peak Flow	7	.072"	Polyurethane	Stainless steel	FEP	No	No
	Sherpa	8	.079"	Polyurethane	Stainless steel	FEP	No	No
	Sherpa Peak Flow	8	.083"	Polyurethane	Stainless steel	FEP	No	No
	Giant Lumen	9	.088"	Polyurethane	Stainless steel	FEP	Yes	No
	Sherpa	9	.092"	Polyurethane	Stainless steel	FEP	No	No
	Sherpa	10	.108"	Polyurethane	Stainless steel	FEP	No	No
	Sherpa 10 Firm	10	.108"	Polyurethane	Stainless steel	FEP	No	No
Schneider	Solid 7	7	.072"	Polyurethane	Stainless steel	PTFE	No	No
	Superflow	7	.072"	Polyurethane	Stainless steel	PTFE	No	No
	Stamina	8	.079"	Polyurethane	Stainless steel	PTFE	No	No
	Superflow	8	.082"	Polyurethane	Stainless steel	PTFE	No	No
	Superflow	9	.092"	Polyurethane	Stainless steel	PTFE	No	No
	Superflow	10	.107"	Polyurethane	Stainless steel	PTFE	No	No
SciMed	Triguide—Elite	6	.060"	Nylon	Stainless steel	FEP	Yes	Yes
	Triguide—Lite	7	.072"	Nylon	Stainless steel	FEP	Yes	Yes
	Triguide—Standard	8	.079"	Nylon	Stainless steel	FEP	Yes	Yes
	Triguide—Intermediate	8	.080"	Nylon	Stainless steel	FEP	Yes	Yes
USCI	Super 7	7	.070"	Nylon	Kevlar	PTFE	Yes	Yes
	Illumen 8	8	.080"	Nylon	Kevlar	PTFE	Yes	Yes
	Super 9	9	.092"	Nylon	Kevlar	PTFE	Yes	Yes

TABLE IV-3. Atherectomy, ultrasound imaging catheters, and stents

Manufacturer	Intracoronary device	Outer diameter*		French	Recommended minimum guide (in.)
		mm	in.		
Atherectomy systems					
Device for vascular intervention	Simpson	2.3	0.091	5.0	0.105
	Coronary	2.5	0.099	6.0	0.105
	Atherocath*	2.8	0.110	7.0	0.105
Heart Technology	Rotoblator	1.25	0.049	3.75	0.076
		1.50	0.059	4.50	0.076
		1.75	0.068	5.25	0.079
		2.00	0.079	6.00	0.092
		2.15	0.084	6.45	0.092
		2.25	0.088	6.75	0.107
		2.50	0.098	7.50	0.107
		2.75	0.107	8.25	0.115
Interventional Technologies	TEC	1.83	0.071	5.5	0.092
		2.00	0.079	6.0	0.092
		2.20	0.086	6.5	0.092
		2.30	0.091	7.0	0.100
		2.50	0.098	7.5	0.107

Continued on page 538.

TABLE IV-3. Atherectomy, ultrasound imaging catheters, and stents—cont'd

Manufacturer	Intracoronary device	Outer diameter*		French	Recommended minimum guide (in.)
		mm	in.		
Intracoronary imaging devices					
CVIS	"Insight" imaging catheters	1.43	0.056	4.3	0.072
Diasonics	Sonicath	1.67	0.065	5.0	0.079
		1.60	0.062	4.8	0.082
		1.00	0.039	3.0	0.063
		1.67	0.065	5.0	0.076
Endosonics	Visions	1.83	0.071	5.5	0.078
Intertherapy	Interpret	1.37	0.054	4.1	0.076
		1.63	0.064	4.9	0.079
Stents†					
		2.0		4.4	0.077
		2.5		4.4	0.077
		3.0		4.4	0.077
		3.5		4.4	0.089
Cook Gianturco-Roubin	FlexStent	4.0		4.4	0.089
Johnson & Johnson		1.67	0.066	5.0	0.079
Interventional Systems	Palmaz-Schatz	2.00	0.079	6.0	0.092

*The dimensions here are based on the following: French size outer diameter refers to the cutter housing diameter, and the millimeter and inch outer-diameter dimensions refer to the crossing profile of the balloon when deflated.

†The dimensions are based on the following: All stents are deployed with a 4.4 F balloon catheter manufactured by Cook, and the millimeter outer-diameter measurements are for expanded outer diameters of the stent.

PERIPHERAL VASCULAR ANATOMY

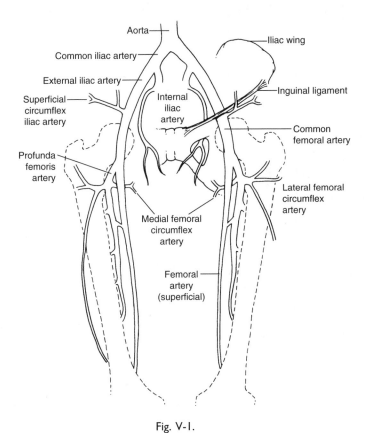

Fig. V-1.

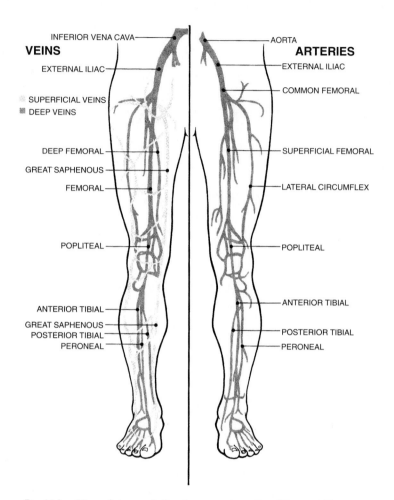

Fig. V-2.   Vasculature of the lower extremity. (From Abbot Laboratories, North Chicago, IL.)

INDEX

Page numbers in italics indicate pages with figures.